WE THE VICTORS

WE THE VICTORS

Inspiring Stories of People Who Conquered Cancer
And How They Did It

Curtis Bill Pepper

Doubleday & Company, Inc.
Garden City, New York
1984

For my brother Jack,
who did not make it.

Excerpt from "Do not go gentle into that good night" from *Poems of
Dylan Thomas.* Copyright 1952 by Dylan Thomas. Reprinted by permission
of New Directions Publishing Corporation.

Library of Congress Cataloging in Publication Data

Pepper, Curtis Bill.
We the victors.
1. Cancer—Patients—United States—Biography.
I. Title.
RC265.5.P46   1984   362.1'9994'0092 [B]

ISBN: *0-385-19122-7*
Library of Congress Catalog Card Number: 83-18481
Copyright © 1984 by Curtis Bill Pepper

CONTENTS

INTRODUCTION

. . . After that, I was another person,
without knowing why or how, and after that,
I lived naked in a new world where the sun
broke through windows to grasp entire families
and crept between trees to wash down streets
without disturbing any object, in a world
where a solitary kiss blew down a door. . . .

Marvin Bell
The Nest

This book contains stories of men and women, many of them quite ordinary people, who have behaved like heroes. Each one has a dramatic tale to tell, and each story differs from the others. Yet they all faced a common enemy, and the familiar course of their battles makes it possible to read them as a variable fable of our time.

Shipwrecked in the midst of life and cast up on strange shores, they are forced to fight the dragons and monsters of cancer. They encounter other untold dangers, and they witness the deaths of companions around them.

Yet, somehow these people survive to return and tell us of their adventures. They speak of their fears, their trembling bodies, their dark despair, and their last-minute prayers or curses. Then they report a sudden turn of events—the arrival of unexpected strength from within themselves, along with support from others who come to protect their flanks and bind their grievous wounds.

So they emerge as victors to tell us how this experience has changed their lives: How they see a bird in the sky, a boat on a river, a small leaf on a tree as a new vision of the totality of life. How they have an increased capacity for unconditional love. How they seem to have been born again with a greater awareness of who they are. How they have less fear of death and less terror of life's crushing forces, which circumscribed and diminished their previous existence.

It is inspiring to see this in these people, and they appear to be more beautiful because of it. Finally, as they describe how all this happened, relating their intimate feelings at the time, we are led to some of the most remarkable testimony to emerge from this survey of one hundred former cancer patients, with thirty-one of their stories included in this book.

For here, from a common group of human beings, from a pool of people freed from the lock gates of disease, we discern something far more universal than individual reentries into life.

It is that these survivors—and, hence, potentially all of us—possess an innate sense for beauty, for goodness, and for truth or perfection. In action, this appears as an active awareness and concern for what is "right"—for themselves and for others. It may be hidden within them, it may alternate with extreme cruelty, cowardice, or treachery. Yet it is inevitably there, and we observe it most clearly in these men and women as they emerge from their crises, after facing the possibility of dying.

We were taught that this existed, of course, and we were told its various names: conscience, honor, or the a priori moral law within. It was said to be a sublime mystery of creation—indeed, integral to it, if one considers the Fall to be a fall into self-consciousness. Yet this occurred so long ago. The teachers are gone, the legends are lost, and the supporting myth-rituals are playing to empty houses in a spreading wasteland of auto graveyards, nuclear dumps, beached whales, and hydraulic sex.

To discover its existence again amid the media-linked millions, to observe it as a life-enhancing reality in the psychic recesses of these former cancer patients, is more than surprising. It is a challenge for us to live as though we, too, came out of a cancer ward—to live as these people do, with rejuvenated lives.

It may not be possible, of course. Most of us probably could never undertake such a profound change without having lived through a similar trauma. To dismantle the protective structure of our lives, the expedient psychic dome wherein we work and play, would appear to be too great a task for anyone who is not psychologically desperate or seriously ill. Some violent storm is needed—and not just a passing one. For there is an element of "permanence" about cancer—the possibility, however remote, of its return—which tends to render more lasting its effect upon those who have had it and are now in remission.

Yet it should be within our reach somehow to obtain a similar renaissance in our lives. For we also possess the determinant factors for it—a

moral sensibility constantly challenged and renewed by a joy in the unfolding of life. These attributes appear to be built into the hearts of human
beings, and so are accessible to all of us in our capacity to dream and in
our need to be heroes. If for no other reason, it would seem that this
makes every single life as precious as any other.

As we discover in these collected stories, the sudden opening up to life
brings with it a sense of euphoria, of expanding warmth, as if these people
had somehow reached the pulsating heart of nature, of all existing life. In
varying degrees, they experience a self-transcendence, such as occurs upon
finding a guiding faith or a great personal love. For some, there appears to
be at hand the missing elements needed to explain the meaning of life.
Others, less explicit, seem to say that all we have to do is witness the event
—and listen.

So we listen now to these voices, to these people who have survived.
They speak of many things, in simple yet profound ways. Like children
finding shells on the beach, they appear to rush upon us without artifice.
They look at life with the defenseless eyes of the innocent. They seem to
move, to turn with a special grace even when disfigured by their ordeal.
They smile and they laugh in a manner that must be familiar to the angels.

They are different now, and they can never go home again—not to lives
once lived. The effect varies, of course. With some people, it is less visible
than with others. Yet all of them, in one way or another, have merged into
a new existence with a greater openness to the totality of life. For some, it
is too much to describe in words. They fall silent, unable to explain it.
Others will take your hand or touch your arm while speaking—a physical
linkage practiced most often by saints and sinners who know that words
alone can never explain or harness the human spirit.

Regardless of any religious belief, they have all experienced a last supper, a personal agape, a shared awareness that the loving substance of their
mortal existence is destined to pass to others. In effect, they can never rise
again from that table of their naked selves. And they continue to experience it, even as they return to their former lives after being considered
clinically cured.

Some seek to hide it, as if it was too private a matter. Yet it remains
visible to those who were with them during their struggle to live. Mary
Wall, one of the social workers, says, "When they return for a checkup,
you can see it sometimes in their faces. It's in the way they look at you, in
the eyes and how they smile and nod—something very private you have
shared with them which they will never forget."

A major question asked in this survey is one that people ask all over the world. It comes up when they meet someone who has survived a type of cancer that claimed a friend or a family member: "How did you manage to survive when other people, with the same cancer, didn't make it?"

In an effort to obtain as objective a reply as possible, this question was not asked directly in the initial interviews. The former patients were asked only to tell their stories—the first sign of illness, the treatment, the eventual recovery.

From the bulk of this testimony, five factors appeared to be determinant in eventual survival: *Love* (being loved or loving—in any form); *Self* (holding on to a sense of self-determination, of central command, asking questions, taking an active part in the treatment at risk of appearing overly anxious, difficult, or downright mean); *Need* (being needed by others for their survival, or having unsettled accounts involving identity, reputation, or honor); *Luck* (unforeseen, inexplicable factors which alone made survival possible); *The Best* (getting the best in medicine, surgery, or clinical treatment at any comprehensive U.S. cancer center—this making the difference where other doctors or institutions had given up hope for any recovery).

Later, the former patients were asked to indicate their order of importance for the five factors, or any other element which they believed may have played a crucial role. A few protested that it was impossible to choose one factor over another. One patient wrote: "Okay, I've got your five factors, but they're all important! It depends on what point you're at in the treatment. For example, for me it began with Luck, in getting rid of that lousy doctor who nearly killed me, and then in finding Memorial. It became Love when I was down on the floor for a long count, and my wife was right there with me. But after the operation, it became Self because that's when you get hold of yourself and climb out of there—or you don't. Finally, if it wasn't for Memorial and getting The Best (especially after that other doctor gave up on me), I'd be pushing up daisies right now! So for me they're all Number One." Another patient wrote: "Your questions are like asking me to intellectualize on breathing."

The vast majority, however, felt we had come upon something important, and the replies poured in. Many contained additional insights into their survival, and some of this is included in prefaces to each section.

The quality of treatment and care, especially with cancer, varies greatly from place to place. To control this variable as much as possible, all the patients in this book were taken from the files of one institution which is generally considered to be one of the most advanced in the world for cancer research and its clinical treatment—the Memorial Sloan-Kettering Cancer Center in New York.*

Almost invariably, former patients agreed to contribute to this work, hoping thereby to help others. For legal or professional reasons, five demurred and another four asked not to be identified. In a final editing of the collected material, those patients were chosen who, in their lives and thoughts, most clearly represented the others. Besides these, staff members of Memorial Hospital—doctors, nurses, social workers—also address themselves to the various categories of survival, and this is interspersed with the testimony of the patient.

This work serves four functions. It provides an in-depth report on people who have survived cancer; it tells us what they believe to have been crucial to their recovery, and how the disease has changed their lives, allowing a broad look at where most of this occurred, in one of the world's most advanced cancer hospitals.

The survey was not intended to do more than this. In scientific terms, it is nonrandom and uncontrolled. We do not know, for example, how many people might have possessed the similar characteristics and attitudes of the survivors—yet did not make it.† To erect such a study, to establish two parallel groups at the same clinical and psychological moment in time, would appear to be far beyond the reach of contemporary science and medicine.

Similarly, we were unable to control or record the laws of chance in each case. For example, the varying ability of each individual organism to turn back cancer—the HD/TA, or host defense–tumor aggression ratio— might well have been high in the survivors, unbeknownst to all observers. If so, this might have been a sixth factor—potentially more important than all others.

We do have, however, the patients and the medical staff telling us what they believe to be crucial in recovery. They take us as close as possible to the heart of the mystery. Once there—in the very private chamber of their inner selves—we witness people of extraordinary courage struggling against immense forces. Some live, some do not. Some seem destined to die, yet they survive. And it is these who now speak to us.

Their voices come to us as from a distant shoreland of memory where

---

* For other major U.S. cancer centers, see p. 13.

† To illustrate this important factor, one patient is included who had all survival characteristics and seemed, more than most, destined to live—yet did not.

the image of home and the objects of love are so precious, so meaningful, that the heart breaks with nostalgia. As one of these patients says upon his return, "You know, cancer patients are like all other people—only more so."

C.B.P.

ONE

THE BEST

It appears to me a most excellent thing for the physician to cultivate Prognosis; for by foreseeing and foretelling . . . the present, the past, and the future, and explaining the omissions which patients have been guilty of, he will be more readily believed to be acquainted with the circumstances of the sick . . . and he will manage the best cure who has foreseen what is to happen from the present state of matters.

Hippocrates
The Book of Prognostives

The fruit of a surgeon's experience is not the history of his practice . . . that he has cured four people of the plague and three of the gout, unless he knows how thence to extract something whereon to form his judgment, and to make us sensible that he is thence more skillful in his art.

Michel de Montaigne
Essays

As will be seen here, increasing numbers of people are surviving cancer. Five million living Americans have been treated for it. More than half of these have lived past the five-year mark, free of any further trouble—and so are considered to be clinically cured.

Now we are being told that many more could be saved. The American Cancer Society, for instance, reports that the 1984 estimated toll of people who will perish from cancer—450,000, or 1,230 people a day, about one every seventy seconds—could be reduced by one third. This would save 400 lives a day and dramatically raise the survival rate from 38 to 55 percent. All we have to do to achieve this—and so save more lives than we lose—is to increase the availability of the newest techniques and protocols used in defeating cancer—especially early detection, prompt treatment, and follow-up controls for those presumed to be cured.*

It's just as simple as that—or so it would seem. Most of us know,

---

* The ACS figures: In 1984, about 870,000 people will be diagnosed as having cancer. Of these, about 326,000 will "survive"—that is, be alive five or more years later. This is three out of eight, or a 38 percent *observed* survival rate. The observed rate is determined by the number of those still alive after five years. When normal life expectancy is taken into consideration (factors such as dying of heart disease, accidents, old age), the figure increases to 48 percent. This *relative* survival rate is a more commonly used yardstick to measure progress against cancer. However, it can cause misunderstanding. For example, Dr. Vincent DeVita, Jr., director of the National Cancer Institute, states the relative survival rate of cancer patients has now reached 48 percent—with current figures indicating it has passed 50 percent. This does not mean—as reported in the media—that 50 percent or more of all former cancer patients have survived at least five years. Only 38 out of 100 are alive today who had cancer five or more years ago.

however, that it is neither simple nor easy. For a variety of reasons, we don't check the disease in time. We reach the oncologist—the cancer specialist—too late. Or we don't get there at all, and we lose someone who might have been saved.

With cancer striking three out of ten persons—and three out of four families—we seem destined to witness an onslaught of the disease, among family or friends. And all too often we hear the guilt-lashed remark "If we'd discovered it sooner, there might have been a chance."

How does this happen? If we can save one third of those who are currently being lost, it would seem to be most urgent to determine why we are not doing it—or, at least, not doing a better job of it.

Many of the survivors in this book believe they can help us, so that we may better defend ourselves and our families. They believe that their dramatic recoveries will serve as lessons in survival—in how to avoid the pitfalls that threatened to claim many of them. These people speak with a hope of helping us avoid the errors and delays that can cost a life. They speak as though of one voice, one spirit which they first displayed upon being asked to participate in this survey. Their replies, which were consistently surprising and of singular beauty, seemed to confirm one of the great mysteries of creation: the existence of a potential for heroic self-transcendence in all of us. It can be experienced in many ways, but it is essentially an innate drive to go beyond ourselves, beyond any individual life or biological death.

Typical of many was the reply from Joan Warshun, a pretty girl with long brown hair and blue eyes, who lost her right leg: "If my story will help someone else, then maybe it will have a meaning beyond just my being alive. Maybe it will help someone else to live."

Each survivor's story seems more incredible than the other. We become aware of impending dangers and want to tell the victim, "No! Don't delay any longer!" Or, "For God's sake, follow your instincts, get another opinion!" Many proceed, as if blind, toward certain extinction. Yet somehow each escapes at the last minute—by luck, by strength of self, by grace or love from an intervening hand—eventually to find the truly qualified specialist or "the best" treatment in time to be saved.

From their experiences, we quickly discern two areas where we can be

---

Still, this is a new high in cancer survival. In the 1930s, fewer than one in five was alive five years after treatment. In the 1940s, fewer than one in four. In the 1960s, and until recently, it was one in three. Now it is three out of eight with the likelihood that it will be one out of two, or even slightly better, for those getting cancer in 1984. Looking to the future, that is the key figure to remember.

sidetracked and so lose the maximum chance for survival. One is within ourselves; the other is in our referring doctors.

Within ourselves, there appear to be two factors capable of causing critical delay—ignorance and fear. The first, when not linked to the second, is usually the result of being uninformed and so unaware of cancer's danger signals. We begin to lose energy, we have a persistent cough, an enlarged mole, a strange lump, a "digestive" problem—to name a few. We have no idea what's causing the trouble, and we attribute it to a variety of causes—resulting in dangerous delay.

MORAL: Learn the warning signals. The American Cancer Society has described them in pamphlets which may be obtained, free of charge, from any local ACS office. If you suspect something, don't be afraid to talk about it, and don't worry about being called a hypochondriac. Go see your doctor and don't be intimidated. You don't know as much about medicine as he does, but in many ways you know yourself much better, because you live in your body and he doesn't. Maybe you're not due a checkup for another six months. No matter, if you feel it's urgent, ask for it. If your doctor doesn't agree, he may well be right, but if you have reason to believe he's not, then get a second opinion from another doctor. An earlier checkup might be just in time—as occurred here for Pat Ciccarelli. And that, in substance, is the first lesson from these survivors.

The second lesson deals with fear—how not to allow it to paralyze us or cause a loss of selfhood. The survivors within these pages show us how it can happen, how otherwise intelligent, self-assured people suffer a personality breakdown upon learning they have cancer.

A successful commercial artist, Albert Moore, considers leaping from his office window. A handball champion, Herman Krevsky, briefly loses control and begins to sob. A New York cop, Pat Ciccarelli, weeps in the privacy of his room.

It was to be expected, of course. For with our gift of self-consciousness, we are unique in the animal world in possessing a foreknowledge and consequent fear of death. It is a universal and inescapable determinant. From the moment we learn we will someday die, we construct our character and our lives to avoid and even deny this. To further ensure it, we collectively erect a cultural system that isolates death and, in exchange for fixed ritual and belief, even promises immortality.

Little wonder then that people react as they do upon learning they have cancer. They imagine that death has somehow slipped past the gates and invaded their bodies. They are instantly disoriented. From feeling in command of their bodies, they suddenly find an alien body commands them. From a familiar world of self-determination where the rules are known, they are thrust suddenly into a battle where there are no given rules and no sign of having a fighting chance against this nebulous enemy within.

Fear of this sort is communicable and spreads rapidly to others. As a result, these patients experience the desertion of lovers, the dispiriting faces of their families expecting death, the skimpy telegrams from absent friends or employers.

MORAL: Fear serves as cancer's ally by blocking action against it. We delay or skip critical checkups, we fail to act immediately on warning symptoms. In this way, fear condemns us to the group who do not survive because they fail to get there on time.

So we are being told that to have cancer does not mean to die—certainly not for the former patients in this survey, although many of them once thought it did. There *is* something you can do about it. You are *not* instantly in a hopeless condition. You *can* and *must* fight back in various ways—and one of the most essential is not to delay in getting the best possible treatment.

The patient's initial physician—a general practitioner or the family doctor—plays a critical role in the course of the cancer treatment. His recognition of a symptom that may be related to cancer can be vital and save a life. We see this occur here. We also see some doctors—a surprising number, in fact—who were not alert to cancer's subtler symptoms and so failed to detect it in its initial phase, when there is a maximum chance for recovery. Or they failed to note the risk factor of a history of cancer in the patient's family, requiring more frequent checkups.

As a result of diagnostic failure by their physicians or specialists, many of these survivors nearly died. Others, though not all, narrowly escaped needless surgery.

A young, substitute doctor tells Estelle Marsicano that her liver is enlarged and should be seen by a specialist—who most probably would have discovered cancer. Her regular family doctor scoffs: "My liver's large, too —want to feel it?" He puts her on tranquilizers for a "nervous digestion" until she worsens, has dizzy spells, and, finally enraged, demands further examination—just in time.

John Alexion is told by "the chief urologist of a major New York hospital" that the only cure for his prostate cancer is surgical castration and radical removal of the prostate—an operation that would have made him a eunuch. Instead, a procedure developed by Dr. Willet Whitmore and associates at Memorial destroyed the cancer with no further bodily damage.

It is easy to become upset with these men because our lives are on the line, and we expect them to save us—or, at least, not to be ignorant of the disease. The fact is, however, that many doctors are not aware of the latest developments in the detection and control of cancer. This should not be surprising. Cancer takes many forms in at least a hundred different diseases. The study of it—oncology—is a relatively new field of medicine, missing from the curriculum of many medical schools. Specialists in this field attack the disease on a rapidly moving, multidisciplinary front— using aggressive surgery, radiation therapy, a changing array of anticancer drugs (chemotherapy), and the harnessing of immunology (the body's defense system) the better to detect and destroy the invading disease.

While all this is going on, the general practitioner and his immediate battalion of specialists are fighting their own battles against a host of other ills, trying to save as many lives as possible. Most of them have little time to read the latest news on the war against cancer, let alone understand its intricate tactics and strategies. Some do manage, however. Recognizing the need, an increasing number of physicians are developing subspecialties in oncology.

None of this knowledge should lessen our respect for any of these doctors. Most of them, though certainly not all, spend their lives in service to the patient, often performing heroically with little or no recognition.

MORAL: Position yourself to get the best possible medical treatment in the shortest possible time, especially if the symptoms persist or are ill-defined. If you live near a major cancer center or hospital, you might want to go there for a checkup—especially if there's no clear diagnosis from your family doctor.† Remember, you have a right to a second opinion. Do not worry about upsetting your first doctor. If you are told that you have cancer—regardless of the outlook—you should obtain a second opinion from an oncologist. Your own doctor, or even just one cancer specialist, may not be enough for your needs. In all likelihood, your physician is a sincere, well-meaning, professional, and wants to do what is best for you. Yet, as we see indicated here, there is no other area of medicine with so great a gap between daily practice and the theoretical possibilities of avail-

† Besides Memorial Sloan-Kettering Cancer Center, in the United States there are twenty other "comprehensive cancer centers"—so designated by the National Cancer Institute as capable of providing up-to-date information and care for all major types of cancer. There are also more than 1,000 American hospitals and medical centers approved by the American College of Surgeons with varying facilities for cancer diagnosis and treatment. To locate the center nearest you—or for free service in your region from information specialists on causes, diagnosis, treatment, rehabilitation, referrals, or other cancer-related matters—call the Cancer Information Service of the NCI, toll-free from anywhere in the U.S.: 1/800/4-CANCER. In District of Columbia call: 636-5700; in Alaska: 1/800/638-6070; in Hawaii: 524-1234.

able treatment. Your goal is to close that gap as much as possible—should it become necessary.

At this point, we have seen the critical importance of getting the best and most prompt diagnosis or treatment, and the ways in which we are dangerously delayed.

We have yet to see what "the best" can do, how a hospital functions as an interaction of dedicated men and women bringing to it their diverse skills, their hopes, their lives—all of it working in an overall harmony as though the hospital itself was one living body, a healthy body casting off sick or diseased cells. When viewed this way, Memorial Hospital is a remarkable creation—as we discover from these men and women who were saved there.

They'd just operated on me, and my daughter was getting married in three weeks. I could hardly lift my arm, let alone go anywhere. But I figured if I could build myself up to walk a mile a day, I'd be able to get out in time to walk her down the aisle of the church.

When they let me out of bed, I went out to the corridor. You know the floor tiles there at Memorial? They're exactly a foot long. So I shuffled down the length of one corridor, counting them, then across to the opposite corridor. I figured the complete turn, down one corridor and up the other, was four hundred eighty feet, so eleven times around would be a mile.

I was working it out with a diagram on a pad when a nurse asked me, "What's that? A plan to break into this place?" "No," I said, "it's a plan to break out."

He's 54, a small figure with light blue eyes, a gentle voice, and quiet manner —possessing also an inner strength and personal resolve he believes was essential to his recovery from melanoma and then cancer in the lung. "Once you get to Memorial, you've got the best. That's most important. But once they've given you the best they have, the ball is in the other court. What counts then is your own input. You've got to fight your way back to where you were. If you don't do it, if you lack confidence, you can lose the game."

Once a month, Jay Weinberg—who has the Avis franchise for Westchester County, New York—leaves his office in Mount Vernon to drive to Memorial. There, he descends to a basement locker room to don a blue jacket with nameplate, identifying him as one of the hospital's 450 nonpaid volunteers. They come from every strata of society and serve in one hundred different areas, including the thrift and gift shops, recreation pavilion, patient library, flower service, admitting office, blood donor bank, outpatient clinics, as well as on the nursing floors and in clinical and research departments.

Jay is part of a small group of ex-cancer patients who meet incoming patients or visit them in their rooms. In an unobtrusive manner, he has told his story to hundreds of people who have clung to it as a living reality of how they, too, can survive.

We are seated in an ice cream parlor near Memorial. With Jay is his wife, Marian, a short woman with soft brown eyes and a pleasant smile. She listens and smiles at Jay's story as though hearing it for the first time. "She's the great one," he says. They've been married 35 years.

I was having a physical checkup and told my doctor, "I think I pulled a muscle in my arm skiing, but it doesn't seem to heal." He pokes under my left armpit and finds a lump. "I think that's the problem," he says. "You should go to a surgeon and have it removed." So I went to a surgeon at a local hospital, and he said, "Look, we don't know what it is, but it should come out. We'll set you up for an operation."

I was worried, and I told him, quite frankly, that I wanted a second opinion. So I went to another doctor who notices a mole on my back, and he tells me, "I think the mole is related to that lump. You should have it biopsied before anything else." Well, I should have known it. About two years before, I went to a skin doctor for something else, and he spotted the mole and said, "I want you to get rid of that." Our family doctor at the time was old-fashioned. "Don't do anything," he said. "It might open up a can of worms. We'll just watch it." So you see, all of this didn't have to happen if we'd been smart about it.

When I reported back to the surgeon, he said, "Oh yes, the mole could be related. We'll take a biopsy of it, and go ahead with the operation." So I went to the hospital on a Thursday to have the mole removed and sent to the laboratory. And the next evening, Friday, I checked into the hospital, to have the lump removed.

The next morning, they woke me up early to get me ready for the operation. I'm lying there, under sedation and really not of this world, when the pathology report on the mole came down—saying it was malignant, and I had melanoma. That's when my wife saved the day and maybe my life.

MARIAN: *(Interrupts)* We'd been waiting for the biopsy report. Jay was sedated, the surgeon was ready, the anesthesiologist was waiting—and finally the report arrived saying it was melanoma. The surgeon came up and said, "Marian, this is going to be much more extensive than anticipated, and after the operation Jay will have to go to Baltimore or Chicago for further treatment." I responded, "Baltimore or Chicago? What's wrong with Memorial Hospital in New York?" To which he responded, "I don't know anybody there." So I asked him, "When did you last do an operation like this?" He said, "About five years ago." I said to him, "If you don't mind, I'd rather go someplace where they did five of them yesterday."

He was very sweet, he understood. So we took Jay out of the hospital and went to an ice cream parlor for lunch. But he was so sedated he didn't know where he was or what he was doing, and he fell asleep over his milk shake. *(Laughs.)*

JAY: That was Saturday, and by Monday we had an appointment with

Dr. Shiu at Memorial in the outpatient clinic.* He's a marvelous Chinese doctor in his late thirties who's now one of our best friends. But at that first meeting, he knocked the wind out of me. After looking at X rays, the biopsy report, and examining me, he calls me and Marian in and puts the cards on the table. "We're going to have to operate on you," he says. He was trying to be pleasant, but from the way he spoke, I knew I was in real trouble—more than I'd realized. I ask him, "How bad is it? What are my odds?" "It's not good," he says. "But the operation must be done. It's the only chance." Can you imagine it? *(Smiles.)* I don't feel sick, I'm an active guy, I've got a good business, a nice family—and all of a sudden I realize I might not live much longer!

MARIAN: It sounded so depressing, so terrible, that I finally turned to him and asked, "Have you ever saved anyone with this?" To which he responded, "Of course!"

JAY: Later I learned that during this stage the doctors generally judge whether they can level with a patient right away, or whether they should give it to him slowly, in different stages. We asked Shiu for the facts, straight from the shoulder, and that's why he didn't mince words. "There's a ninety-five percent chance the mole and the lymph node are related, and the melanoma has gone at least that far—though we still have to prove that with a biopsy. I hope it has gone no further, but we can't know that until we have operated and determined the extent of its involvement."

For the next ten days, I nearly went crazy. I'm not an emergency, so I have to wait, and I'm having nightmares all day long. I imagine the cells spreading through my lymph system, I feel like I'm dying every day, and I'm also angry. Driving through the Bowery sector, I see drunken bums lying in the street, and I ask myself, "Why me and not somebody else?"

I later learned you go through six stages with cancer. The first is disbelief. You say, "It can't be me, the doctors are wrong." Next is what I was experiencing then. It's pure anger. You ask, "Why me, dammit?" After that, just before the operation, it becomes fear of the unknown when you ask a million questions. Then, after the operation, there's despair because you've hit the low spot. You're hurt, sick, fragile, and the future looks dim. Finally, there's recovery when the driving out makes all the difference.

Then one day, while I was still in the anger stage, I was working in my office when the hospital called, saying the bed was ready and I must come within two hours. I called home, but Marian was out somewhere. So I

---

* Man Hei Shiu, M.D., associate attending surgeon, Gastric and Mixed Tumor Service, Department of Surgery, Memorial Hospital.

went without her. I drove alone into the city and up to the hospital. By this time, I had left the anger stage and was into the next one of fear. This was it. I was on my way to the big operation and the unknown.

Well, it was April first—April Fool's Day. I get to the entrance of the hospital, and I see a dollar bill on the sidewalk. I think, "It can't be, it's got to be fake, somebody's waiting to laugh at me." I started to go by, then I think, "What if it's real? Maybe I'm scared of this cancer, but I'm not afraid of a lousy joke!" *(Laughs.)* So I decided to bend over and pick it up, telling myself if it was real, it'd be a sign that I had the cancer under control, that it had not spread through my body. So I picked it up—and it was real! *(Laughs.)* Sounds silly now, but at the time it was like getting a word from God. I walked into the hospital telling myself, "You've got it made, Jay, you're going to lick this."

Believe me, I needed something like that, especially after they'd run me through all the tests. My surgeon, Manny Shiu, had me sign papers granting permission for radical surgery if necessary, including resection of the neck area that might have left me scarred and with muscular weakness. I put that dollar bill up on the wall and used to look at it to remind me that I was going to win this one—I had to.

By the time they took me down to the operating room, with no idea of how much they were going to cut away, I'd made up my mind that this was like a plane flight. Most people who are afraid to fly don't realize the pilot is just as anxious to come out alive as you are. Dr. Shiu was my pilot, and I was sure he was going to deliver me in one piece—and he did. He found the cancer had not spread beyond the lymph nodes under my arm, and since he knew I was a tennis player, he dissected with special care to preserve my muscular ability. He also removed more from my back where the malignant mole had been, then applied a skin graft from my thigh to close it—a beautiful job.

I was just coming around after the operation when this guy strolls into my room. I know he's one of the volunteers because he's wearing a blue jacket. It was Kal Eisenbud, one of the old-timers, whose technique I now use myself. You sort of look around the room for clues to what the patient is interested in—photographs, postcards, get-well greetings, a book maybe —anything to help you draw the guy out, to start him talking about himself, or whatever's bugging him.

Kal sees a photo of my daughter, who is getting married in three weeks, and all of a sudden, I'm telling this stranger in a blue jacket how I intend to get out in time to walk her down the aisle. I remember him saying, "I bet you'll do it, that you'll make it. Will you let me know how it goes?" I said, "Okay, I will," and shortly after that I got up and began to count those floor tiles up to a mile.

MARIAN: *(Laughs)* We did all the planning for the wedding from the hospital. With Jay's trouble, we'd delayed the invitations, and they were sent from Memorial after we knew he'd be all right. He'd lost a lot of weight, so we ordered a new suit over the phone from Saks. The tailor came to fit it, then came back again to make sure it was right. He was a terrific guy, an Italian. Jay wanted to give him something for his trouble, but he refused it, telling us, "No, this is my part of the wedding."

Then my dress. I'd bought it in about five minutes and was anxious for Jay to see it. So I come over to the hospital and put this dress on. I'm parading up and down the halls, showing it to everyone, and we decide that's it. Then I'm in the room, pulling the dress over my head to take it off, when the door opens and in walks Manny Shiu. He said, "Oh, excuse me," and left. He didn't know what was going on, but he had such terrific respect for Jay after that—I mean, a man in his condition! *(Laughs.)*

At the wedding, Jay walked his daughter down the aisle. Everyone thought it was a beautiful day. Shortly after that, Jay and Marian went to Lake Placid. The local Avis franchise was for sale—because of poor business— and Jay bought it. "I picked it up for very little, and the guy was happy to get rid of it. Then they announced the winter Olympics were going to be at Lake Placid, and I told Marian, 'Everything's going our way—the operation, the wedding, and now this bonanza.' She said, 'Bite your tongue.' I didn't, and maybe I should have."

On the fourth of July, I got a chest infection. We went into Memorial, and the physician on duty aspirated a great deal of pus. He murmured something like "This usually occurs when there's a lung involvement." He took some X rays, and I went home.

A week or so later, a letter came from Memorial. They didn't like one of the X rays and wanted it done again. So I went in, and the new ones showed a spot on the lung. I thought, "Oh God, this is it. Lung cancer is a killer." Manny Shiu tried to encourage me. "This isn't the end of the world," he said. "We can probably lick this one, too. I could do it for you, but there's somebody who's better at this than I am. He's a specialist in thoracic surgery, and I'd like you to go to him."

That's when I met Dr. Cahan.† You could pick him out in a crowd

---

† William G. Cahan, M.D., attending surgeon, Thoracic Service, Department of Surgery, Memorial Hospital.

anywhere—a handsome guy with white hair, very friendly, and immediately I felt secure with him. He explained this wasn't cancer *of* the lung, but rather *in* the lung, meaning it didn't start in the lung as it does with people who smoke. I've never smoked. He thought it was a solitary metastasis, coming from the mole melanoma, and the best way to attack it was to take out an entire lobe of the lung. At the time, this was a relatively new technique. He had made an intense study of it, and he told me, "If we just take out a piece of lung, where the cancer is, we might not get it all. If we take out the entire lobe, it's still a gamble because you never know with cancer. But I think you'll have a far better chance that way." I said, "Okay, let's do it." Right off, I trusted him, and I knew I was going to lick this one, too.

MARIAN: *(Interrupts)* I didn't. I thought that everyone who got lung cancer died of it sooner or later. So this time I was really scared. I figured that melanoma had gotten loose and was spreading all over his body. But would you believe it? All I hear is Jay babbling away about his new Lake Placid franchise and how much fun we're going to have in the 1980 Winter Olympics—six years away! *(Laughs.)* I thought, "The man's crazy. He's talking about 1980 as if he's going to be there." I never thought he would.

JAY: The second time you go back to Memorial, it's like going into the Army again. You know the ropes, where before you felt exposed to an unknown terror, afraid of losing yourself, your identity—if you know what I mean. The second time, you're better able to hold onto yourself, and you have less fear. You also know the ways of the hospital and that you can get passes to go out to dinner, if the doctor okays it. We checked in Sunday afternoon and, since Dr. Cahan wasn't there, I figured I had to wait several days for the operation. So I asked for a pass, and we went to a lovely restaurant with some friends and came back by nine o'clock.

In the meantime, Dr. Cahan had been looking for me, asking "Where's my patient?" He was absolutely furious that I'd been allowed to leave. The next morning, when they rolled me into the operating room, he looks down at me and says, "Where'd you run off to last night?" I was heavily sedated and groggy, but I recall saying, "I was busy." "Busy?" he says, "What's more important than this?" "Just one thing," I said, "having a layman's last supper." He laughed, and then I passed out—but it was the beginning of our friendship.

He took out the lower lobe of the left lung, leaving me one good lobe there, and the usual three lobes on the right side. After the operation, he said it went okay, and I told him I had to attend an important Avis convention in Vancouver in two weeks. He said, "No way. You've had major lung surgery." He smiled and said, "Why don't you cable them, 'At Memorial, they try harder, too'?"

Well, I started walking down that corridor again. It was a lot harder this time, but I kept at it, and I kept nagging Cahan, telling him about my lap time getting faster and faster until he finally let me go—all wrapped up and with strict orders to take it easy.

That was nine years ago, and since then I've had no trouble. In the beginning, they gave me some immunological boosters but after that, nothing. At first, I couldn't swim three laps without wheezing. Now I do forty every morning before work. I ski and play tennis—and, once a month, instead of tennis on Sunday, I come into Memorial as a volunteer.

What do I get out of it? I feel that I'm helping some people who are in desperate need of knowledge. I know because I lacked that knowledge when I came here. This whole place was a mystery to me, and it's a mystery to most people when they come to a cancer center—what's going to happen? where are they headed? All their lives, they've heard, "Cancer —boom, that's it. You've had it." They need extra hope, the charge that they are going to make it. Doctors can give all the medical help that's possible, and nurses and social workers can take care of your immediate needs, but if the patient sees somebody who's been through it, who's had cancer and has come out of it okay, it can give them that extra push they are going to need.

I didn't have it when I came in. I got it when I was here, when Kal Eisenbud walked into my room and got me to talking about my daughter's wedding and gave me a goal, the extra push. I suppose that's why I keep returning here—to give back some of what was given to me that day.

POSTSCRIPT: Two years later, Jay Weinberg was trying to give even more. With Priscilla Blum, another former Memorial patient, he had recruited 230 business corporations into a rapidly expanding Corporate Angel Network (CAN), which utilizes empty seats on flights of corporate aircraft for the travel needs of cancer patients, homeward bound or en route to specialized care hospitals like Memorial. For many, it can be crucial. Travel costs are not covered by Medicare or private insurance. A CAN flight is free. Patients must be ambulatory and coordinate their schedule with the corporation's. The idea originated with "Pat" Blum, 57, a free-lance writer and licensed pilot, who was cured of breast cancer fourteen years ago at Memorial. An independent, non-profit entity, the expanding network of five hundred planes has linked up corporate aviation across the United States. Tel: 914/328-1313.

He is pacing back and forth in the living room of his riverfront home in Harrisburg, Pennsylvania. Above him, on a bookshelf, is a gleaming row of silver tournament cups, won at handball. It is the lack of one more cup that irritates Herman. He has just lost the final match for the U.S. Handball Championships—in the over-60 category.

We had met to talk about another victory he had won, against cancer of the colon, after a Harrisburg surgeon had given him less than six months to live. At the moment, however, he is too angry about losing the national title to talk of anything else. "I had that guy. I can beat him or anybody else over sixty. But I blew it. Would you believe it?"

Herman sinks into a sofa chair. He is 63, with a powerful body, thick arms and legs, and an oversized stomach. His wife, Fannie, sitting on another sofa, explains: "He's a chow hound. He eats anything." Herman's reply is a solemn oath, delivered with his eyes closed. "I'll get him. I'm going to live a long time. Sooner or later, I'll run him into the ground."

My father was an Orthodox rabbi. Ever since I can remember, my parents instilled that drive to get as close to perfection as you can. Whatever you do, do it right. When we were kids, I'll never forget, I said to my mother, "Why can't I go outside without a shirt? My friend Charlie's doing that." She said, "Your friend Charlie isn't Jewish. They won't say anything if he goes out like that, but if you go without a shirt, or don't look presentable, they'll say, "There goes that goddamn Jew." She didn't use that exact word, but the inference was there.

FANNIE: *(Interjects)* He's also stubborn and has an ego as big as this house. If it weren't for that and losing those handball games, he'd probably be dead today.

HERMAN: The first time I realized there was something wrong, I was working and felt I had to break wind. I was by myself, and I noticed a little wetness there. I said, "Oh, my goodness, did I have an accident?" So I immediately headed for home, and upon examining myself, I found that it was blood.

The next day I went to a doctor. He checked me out and said, "Yes, Herman, I can see that you have a bleeding hemorrhoid." So for about four months I was afraid to break wind because every now and then I would have a little accident. Also, when I would go to the bathroom, there would be blood in the commode. I took it for granted that all this came from a bleeding hemorrhoid.

I'm a tournament handball player. I play competitively four or five times a week. The top players from the city play among themselves. It's like any other sport. You play with your peers. If somebody doesn't give you competition, you don't play with him. Well, gradually, I stopped playing fellows on my level and began dropping down. I would stand up against the wall, gasping for breath. I couldn't understand what was happening.

One day, I'm playing a fellow, and he jokes about it: "Herman, you hardly ever talk to me. Now you're not only talking, but you're even willing to play with me!" Then he beat me badly. The next day a fellow beat me who I normally would never play with. He's a doctor of philosophy, and he said, "Herman, something is wrong. For me to beat you, twenty-one to one, you must be sick. You should see a doctor."

So, on the way home, I stopped in to see Dr. Brenner. At first, he was furious and said, "Herman, Fannie made two appointments, and you canceled." I said, "Lou, why do I have to come to see you? You told me I have a bleeding hemorrhoid, and so I bleed a little bit. Isn't that what happens?" He said, "Yes." So I said, "You might think this is ridiculous, but you know I play handball. I should be in tremendous shape, but I don't have any stamina. After one or two points, I'm breathing heavy. Guys I don't normally play with are running me into the ground."

He was a little upset at this and sent me out for an X ray. The doctor's nurse, Mary, who's a personal friend of ours, called the next day, and she's concerned. They'd found a spot, and Dr. Brenner wants to see me. So I go to him, and he says, "Herman, you have to go to the hospital." Up until this time, I'm quiet and composed, but this is too much. I can't go into any hospital at this time.

He's in the installment business. In New York, they call them customer peddlers. "I do direct selling to people I've been doing business with for years. Whatever they want, I give them. They pay me a minimum down, and the rest later. I used to have a big operation—forty salesmen, fourteen collectors. With my brother-in-law, we did about seven million dollars a year. But the more business we did, the more we went into debt. It was just a horrendous situation. My accountant said, 'Herman, you're a rich man.' I said, 'Show me a little cash.' Finally, I cut back, little by little, until today it's a one-man operation. I'm doing one twentieth of what I once did, yet making a tremendous profit."

I can't go into the hospital because it's Thanksgiving, and my big time is coming up. Ninety percent of my business is in December. To get ready for that, I buy all year and have a warehouse full of stuff. So I told the doctor, "Okay, whatever you say. Just let me finish my Christmas business. How's about December twenty-fourth or twenty-fifth?" He said,

"You misunderstood me. You have to go now." I said, "Lou, it's easy for you to say, but everything I have is tied up in that warehouse. If I don't unload now, I won't have anything to collect later." He shook his head and said, "Herman, it all depends on your priorities. Do you want to have a business and be dead, or do you want to go to the hospital and be alive?" I said, "You don't give me much choice, do you?" He said, "No, I don't. Either you go, or I'm not your doctor." I knew I had to go. But it's the day before Thanksgiving, and how am I going to break the news to Mother? We were having our usual big family affair—about forty people. So I don't tell her or mention it to anyone.

FANNIE: *(Interrupts)* I knew. You came in and broke down. *(Herman shakes head in disbelief.)* Even so, I'd have known it. With a wife or a mother, there's some kind of divining rod, so you're sensitive to every little nuance. It's a different kind of love than passion. It's a very caring love and a very worried love. Besides, I'd already called Mary, and she'd told me they'd found something, a little larger than a pinpoint.

Herman was choked up. He said, "Why'd this have to happen to me now?" Then he broke down. But it was the only time I saw him like that. From then on, he was pretty composed. I was the one who broke down next. I took to my couch and said, "God almighty, you've got cancer and that's it."

HERMAN: We didn't know I had cancer at the time.

FANNIE: You didn't *think* so, but you had every classic thing. What I noticed was your color. It was almost gray. And you were chilled all the time. In the summer, you used to sit with your sweater on.

HERMAN: *(Sighs, looks upward)* Maybe that could be, but I insist I went to the hospital a well man. I was short on stamina, but I didn't feel sick. I went in on a Sunday. . . . *(Laughs.)* I told Fannie, "They won't let you come." So my local doctor and my surgeon took me into a room, told me bend down with my head on a pillow, and then started probing with a sigmoidoscope. I let them go as far as they could, and when they released me, that pillow was soaking wet.

Dr. Waltz, the surgeon, said, "Herman, we can't see anything, which is a good sign. You have an obstruction further up, but from what we see, I don't think you'll need a button." I didn't know what a button was, and he explained it was a colloquialism for a colostomy, which was the furthest thing from my mind because I'm still feeling good.*

---

* An operation in which the large bowel is brought to the abdominal wall and given an opening there, with feces passing into a plastic bag attached to the patient. There are two kinds: reversible, or temporary, and permanent. Colon-rectal cancer will be diagnosed in about 120,000 Americans this year and 54,900 will die of it—second only to lung cancer in

They operated the next morning, and the first thing I know a girl is waking me up, "Mr. Krevsky . . . Mr. Krevsky, you have a colostomy!" That brought me to my senses fast, and I let loose with a tirade in a language she never knew existed. Then I passed out again. Fannie can tell you what Dr. Waltz said after the surgery.

FANNIE: That morning, I went to the hospital very early and found my sister and my niece waiting for me, and we went to the coffee shop. I had lost some of my apprehension because the doctor had said, "I don't think he'll have to have a button." But there was always the fear in the back of my mind, and I thought, "Please God, don't let him have to have it." Then I hear my name on the intercom, "Mrs. Krevsky . . . Mrs. Krevsky." Dr. Waltz wants to see me, and right away I know something is terribly wrong. He is waiting for me at the nurse's station and says, "Mrs. Krevsky, I'm sorry to tell you, he has an invasive tumor blockage and I couldn't remove it." He's walking down the hall with me, and he says, "If he had come to me six months sooner." I tell him, "He wasn't sick six months ago." He shrugs his shoulders, and I ask him, "How long do you think he has?" Very matter-of-factly, he says, "Three to six months." With that, I went into Herman's room and sat down on a chair. I don't know how I got home. My sister, Sylvia, says she took me.

I didn't cry. I was very wooden and didn't cry at that time. I remember thinking how terrible life would be without him. That's all I kept thinking. So I came in the house and picked up the phone. He has three brothers who are doctors in Detroit. I called one, who is a pediatrician, and blurted out the whole story, and he said, "Okay, I'll get right back to you." After that, the other two brothers, another pediatrician and a gynecologist, called to say they would get in touch with Herman's doctors.

Then Dr. Brenner said he wanted to see me, and I was devastated. That was the end, I knew, because a friend of ours across the street had had a brain tumor, and Dr. Brenner had called his wife to tell her the bad news. *(Pauses.)* So I went to him, shaking and teary, and he said, "Fannie, we're taking Herman to another hospital." I said, "Why? If he's going to die, just let him get finished in a hurry." "No," he said, "I don't agree with Dr. Waltz's opinion."

HERMAN: There was never a moment when I didn't think I was going to make it. Chalk it up to ignorance—or maybe my brothers. They were talking to me constantly and assuring me that everything was going to be

---

its occurrence rate and claiming more lives than breast cancer. From 75 to 80 percent of these cases could be cured by early diagnosis and treatment, since these cancers are usually slow-growing and remain localized for long periods. A high-fat diet that is low in fiber or roughage is believed to help induce colon cancer.

okay. *(Shakes head.)* Their telephone bills must have been staggering. They called all over the country to determine who was best for this particular operation. As medical men, they had access to more people than the average individual, so I guess I had that going for me, too.

After a while, Dr. Waltz and his partner, Dr. Kistler, became annoyed with my brothers' phone calls. Dr. Kistler is a TV version of a doctor: over six feet, built like an Adonis. When the nurses see him coming, they swoon. He finally told my brother Dave: "Herman's got three months to live. Why don't you just keep him comfortable and let him go?" My brother said, "What would you do, if it was your brother?" Dr. Kistler replied, "You're right. I'd probably be doing the same thing." Also, I have to hand it to Dr. Waltz. He was very honest. He said, "Quite frankly, we don't have the possibilities here to remove your blockage, but there are specialized cancer centers where it might be possible." Later, I learned that Dr. Waltz had actually saved my life by not cutting into the tumor and spreading it. He knew when to stop, and he fixed me up with a colostomy to give me time to have it done elsewhere.

FANNIE: If he'd gone on cutting, Herman would be dead today. So we're not putting him down, but I think it's important to talk about this and not hide anything, so that people in places where they don't have cancer specialists, where the surgeons aren't cancer surgeons, can say, like Dr. Brenner did and like Herman's brothers, "Hey, wait a minute, we want a second opinion, we want a doctor or surgeon who handles ten of these every day, not ten in a year."

HERMAN: That's right, and that's when my brothers called and said, "Herman, if they ask you where you want to go, tell them Memorial Hospital."

FANNIE: *(Interjects)* It was a choice between two surgeons at Memorial —Maus Stearns or Dr. Quan—and whether or not they would take Herman. Dr. Brenner had long talks with Dr. Stearns, who finally decided there was a fighting chance.† Before leaving, I bumped into Dr. Waltz in the corridor. I was probably at my worst because I felt he'd been so cruel to me. He said, "I hear Herman's going to New York. The treatment they're going to give him there is what I wanted to do here. But when I opened him up, there was so much inflammation, I couldn't discern the actual tumor."‡

HERMAN: Yes, but Dr. Stearns knew how to do it. When I came to his

---

† Maus W. Stearns, Jr., M.D., attending surgeon, Rectal & Colon Service, Department of Surgery, Memorial Hospital.

‡ As events transpired, Dr. Waltz's surgical caution at this point actually saved Krevsky's life.

office the first time, it was an experience in itself. You think you're coming as an individual, a big shot maybe from a small town. You come in with your X rays in that brown envelope, two by three feet. You sit down and look around the room, and there's a big landowner from Rio de Janeiro, somebody from Paris, a family from India, another from Italy—from all over the world, waiting with their big brown envelopes.

Finally, Dr. Stearns looked at my X rays. He's very low-key, and he said, "I think we can help you." Then he said to not bad-mouth Dr. Waltz, "Your Harrisburg surgeon probably saved your life by not going further. He gave you a colostomy that cut off blood supply to the tumor. He did not cut into it or disseminate it. So now we can begin cobalt treatments— twenty-five, starting tomorrow. When that's over, we'll go from there."

This news was a shock, because I pictured my neighbor who had just died. He took cobalt and turned yellow. His hair fell out. I said, "Do I have to go through all that and then die? I'd rather not, really." He said, "No, the cobalt is not a cure-all. What it does is harden the tumor. If you touch a rotten peach on a tree, it will disintegrate in your hand. If you wait until it becomes ossified, like a stone, then you can touch it. That's what the cobalt treatments will do for you. It will help make the tumor manageable."

To show where I was to be radiated, they painted my back like a cross-word puzzle and Stearns said, "Don't wash that off. Leave it on." So it began, every morning—the cobalt radiation. We were in an apartment on Sixty-third Street, one of those buildings designated for patients taking treatment at Memorial. The radiation gave me a terrible itch at the top of the crack in my behind, at the coccyx bone. It was just awful. You wanted to tear the itch out of your body. Otherwise, it wasn't too bad. My participation in sports helped. Dr. Stearns said, "You have good muscle tone, which is a good sign."

His worst trouble was in handling the colostomy opening. At first, in the Harrisburg hospital, he had refused to look at it, and the nurses had cleaned it. There wasn't much fecal matter, anyway, because he was being fed intravenously. "Shortly before I was released, two nurses came in and said, 'You're going home in two days, and you don't know how to take care of your colostomy.' I said, 'No, frankly, I haven't touched it.' I guess the problem is the same with everyone. You don't want to recognize it, so you ignore it. This one girl says, 'Okay, we'll show you. Hubert Humphrey had one, and even Fred Astaire had one while he was dancing.' I didn't know whether she was telling me the truth about Astaire, but it does make you feel better to know you're not alone. The other nurse was more direct. She said,

*'Either you learn how to do it, or you can't go home.' So I tried it, while still
in the hospital, and at first it seemed I could manage."*

But when I got to New York and began to move around, I ran into
trouble. You see, you have this hole in your stomach and a bag over it,
which is supposed to collect whatever comes out. But I'm slightly obese, to
put it mildly. So with the fat and blubber moving, most of the time the bag
wasn't in position, and it would go down my clothes—and that was the
most awful thing that I've ever experienced in my life.

Every day you have to wash yourself, a kind of enema through the
colostomy opening, called irrigation. You're supposed to do it regularly, at
fixed hours. So I used to get up at five or six A.M., and at first it was a two-
hour job. I would sit in the bathroom and read until I felt it, and then I'd
go over to the commode and try and regulate myself. But then later, it
would unexpectedly come out. That's the most embarrassing part. What
can you do? You have to excuse yourself and leave.*

One afternoon we went over to Broadway to see a matinee of *Pajama
Game* with Diahann Carroll—an unusual show, with black and white
costars. After the show, we went to Howard Johnson's, and she came in
and sat near us, and I said, "Just saw you, Diahann, and thought you were
great." She laughed and thanked me, and then I felt my bag overflowing.
That meant I had to take water right away to clean out the bag and
irrigate myself. A water glass would do it, but I didn't have one. So I said
to the waiter, a Puerto Rican kid, "Give me a glass of water, please, I must
go to the toilet." He refused, and I wasn't about to start explaining. Finally, he brought me a paper cup, and I head for the bathroom, feeling it
coming down my pants. Fortunately, Howard Johnson's has a stall with a
sink close to the commode, so I could maneuver.

When I came up, I told Fannie, "Honey, let's go." She says, "Herman, I
can't stand." I couldn't believe it and said, "You didn't have a drink,
what's the matter?" She said, "I don't know, I just can't walk."

Well, unbeknownst to me, Fannie has been popping pills—Valium and
phenobarbital. She sees me go down, she sees me go up, and she gets upset.
Whenever my back's turned, or when I'm in the bathroom, she takes the
pills without my knowing it. Now I see she's stoned, and I'm barely able to
get her into a taxi and home.

FANNIE: I felt sorry for him as a human being because this was all so

---

* Herman Krevsky's difficulties were exceptional. Most colostomy patients soon learn to
regulate themselves and do not experience similar troubles. This is, however, one of the
most instructive features of this case, further defined in the survival factor, Self.

degrading. We went to a party one time, and the pouch overflowed into his pants. The feeling I had for him at that time was pity, just pity. We flew to New York because we thought it would be easier, and we wanted to get there as fast as possible. Then in the limousine, he had an accident. The stench was horrendous. When we finally got to the apartment, I began washing his pants.

I'm going to tell you how I really feel about this. Why am I washing his pants? It's because I finally know about pity and love, and I kept saying, "I don't care what happens, I'm willing to undergo it." I was thinking of myself, treating this thing, living with it, washing his pants. "Just let him live, God. Please God, if he lives, I can exist with him any way it is." My girlfriend Sylvia stayed with me, and the doctor said we had to clean his colostomy. He refused to deal with it at first. He said, "I won't do it." So I said, "I'll do it."

HERMAN: I couldn't reach it. Someone had to help me with it.

FANNIE: Aside from the difficulty of doing this physical thing for him, I had so much respect for him. I think at the time I admired him more as a human being than anyone in the world. Everytime we went someplace, if he went to the bathroom and wasn't back immediately, I'd go down. It's a men's room, and I look in there, and he's standing at the sink. That's where he had to do it, wash himself, with anybody looking at him. And the steps, the long steps down. Then the Puerto Rican kid told him he couldn't have a glass. It was so uncalled for, you know. What does a guy want a glass for? The tiny little things you take for granted. The kid wouldn't give him a glass, just a paper cup.

He was the happy one, the strong one—all those things—and I admired his spirit. For radium treatments, he went alone. If we took a walk or went to a movie, he was the one that got us moving. I just kept sinking deeper into this kind of never-never land, like I didn't want to do anything. I stopped eating. I was a total, total mess. I've been sick a lot of times, real bad sick, but I really hit the bottom on this. "Boy," I thought, "he has so much spirit, and look at me, I don't want to do anything."

HERMAN: The pill popping had me really worried. The pressure was getting too much for her. When our son George came to visit, I tried to send her home. I said the apartment was too small for all of us, but I really wanted her to get some rest and pull herself together.

FANNIE: (Interrupts) They wanted to ship me out. Our son was trying to help, but he only made matters worse. He asked me, "Do you ever think about dying?" I said, "I think about it a lot, George. What are you trying to tell me? Something about Daddy that I don't know?" He said, "No, Mother, only that you should prepare yourself for that eventuality."

I turned on him angrily. *(Voice falters.)* "You are so brutal, so hard, George. You see me going through all this. Why bring up this business of dying right now?" *(Pauses.)* Looking back now, I see that George was good for us. But when he stormed out of the house that night, leaving me alone with the Terrible-Tempered Mr. Bang, I wanted to be as far away as possible from the two of them. Then it passed, and, next you know, Herman doesn't want me to go anywhere except—he wants to make love, and I am too worried to do anything.

HERMAN: I thought I was ready, but she was afraid. So she called our nephew, the orthopedic surgeon. He said, "That's an excellent sign. Very good. Go to it. Do what you like." I felt I was going to make it then. I always believed that, believed in Stearns, but . . . *(Pauses.)* I've never told this to anyone. I had to wait a short while outside the operating room. They had rolled me down there, and I was alone, in a dark area, waiting for them to take me in. I'm prepped for the operation, and I'm old enough to realize this is the most momentous occasion of my life. I'm going to have a tumor removed. Do I live or do I die? I hate to say this in front of my wife and my close brother. *(His brother Jay has joined us in the living room.)* Also, I don't want it to come out the way it sounds. That's why I'm prefacing it . . .

FANNIE: *(Interrupts)* Then don't say it.

HERMAN: You're talking to somebody who is close to being an atheist or an agnostic. I live the life of an Orthodox Jew because I want to. I was brought up that way, I do it for my children, I do it out of respect for my wife. But there are a lot of unanswered questions. I want to emphasize this because what I want to say might be a little . . .

FANNIE: *(Apprehensive)* Maudlin.

HERMAN: Not maudlin. You're lying there, and there's nobody with you. You're half-doped up, and you've gotten the shot that's going to put you out in a few minutes. Dear God, what do I do? I say, "Dear God, please make it come out." I'm not used to praying, so what do I say? I say, *"Sh'ma Yisrael adonai elohenu adonai echad* . . . [Hear, O Israel; the Lord our God, the Lord is one . . .]." I've never repeated this to anybody . . . *(Sobs, unable to continue.)*

FANNIE: Do you think that helped pull you through?

HERMAN: I would think so. Dr. Stearns and God. Not God alone—Dr. Stearns, too. He's life to me—one God, one Dr. Stearns. My mother brought me, Dr. Stearns kept me. Where were we? Yes, I'm finally in the operating room. Dr. Stearns has a green hat on, and at first I don't recognize him. He looks at me. We wink at one another, and I say, "You can do it." That's all I remember. *(Pauses.)* Now, I'm embarrassed. I don't know why you made me go into all this. It's the first time I've thought of it since that time.

I had asked Dr. Stearns if my brothers could stand in at the operation, and he said, "Absolutely." So it was Harold and Seymour. They washed and dressed and stood at the head of the operating table. It started at eight in the morning and went to four in the afternoon—eight hours. Harold told me that, as the doctor cut the tumor from its area, they would periodically send a piece up to the lab to see if it was malignant or not. After a few minutes, over the loudspeaker would come back whether the last piece was positive or negative. If it was negative, it meant they had cut away enough to be free in that area. He could see my heartbeat on the screen, and he listened for a sign of weakness, but it kept thumping on, solid and strong. The first time Harold saw the tumor clearly was when it was lifted a little way out of its cavity. My brother started saying to himself, "Come, baby, come," as it got higher and higher, until finally Dr. Stearns says, "The tumor is removed in its entirety." Everybody gave a sigh of relief, and when I was closed up, Dr. Stearns went to call Fannie.

FANNIE: He told us to wait at home, not at the hospital. He would call us. So Sylvia, my girlfriend, and I had been tippling a bit—you know, with the strain and the waiting. Finally, the phone rings, and I hear, "Mrs. Krevsky? This is Dr. Stearns. I'd like to tell you that the operation was successful. We have removed the tumor in its entirety, and there was no fragmentation." Well, I started to scream I was so delighted, then I made him repeat it. Sylvia took the phone, and I think she fell over. I remember him telling us to pull ourselves together. But wasn't that real human of him to call us right away?

HERMAN: They took me out to the recovery room, then up to my private room. My sister got through on the phone, and I was very groggy. "I didn't mean to wake you," she said. I said, "No, I'm glad you did. I have to pee." So I called the nurse, and she brought a urinal. I said, "I can't do it in that, never have been able. If you get me out of bed, I can manage it." She said, "I don't know if I can, you've just come up from the operation." I said, "Just stand me up, I won't move." I had a lot of tubes attached to me, and they had closed the first colostomy opening with another temporary colostomy between my stomach and my chest. The nurse stood me up, and I urinated and went back to bed. That was some nurse, a gorgeous Filipina. I knew I was getting better when I noticed her.

FANNIE: It's known as a quickening of the loins.

HERMAN: Not right away. After an abdominal operation, they want you to cough up gas. This nurse used to work with me. She was a perfect size five, real gorgeous, and she wore miniskirts.

FANNIE: He has minor orgasms.

HERMAN: The only way I could cough up a little bit was for her to push on my stomach with a pillow. However, she couldn't reach me. She was petite. So she used to climb on the bed to push on my stomach. When I noticed that, I knew I was really getting better.

FANNIE: *Mon dieu.*

HERMAN: Then there was a third operation, closing the temporary opening, and finally everything is wonderful. I'm just putting in time there, to be sure everything is okay.

People I don't know began coming over to me. "Oh, Mr. Krevsky, I heard you had a colostomy and that you were reconnected. How do you feel? My husband is going through this, too." So they saw me. I had made it, and they were seeking some hope. I talked to all of them, saying it would be all right. There was a couple from London, and she said, "I don't know what to do with my husband. He's a baby. He won't even butter his bread. You can't imagine how I wait on him hand and foot." I said, "Don't worry. Everything will be okay. If I made it, he's going to make it." And she said, "You don't know how much it means to hear that. Thank you so much." The day I'm finally leaving the hospital, I come down just before visiting time. People are congregated, waiting to visit the patients, including many of those from our floor. When they saw me, they started to applaud as though I had won a race. It was a most memorable day.

Before my release, I asked Dr. Stearns, "Is it all right if I play some handball?" He said, "I see nothing wrong with that. Just don't overdo anything. Don't go out and lift pianos." So I'm home finally and my brother Harold calls. I say, "Isn't it wonderful? Dr. Stearns says I can play handball." Harold can't believe it and makes me repeat it. Then he says, "Herman, that dumb SOB doesn't know what handball is—not your kind, anyway. You feel good outside. Your scar is healed, but inside you're still raw." Then in Hebrew, he said, "In the name of God don't you dare." With that, I knew this was very serious. "When you're ready, I'll let you know," he said. "If you want to jog a little bit, that's okay. But don't overdo it." He no sooner hangs up, and David calls. "Herman, don't you dare! Harold just told me. I can't believe it!" He hangs up, and twenty minutes later, Seymour calls. Clearly, this is an emergency. "Herman, don't be insane. It's April now. In six months, maybe you can play handball. Yes, you can jog—but take it easy."

It's also six months since Thanksgiving when my trouble began, and I really feel good. As they say, I'm full of piss and vinegar. Across the street, along the river, there are joggers galore. So out I go, and since it's the first day, I plan to only do five or six blocks. Not push it too hard.

I started off, not too fast, but after fifty yards, I said, "Herman, just get to the end of the block." When I got there, I was sucking wind like I used to do when I was smoking heavily. I didn't think I could make it back—walking. Across the street from our house there's a cement sewer outlet. I sat down there, and I was saying to myself, "Is this the way it's going to be?" I didn't realize that Fannie is watching me from our patio.

FANNIE: He was gone so long, I had visions of him lying out in the street. There was a siren, and I said, "Oh my God, that's for him." Then I looked out and saw him sitting on that pillbox. The perspiration! There was a pool of water under him.

HERMAN: I realized I had to build up slowly. So the next day I jogged down to the corner and walked back. When I say "jogged," I mean very slowly. I did this for a week—to the corner and back. A week later, I went half a block further and ran halfway back, building up.

I didn't know how popular I was in this city. I'd be going down Front Street, dragging my legs, and people would blow their horns to urge me on. I'd give them a V sign and keep on going. As I built it up, I was running down into the city—six miles a day. I did it for six months, come rain or shine. People used to laugh at me in town. They'd say, "Herman is running." At New England Life, Judson Pettis, who's on the board, used to call to people in his office, especially during a rainstorm: "You'll never guess who's running outside." They would all crowd to the window, saying, "Herman's here!" People I didn't even know. I think they liked to look at me because it made them feel better. Life isn't easy for anyone, even if you're well. And to see someone else, a condemned man who was supposed to be dead, climbing back up into life, it made them feel better somehow.

POSTSCRIPT: Herman made good his vow one year later—winning the YMCA U.S. Handball Championship in the over-60 category.

She was 15 when her left leg was amputated at the hip. Three lung opera-tions followed, as surgeons tried to stem the spreading disease. Walking on an artificial leg, she returned to high school—only to be shunned as a freak by her schoolmates. In college, after she had finally found friends and love, the lung cancer returned.

Today, fifteen years later, she is a successful photographer, has published a book on the major fashion designers, is happily married, and has had a baby girl named Jersey.

The leg made me everything I am today. It instilled in me something very strong, and what I have been doing up to this point is proving who I am. I had to prove that I could do it, that I could succeed better than any of those people I went to high school with. None of them thought I could make it because of the lung cancer, the fake leg, and having a limp. *(Laughs.)* You know, everything was "How's Barbara?" or "Poor Bar-bara."*

We are sitting in her spacious Manhattan loft, designed by her husband, Kevin Walz, an interior designer, who joins us periodically between phone calls. Bartok is heard on the hi-fi, and an Irish wolfhound lies nearby. Sunlight pours through a tall window. At 29, she has a slender figure with tousled blond hair, delicate hands, high cheekbones, and a face without lines other than down-sloping shadows beneath gray eyes. She smiles often. Kevin says, "That smile somehow keeps you looking at her face."

She walks with a body swing that brings the artificial leg forward. It appears precarious, but Barbra claims it doesn't impede her work on photo assignments. "I lug around thirty pounds or more of equipment. Crazy! But that's how it goes."

I can do a lot of things, like riding a horse or a bicycle. *(Laughs.)* Once last year, my car was being fixed, and I had a lot of stops uptown—just ap-pointments. Instead of taking seventeen cabs, I took my new bike. It's tricky with the balance. You have to be careful with curbs, but I manage okay with the right leg. The left pedal is off, so the bad leg can hang down. *(Laughs again.)* On the way uptown, I'd stop at red lights, and truck drivers began yelling at me, "Hey, lady! You've lost your pedal!" "Hey,

---

* At college she altered the spelling to Barbra.

Blondie! Who's got your pedal?" I told them, "I went too fast, and it fell off!" It was a laugh.

As a girl, she grew up in Wayne, New Jersey—a town of 50,000 on the Passaic River in the north. Its residents largely commute to New York or are employed in nearby administrative centers of half a dozen major industries. Her father, Stanley Turner, works at an aviation plant owned by the Singer Company.

I used to skate a lot. There was a pond in the woods behind my parents' home, and in the winter time after school, I would take my skates and run through the woods to the pond. It was so beautiful there. Then, all of a sudden, I had a charley horse in the left knee. Everytime I bent it, you would hear a chink. So I went to our family physician, and he said, "Don't worry about it. You must have sprained it. Come back in a month if it isn't gone." So I remained active and went to gym classes. We were jumping over wooden horses then.

I still had it a month later, and he sent me to a bone doctor, an orthopedist, who took an X ray and said it showed a lump on the knee, a calcium deposit. For this, he put my leg in a cast. A week later, he called my mother at night to say he just happened to consult the first X rays and found a lump that had been overlooked. Evidently something was growing, perhaps a tumor, and he wanted an immediate biopsy. So I checked into the local hospital, and they did the biopsy. I was only 15 then, and it was so overwhelming that I simply blanked it all out.

The next evening I was in the hospital room, watching *Lost in Space* on television. It was my father's bowling night, and my mother was alone with me. About seven-thirty the same orthopedist comes in, and he looks very grim. He doesn't even bother to turn down the television. He simply says, "We've got the results of your biopsy, and we're going to have to send you to Memorial Hospital in New York because you have cancer, and your leg's going to have to be amputated." Just like that! Would you believe it? Telling a girl of 15 point-blank that she was going to lose her leg! My mother went into shock, and I went numb. I didn't cry or get hysterical. I just went tight inside, and maybe it was then that I began my inner defense against this.

My mother got on the phone, and it became a strange night. Relatives came from all over, including our aunts and uncles from Long Island. They stayed until very late, and they were all very sad. I was crazed and numb, and finally they gave me a sleeping pill.

The next morning, my parents took me to Memorial and I met the great

Dr. Marcove,† who was furious with the orthopedist for saying I had to have an amputation. He didn't tell me then, but nothing was certain at that point, including whether or not he could save me, even with an amputation. Just the same, I knew I was going to lose my leg, and for some strange reason, I resigned myself to it.

"After the second day at Memorial, I had complete confidence, I didn't worry about the possibility of dying, of the cancer traveling elsewhere, of not being able to cure it. I had cancer, the leg would be amputated, and I would be fine. It's funny, I envisaged the fake leg as being perfect as a normal leg, probably because I had to build up some kind of fantasy in my mind to get rid of the whole thing, a fantasy of being completely normal. It was in the midsixties, with short skirts and textured panty hose. I was really excited, because I saw myself wearing short skirts and looking real good. I had a nice aunt who promised to take me shopping for a whole new wardrobe when I went back to school.

"It was also a tricky age for me—before any type of development of the mind, any self-identity, because at 15 I didn't have anything there. I was just a sophomore in high school. I'd have a crush on somebody and dream of him—that kind of thing. What I really wanted, more than anything else when I went back to school, was to be completely normal." (Laughs.) *"You know, that means being like everyone else—the straight line, the same clothes, the same color hair, the same flip—especially back there in the sixties, before the bubble exploded. You know what I mean?"*

When I woke up after the operation, I felt my leg was still there. There was a pain, mainly in my foot, but when I felt for it, the leg was gone. I still have it, this sense of a phantom leg. At first the pain drove me out of my mind. There was nothing I could do about it, except take sleeping pills. After a month, it went away. But I still have this ghost leg. Right now, if I think about my left leg, I can feel the toes, the foot—everything. It can go on all the time if I let myself think about it. I feel the foot most. Maybe those nerve ends are the most sensitive. It's almost as if I could move my toes, if I tried hard enough.

Five days later, I went home, and my teachers came to my house to tutor me for three weeks until the end of the school term. After that, I had to wait three months for my leg to be fitted.‡ So that summer I just stayed

---

† Ralph C. Marcove, M.D., associate attending surgeon, Orthopedic Service, Department of Surgery, Memorial Hospital.

‡ "In event the disease should spread, usually to the lungs, we routinely imposed a waiting period before acquiring an artificial limb."—Dr. Marcove.

home. I never went out on crutches, and no one came to see me, except a couple of girlfriends. No boys called. I kept telling myself, "It's going to be different when I get the leg. I'll be more normal."

Finally, in August, I went for my final checkup with Marcove before being fitted for the leg. He took some X rays, and then we went into his office with my parents. I knew something was wrong, because he was acting weird toward me. Then he told me they wanted me to check back into the hospital—nothing serious, just a few more tests before I was fitted for my new leg.

"All of a sudden, I was meeting a whole new set of doctors—Dr. Beattie's team. * Marcove didn't come around until two days later. He sat next to me on the bed, and I asked him, 'So when can I go home?' He sort of put his arm around me and said, 'We have to do another operation—in your lung.' I couldn't believe it, because I didn't have any pain there, as I'd had with my leg. But then I told myself, 'Okay, I have to have another operation. I'll survive this one, too.'†

"I loved Beattie, and I had great confidence in him. He operated on the left lung and took out five growth nodules. Two weeks later, he came in, and I asked him, 'So when can I get out of here and get my new leg?' He sat next to me and said, 'Barbara, we have more trouble—in the right lung this time. We have to do another one.' It wasn't the end of it either. Two weeks after that, they let me go home, but I had to come back four months later for a third operation—again in the left lung."

During all this, my parents kind of freaked out. They said the town newspaper wanted to raise a fund for me. I said I didn't want it, I didn't want my name in the paper. But they did it anyway, and when I came home, they showed me all these clippings.

---

* Edward J. Beattie, Jr., M.D., formerly attending surgeon, Thoracic Service, and Chief Medical Officer, Memorial Hospital. Professor of Surgery, University of Miami School of Medicine, Division of Thoracic and Cardiovascular Surgery.

† Dr. Marcove, upon examining Barbara Turner's X rays, found the bone cancer had spread to her lungs. Medically, she had multiple pulmonary nodules of osteogenic sarcoma. He had acted "weird" in his office because he realized this young girl would soon be dead —unless something was done. The stark statistics: 50 percent dead within three months of diagnosis; 95 percent dead after three years. Despite this, at that time there were few attempts to save such patients through surgery. Determined to rescue Barbara, Dr. Marcove went to Dr. Beattie: "I told Ted Beattie we ought to give this a try, and he agreed. As a result of his surgical skill, we have since saved many others at Memorial."

An old bulging scrapbook in her files contains clippings from the hometown paper, Wayne Today, *reporting her struggles—the loss of the leg, the lung operations, then a drive to raise money for the Barbara Turner Fund, culminating in a front-page tally of $20,000 with a photo of "the brave Wayne girl saying a grateful farewell to doctors and nurses at Memorial Hospital."*

(Barbra points to the photo.) Look at that! Did you ever see anybody so lost and confused? *(Laughs.)* Poor little thing! I was a mess, a total mess. I was grateful for people wanting to help—and still am. But this was turning me into a famous freak when I wanted to be normal, not different. I told myself, "When I get my leg, I'll be able to walk without help from anyone. I'll be a high school student like all the others." I had no idea of what lay ahead.

Finally, in November, I was able to go to Mary Dorsch in New York, for my leg. When you're fitted for these things, you're suppose to have intensive therapy. You go away somewhere for a month to learn how to walk. But I was so excited, I decided to throw away my crutches right there and go back to school the next day.

The leg was brought out to me. I put it on, took a few steps, and then started walking around in the back of her place, where there was some space for me to move. Then I walked out of there—no crutches, no canes, no walkers. *(Laughs.)* I just walked out of that place, and I went to Marcove at Memorial for approval of the leg. Then I went home, and that night I walked some more. The next morning I got up at seven thirty, walked to the bus, and went back to school.

She soon realized that her dream to appear normal, to be like everyone else, was not possible. The newspaper had front-paged her pending return to school: "Brave-spirited Barbara says 'I don't want the board of education to provide special transportation. I want to be treated like everybody else, like all of my classmates.'" Her classmates, however, felt otherwise.

At school, everyone was scared of me. I didn't have any friends—no girl-friends, and God knows, boys wouldn't come near me because I was a freak. When you're in high school, you're really popular if you're just like everybody else. So who wants this freak girl coming back with all the publicity and with her little limp after going through hell? See what I mean? They couldn't cope with me.

I struggled to look good. I'd come home and sew new clothes. My mother would buy me new pants, and I had cute miniskirts. But it didn't work. Nothing worked. I tried to make friends, but nobody wanted to like me.

I had lots of fantasies, though. I'd like this boy or that boy, and I'd fantasize about them—but that was all. Weekends, I'd sit home with my mother. And I was still sitting there when the senior prom came along. Nobody even asked me if I was going to it. It was a real bum two years. Did I cry? Yes, I guess I did—especially inside. I cried a lot inside. At that point, all I hoped for was to go to college. *(Laughs.)* I told myself nothing could be worse, so it just had to change there. And you know, it did!

Fortunately, I went to an art school—Pratt Institute. The first thing it did was to put me on my own. At home, I had had everything taken care of. I had this terrible thing, so I was pitied by the whole family, and I got everything I wanted—even a car for graduation. Then, all of a sudden, I'm in a dormitory, and if I want a glass of milk at ten o'clock, I have to go out to the store and buy it. I can't tell my father to go and get it, or call my mother. I have to walk everywhere, to classes and to the food service.

Also, I was a freak in high school, a little dot somewhere else on the page. But at college—and especially at Pratt, an art institute—all the freaks are blossoming flowers. So a miracle happens. I begin to have boyfriends and girlfriends. It was fantastic. By Thanksgiving, when I came home for vacation, I'm a whole different person—or beginning to be one. Then Kevin and I began to see each other, and by the time I came home that summer, I was in full rebellion. I understood what had gone on in high school, and I really felt that I had been fucked over.

I got a summer job working in the local department store, where I began seeing kids I'd gone to school with. There were two groups—the popular group and the semipopular group. Both of them had been particularly vicious to me, but now they didn't know what to make of it. They would see me in the store, and they didn't know how to take this change in me. I was starting to look better physically, and I had confidence. When I told them about my college boyfriends and what I was doing, they were a little surprised. I thought, "You haven't seen anything yet, brother. Just wait, I'll show you a lot more."

In my second year, I got interested in photography and became career-directed. Coming home for vacations, I'd take my camera and roam around department stores or shopping malls. You take artistic pictures when you start in photography—your family, your wife, your lover, or whatever is around you. So people saw me with my camera around my neck, looking like a rebellious college student, and they'd say "Gee! You've changed! You must be doing fine!" But in their eyes, you could see they were really saying something else: "Who does she think she is? How can she go anywhere, especially as a free-lance photographer? Who's she kidding?" And I thought again, "Just wait, you haven't seen anything yet!" *(Laughs.)*

Everything seemed to be going her way. College was all she hoped for. "Everyone liked you for what you were, and if you were different or special, you were better than normal." She was deliriously in love with Kevin, and they decided to share an apartment off campus. Before they could move in, however, she went for her regular two-month checkup at Memorial. "When I saw Beattie's face, I knew something was wrong. I could tell because he was always happy for me. He said, 'Barbra, I've got to put you back in. You've got one more tumor on your left lung.' He said he'd been watching it for some time. So it wasn't a new one, starting up again. This gave me confidence."

But I was really pissed off. School was starting again, I was anxious to move into the apartment with Kevin—and now I had to go back into the hospital. I told my friends, and they were all upset. Unlike high school, they all related to it. Instead of running away from me, everyone was coming to me. *(Laughs.)* I also told them I'd made a bet with Kevin that I'd be back at school in seventeen days. I don't think anyone believed me. It seemed impossible.

My parents picked me up at the dormitory on Sunday, and I had the operation on a Tuesday—the same operation as last time, opening it up from the back. I told Beattie when I checked in that I had to be back at college in seventeen days, and I wanted to go home three days before that —on Friday.

By Friday I wasn't physically ready to go home, but I was going, anyway. Beattie used to come by my room around five o'clock, so I decided to get all dressed and wait for him by the bed. He came, and I said, "I'm going home. You promised me I could go." So he let me, and I stayed home that weekend. On Monday, the seventeenth day, my mother dropped me off in front of the school, and I ran into Kevin in the hallway. . . .

Kevin interrupts: "When I found her, she'd lost twenty pounds, and she couldn't walk straight. It makes me want to cry, just thinking about how she could hardly stand. She had to lean on the wall when she walked. But she had this big smile on her face. I thought, 'What's going on here?' Looking at her face is one thing, with the big smile, but her body is telling me something else. I mean she doesn't allow you to look at what the problem is. She makes you look at her face."

After that, there was no more trouble, and Kevin and I decided to get married. The first time I took him home to meet my parents, I was so nervous I crumbled my contact lenses. *(Laughs.)* We went to Europe, then we graduated—and finally we got married. A priest I had met at Memorial did it for us—Father Peter Elder, a wonderful man. I didn't want it in a church, so he did it in my parents' backyard. We had a lot of people, and it rained, but Father Peter said that rain on the bride brings good luck—and so far he's been right.

She began her career with photographic studies of top designers of high fashion. Eventually, fifty of the most famous ones were gathered into the book, The Fashion Makers. *In it, many of her subjects state that Barbra Walz has an unusual ability to penetrate into their inner selves. Barbra does not know how she does it.*

When I go out to photograph people, there's something about me, an ability to open people up. They are drawn to me, I don't know why. I hope this doesn't sound egotistical, because I don't mean it to, but there's something different about my makeup, why I'm such a survivor. I get what I want on a scary level. I don't really understand it myself.

After the book came out—with good press reviews, displays in major department store windows, and a talked-about celebrity party at Studio 54—Barbra got her long-awaited chance: a tenth anniversary reunion of her high school class at Wayne, New Jersey.

Nothing could have made me miss this one—not even a summons to the White House or Windsor Castle. *(Laughs.)* My time had come, and I was prepared for it. I wore a plunging Kamali blouse, very low-cut, with tight, white pants. My hair was platinum blond and frizzed like crazy. I was very confident and couldn't wait to see what was going to happen. It was at some horrible drive-in place. . . . I walked in, and what I noticed first was their eyes going down to the leg, as they used to do in high school. But they couldn't connect the face, because it had completely changed. Look at it. *(Points to photo in scrapbook.)*

Kevin: "When they realized who you were, it was like seeing a ghost."

The boys didn't come near me, they were still afraid *(laughs)*—but this time on another level, because I was powerful. I walked right into the place with more confidence than anyone else. They felt it, and those girls I hated so much, who would never speak to me, came up and said, "Gee, you look great!" They were surprised I was still alive, surprised at the way I looked. Some had read articles about me. "I saw a piece on you in the *Times,*" or "I read you're doing great photography." I'd brought my book, and when they saw it, it was like there were three hundred kids, and I was the only one who had grown up.

Suddenly, I felt different. I had expected to be real hostile about the whole thing. After all, they had made me miserable for two years. I never had one kind word or a simple, generous gesture from any of them. I should have rubbed it into their faces. I should have relished making them squirm. But I only felt sorry for them. They had never had the chance to be more than what they were. They never had to reach out for something. They were sort of standing still and growing old without growing up. I realized then that I'd been lucky—luckier than most of them. And finally I was free of what they had done to me.

It was a weekend in November of '76. I woke up and noticed I had double vision. It appeared like that, overnight. I went out to play touch football, and when I looked up, I saw two footballs coming at me. It was very strange. The area in front of me was fairly clear, but as I glanced to the side, it doubled up badly. For a couple months, I let it go at that—seeing clear in front, but double at the side—until I started getting headaches.

He is 32, and his wife, Esther, is three years younger. Rod is seated at one end of a sofa, and she sits opposite, in an armchair, watching him as though he were on stage. He holds a white slip of paper on which he has written the principle dates of his battle against brain cancer. "It's not that I can't remember," he explains. "I just want to make sure it's right."

We are in a small living room of an apartment on the top floor of a two-flat house in Bayside, Long Island. In the corner is a child's dollhouse and, above it on the wall, a print of Van Gogh's Sunflowers. *From outside, there is the muted rumble of traffic along a nearby expressway with the occasional wailing of an ambulance or a squad car siren.*

I went to an eye doctor who referred me to a neurologist in Queens who gave me a CAT scan.† It showed no trace of a tumor. So he suspected a viral infection and sent me to another brain specialist at a major New York hospital. I will say frankly this was not a sympathetic doctor.

ESTHER: *(Interjects)* He's supposed to be one of the finest neurologists around, but he treats you like dirt. After two days of tests, we knew nothing, and I had to corner him in the hall, asking him over and over for the results. "What does my husband have?" He had a group of young doctors around him, interns and residents, and he replied, "Do I really have to tell you now? Well, I think it's meso—something or other. Does that make you feel any better now that you know the name of it?" He looked at the other doctors, and they began to giggle and laugh at me.

ROD: *(Shakes head sadly)* They see so many really bad, hopeless cases. Maybe they're driven to build up protective barriers against caring. But it

---

* Identity of patient and wife have been altered.

† CT or CAT, for "computerized axial tomography," focuses multiple, narrow X-ray beams on a specific level or plane of the body. These are then fed electronically into a computer, revealing the density of tissue. Bone, of highest density, comes out white. Liquids and air, of lowest density, appear black. Shades of gray in between represent various organs, tissues. A CT of an entire head, chest, or abdomen takes several minutes, but the total amount of X-ray exposure is less than one old-fashioned X ray.

makes the patient feel like he's no longer a human being. Finally, they sent
me home, saying it was probably a virus to be cured by medicine. But my
headaches got worse, and I also began to throw up my food. I kept going
to work—I'm an office supervisor for a construction company—but my
work was deteriorating. My boss saw it and suggested I try another hospital. So our family doctor sent me to a specialist in viral and infectious
diseases, Dr. Kelly Smith, at North Shore Hospital. They took more tests
and found I was developing hydrocephalus—excess fluid on the brain—
and their neurologist, Dr. Jeffrey Kessler, put in a shunt to reopen the
blocked passage of my brain fluid, allowing it to flow back into the spinal
column. *(Bends head to left, pointing to spot behind ear.)* Here, you can feel
it.

*The shunt, a small tube, can be felt behind Rod's right ear, descending
along the right throat into the chest from where it finally spills into the
abdomen. His headaches lessened, and he improved sufficiently to show up
for work in October 1977.*

We couldn't make it on the medical benefits they were paying. So I had to
go back and work at least one more month to have five years with the
company in order to draw two thirds of my salary on sick leave, rather
than one half. I made it barely through the month when the shunt clogged
up, and I became a zombie. They took me back to North Shore and put in
another shunt, but this time I came home helpless. I had trouble walking. . . .

ESTHER: *(Interrupts)* His condition was so bad, he couldn't even get the
spoon in his mouth. He was walking stiff and sideways like a zombie. Dr.
Kressler said, "This is a disability you'll have to learn to put up with." I
refused it and told him: "I'll just have to see another doctor. Can you
recommend one?" He said: "I can understand your feelings, and I'm fairly
good friends with one of the best neurologists in the U.S., Dr. Posner at
Memorial Hospital."‡

ROD: Posner saw me and said he suspected it was a tumor—not a virus
at all. They did another CAT scan, and, sure enough, he found a pea-sized
tumor deep in the brain—too deep for surgery. He believed, however, that
it was a type that would be susceptible to radiation. It was near the pineal
gland that controls a lot of your characteristics, as well as your vision.
That's why my vision was being affected. Posner knew all this, even before
the CAT scan was compared with earlier ones, which showed it was grow-

---

‡ Jerome B. Posner, M.D., chairman, Department of Neurology, Memorial Hospital.

ing very fast. So if I had not gone to the best man in the country, I would be dead today.

For the next month, I was hospitalized and got radiation treatments. They directed them behind each ear. I also had two new shunt operations because they kept getting clogged with brain cells breaking off and stopping the flow of spinal fluid.

After a month, the tumor was gone, and they started me off with a physical therapist, who had me using a walker up and down the halls. About a week later, I was discharged. But I was like a real dummy around the house. I couldn't work or anything. Just get up, go to the table and eat, then sit in my big chair and watch people go by, like an android or a robot.

ESTHER: He didn't speak to anybody. That was the scary part.

ROD: I didn't speak unless spoken to. Then I'd give an answer that wasn't worth hearing, anyway. Finally, Dr. Posner gave me a very mild prescription of amphetamines, thinking maybe it would jump me up a little bit. Within two days, I was turning around like a top, and I felt great. It was a mild dosage, but I was driving Esther crazy, cleaning this and that. Every time the kids* took out a toy, I'd grab it and put it back. Real weird. As soon as they'd go into another room, I'd grab the toy, and they'd come back and find it put away. Dr. Posner said the amount of amphetamine could not have made me that much more vibrant. He says my body was just ready to go, and it triggered me off with a lot of pent-up energy.

I started back to work part-time, and I was improving. Then my father phoned me in the middle of the night—it was January, '79—saying my mother had died of cancer. My brother had also died from cancer of the lung—and now my mother. The next morning, I was in a coma, my shunt clogged again with brain cells. They took me to Memorial again, but it cleared up, and I didn't need another operation.

As I came out of the coma, the doctors were asking me if I knew my name. I said (speaking slowly, like a robot), "My name is Charles Fitzgerald. They call me Rod Watson, but I am really Charles Fitzgerald." (Laughs.) Now we kid around with it. Did I have a prior life or something?

ESTHER: (Interjects) I don't know what Dr. Posner would say about this, but each time Rod's shunt clogged, I noticed a difference in his personality. He would change in a certain way. The last time it happened, we were in Florida, and he took another man's bathrobe and walked all over the hospital. They'd put him back to bed, and he'd get up again and

---

* There are two daughters, ages 6 and 12.

start off. He said there were three Rod Watsons in the hospital, and he wanted to find the right one in the phone book. Also, the minute he came out of surgery, he was joking. He'd never acted like that before. I remember complaining to Dr. Posner that Rod never smiled, never laughed, never did anything to bring him joy. Now everything is a joke, and believe me, some of them are pretty silly.

ROD: That's because you don't see things the way I do. *(Laughs.)* I'm still without peripheral vision, but I've gotten used to it. I didn't think I could play football or basketball anymore, because you gotta catch passes from the side. But I was able to adjust to that. I turn my head all the way around to pick up balls or passes coming at me or look straight at the basket to shoot. If I turn my head *(turns away),* I see a double image of you, one here and one up in here *(indicates two horizontal areas).* If I concentrate, I can usually tell which is the real one and which is the fake image, if you want to call it that. *(Pauses.)* I don't really call it anything, I just accept it.

My biggest problem has been my memory. It started to really bug me. I mean my wife will tell me something, and maybe three minutes later I go in, and I'm asking the same question again, and I hear her say, "Rod I just answered that question." I say, "Well, hit me with it again." I go out feeling really dumb. The kids know it and get at me. If anything is missing, they say, "Daddy lost it, he can't remember anymore."

It was okay being corrected at home, but at work it really pissed me off and made me mad. The boss says, "Rod, you forgot to do this or that." And some clerk says, "You didn't mark the form right." It got to me. I hated going to work, and I hated myself. I'd break into tears and hit the walls—but never in front of Esther. I'd do it by myself. On the old closet door or something. On the wall, in the bathroom, on the tiles, a couple of cracks. I mean, as soon as it happens I don't go "Grrr!" like a raging maniac. It's inside, in my gut, and as soon as I walk away, out of sight, you know, I slam my fist into something. That's how I get rid of it, because she doesn't necessarily see the rage that comes out.

ESTHER: But I could feel it inside him. Then one day he came home in tears from frustration, and I called Dr. Posner who arranged for Rod to see the chief psychiatrist at the hospital, Dr. Jimmy Holland.† I don't know what happened between them, but it changed him.

ROD: It's difficult to describe the communications we had. She had me talk about my past with the company and how things changed after I had

---

† Jimmie C. B. Holland, M.D., attending psychiatrist and chief of Psychiatry Service, Memorial Hospital.

a tumor. Also, what was happening in my private life, like my mother and brother dying at the same time of cancer and how it affected me. Then she went into a whole thing about how other people make mistakes, too, but don't get down on themselves. How normal people, who have no brain tumors, can also forget. The clearest, untroubled brain can lose its memory if it's subjected to continual stress, lack of sleep, or people saying, "You are forgetting, you can't remember anymore." It can slip away then because the memory is really very fragile and elusive, and nobody really understands it.

Just talking this way, about what was bugging me, Dr. Holland was able to get me calmed down and not so strung out. Now if I make a mistake, I tell myself that others do, too. If my boss says, "You forgot that, Rod," I say, "Okay, I'll change it"—without getting mad at myself.

Also, I'm fighting back in another way, now. I carry around a little pad and pen, and I write down answers to all my questions. If I think I haven't asked the question, I can always look at the pad and see that maybe I've already got it. That's what I do at work. When I get information that I can't put directly into the file, I make a little memo and stick it up with a paper clip. I have them all over my desk.

The one problem we haven't resolved is my sex drive. I don't have the same urge for women anymore. On the subway, the bus, a woman walks by who is another Raquel Welch, and it doesn't turn me on. Dr. Posner thought the amphetamines might boost me up a little bit. And I knew that Esther was, you know, getting very upset that I wasn't feeling sexually attracted to her again. I said there was just nothing I could do about it. . . .

ESTHER: *(Defensively)* I was okay. I think I'm a pretty strong person. I'm not a weak, retiring little woman-type who falls apart or anything like that. I mean, I can handle being his mother for a while, but I don't want to be his mother forever.

ROD: I think about it in the evening when I'm sitting there. I look at Esther and think about, you know, having sex right now, going to the bedroom, but unfortunately I can't because the kids are still up. And as the night goes on, I get tired and more tired until my drive seems to level off and take a dip.

Driving to the train without Esther, Rod continued to talk about his sex problem.

There's something wrong with my head. It's empty of sex. On the bus or subway, those girls in tight pants do nothing to me. We tried it a few weeks ago. Esther began to make up to me in bed, trying to get me up. But I couldn't do it, and she got out of bed and ran into the living room. I went to her, and she was leaning on the windowsill, looking out at the street. When I put my arm around her, she said, "Don't you cry, Rod. It's my turn now."

He began tearing in the right eye as he drove. Then he wiped his cheek dry and apologized.

I get this way when I think back to the hospital. I would lie there like a zombie, but I could hear everything. I remember what people said, and I could hear all the words to the rock songs. I took it all in, but nothing would come out, like a part of me was prisoner inside myself. That's why I say this sex problem is all in the head. It hasn't been set free yet.

POSTSCRIPT: A year later, the sex problem was less urgent. Rod and Esther were making love more often, more easily, though it was still not enough for Rod. "As far as quality is concerned, everything is fine. But quantity—that's where there's still some problem.

"But my relationship with Esther is now much deeper, more secure, more solid. When I was in the hospital, she gave so much of herself to me. I was an idiot, a zombie, but something happened to us, deep inside both of us. It may sound weird, but it brought us so close that I can't think of anything that would break us apart now."

The taller the tree, the lower it bends. You have these little pipsqueaks, the little trees, and when a big wind comes, they don't bend. A tall tree will bend as low as it can to give in to the wind with humility. It takes a big person to say, "I don't know." That's the difference. At Memorial Hospital, they say, "I don't know, I'll have to check it out." They test you over and over until they have their findings. Then they start treating you. They don't just cut you up, or send you away, saying it's nothing, or it's to be expected because you're a woman in her forties and over the hill.

She is 49, an executive secretary for a major New York investment firm, a tall and handsome woman with dark hair and gray-blue eyes. Her parents were German and her father was a country doctor—origins reflected in her phrasing of English and also in the paintings, ceramics, and decor of the Freund two-story home on a quiet, tree-lined street in Teaneck, New Jersey. We are seated in the kitchen with her husband, Peter, who is a vice president of Marine Midland Bank.

I started to become aware of mastectomies through Mrs. Ford and, shortly thereafter, through Happy Rockefeller. The *Times* and other papers were full of details, and, like every other woman, here I was, 44 years old and very interested. All the girls were interested. It was the beginning of '74, and everywhere there was a run on mammograms.

I was sitting, watching TV, when the Cancer Society showed viewers how to examine your breasts. Peter was away traveling, and I was in my nightie, and I said, "Well, I'll mimic it and see what happens." I found something there, and I said, "It can't be real. I have cystic breasts. It's nothing." Then on TV they said, "When you take a shower and soap yourself, do the same thing." So, I did, and it didn't go away. I figure it's because I'm before my monthly. Then after my monthly, it stays. I began to worry, but I didn't say anything for a month or two. Then I called Peter over and said, "Do me a favor, do you feel something?" He said, "Yes, I feel something. You better have it checked out."

My doctor called a gynecologist, but it was the day after Mrs. Rockefeller had her mastectomy, and you couldn't get an appointment anywhere. Finally, a few days later, I had a mammogram, and the report said I had fibrous cysts in both breasts, especially the left. It didn't say they were malignant—just cysts. So I said, "Maybe I've had cystic breasts all my life. Maybe my doctor is right. Don't be such a worrywart." Also, I had never been ill in my life. So I forgot about it until June, when I lifted something and had a little pain right here—in my groin area.

A gynecologist at Fort Lee also detected a lump in her left breast, but dismissed it upon seeing the earlier mammogram report that it was only a fibrous cyst. He did find her ovaries were enlarged, however, and put her into Holy Name Hospital for a D&C.* When it was completed, he gave her a clean bill of health.

I asked him about the lump in my breast, and he said, "Don't worry about it, especially a woman of your age." That really annoyed me. "What do you mean?" I asked. "You hit 40 and you're over the hill? I thought life begins at 40!" But afterwards, I began to think maybe he's right. Maybe I'm getting the middle-age blues. You know, they brush you under the rug.

That was in June, and I let the summer go by. I went swimming, and I got very depressed because the lump didn't go away, and the little groin pain didn't go away. Come October, and I said, "It's been a year since I had the mammogram. Better have myself checked out again." So I went back to Holy Name Hospital, and they gave me another mammogram. It showed something, because several different doctors came to me. One of them, a surgeon, said, "We can't let you leave. I'll have to do a biopsy, and probably I'll have to go further." I thought, "Oh no, you won't." But I only said, "Let me think about it." It was like being back in the war again, when I had to escape from the Russians. I told myself, "I'm going to run away from this place, too."

She was in a private school in occupied Poland during World War II when the Russians began to advance upon them. "They came overnight, and I started to walk to Berlin with my cousin. We walked six hundred miles, always between the front lines. When we got to Berlin, they began closing in there, too, and I ran away again. I went to a town near the American front and waited for them to come." It was April 11, 1945. "I spoke English and was very lucky. I met General Walter Grow of the Sixth Armored Division. He helped me because he said I had walked away from the Russians long enough. I was 15 at the time, but I told them I was 18, and they gave me a work permit as an interpreter. That was marvelous, but when I was 21 and wanted to emigrate to the U.S., my papers said I was 24. I knew I had to do something because later who would believe me if I took off three years? By a miracle, I found my birth certificate and went to a police station. A very

---

* Dilation of the cervix and curettage, or a cleaning out of the lining of the uterus with an instrument called a curette—a common, minor operation experienced by one in seven women who undergo surgery.

kind policeman said, 'Can I help you?' I said, 'You most certainly can. I have to get my papers straightened out. I'm going to the United States, and I did something terrible. I made myself older.' He started to laugh like there was no tomorrow and said, 'You know, I've been a policeman for thirty years. I have seen women make themselves ten years younger, but never met one who made herself older, especially one looking the way you do.' He fined me only five marks for changing the document."

So I was lying in the hospital, trying to decide what to do when my boss came to visit me. I told him what they wanted of me, and he said, "Why don't we call Rockefeller?"—meaning James Stillman Rockefeller who is on the board of Sloan-Kettering. I used to work for him at Citibank. I said, "Anson, please do me that favor. Get his opinion. Tell him there is a slight chance of malignancy. Am I all right here, or should I go there?" After that, Peter called me and said, "He says don't do anything. Don't have her operated anywhere except Memorial Hospital. Cancel whatever is scheduled. If there's a chance of malignancy, get the best." They tried to get Dr. Urban for me, but he was traveling, so they got Dr. Ashikari who is also a breast man at Memorial.†

When I told this Holy Name surgeon that I didn't want him to operate because I was going to Sloan-Kettering, he said, "Who's going to be your doctor?" I said, "I know a trustee, and he's trying to reach Dr. Urban, or somebody else at the hospital." He asked me, "Who's the trustee?" I said, "It's Mr. Rockefeller, I used to work for him." The surgeon thought I was joking. "You've been reading too many papers, too many novels. You'd better see a psychiatrist or something."

When I checked out, they made Peter and me sign a hundred papers, not holding them responsible for whatever happened to me. Then we drove into the city and I walked into Sloan-Kettering, my first visit. In Dr. Ashikari's office there is this little old lady, saying, "Doctor, doctor, am I dying?" He said, "Don't worry about it, we all do from the day we are born, but you are not going to die now." I thought, "Now here is a place where no one is going to hide anything from me. I can trust them." Dr. Ashikari examined me, then took us both aside and said, "Look, it's fifty-fifty. We have to operate." He meant fifty-fifty it would be malignant. That's a nothing chance, almost positive. But I felt good about him. I said, "If anyone can do anything for me, it's right here."

Going home, I told myself to be brave and not think about it. But I

---

† Hiroyuki "Roy" Ashikari, M.D., formerly associate attending surgeon, Breast Service, Department of Surgery, Memorial Hospital.

couldn't help myself. It never left me. I remember sitting in the bathtub, looking at my breast, and saying, "Well, you know, my twins, this one is going to be gone." I wondered what was it going to be like without it. Would I be able to be myself, my usual self, before my husband and other people? No matter how I felt, how would they see me?

The next day I checked into the hospital, and I had a fabulous roommate, a little Jewish woman from Brooklyn. She woke up with four-letter words and went to bed with four-letter words. Her name was Ida. When I walked in, she was deathly ill from a difficult operation. She said, "What are you in for?" I said, "I probably will have a mastectomy." She said, "That's nothing. I had one and lived with it for thirty-six years. It didn't make a bit of difference. I'll tell you, the world is divided between two kinds of men—the real ones and the tit men. If I see your husband, I can tell you whether you're safe or not. If he's a tit man or a real man, that's the only problem you'll have." *(Laughs.)* What a down-to-earth, real woman! Then Peter walked in, and she winked and nodded like saying, "You don't have to worry about it, he's okay." We started to laugh, and Peter didn't know what was happening. We were like a comical team. She was little and short, and I was tall. She was so funny, she took the fear out of me, and I loved her. I said, "Really, if my life were to be dependent on this one part of my anatomy, I would really be lost." When I checked out after a week, we were the best of friends. And the gift she gave to me, I must now in some way give to others.

The next day, I was operated on. When I woke up, Dr. Ashikari said, "I have good news, and I have bad news. Let me tell you the good news first. I took out twelve glands, and they were all negative—but I had to amputate your breast." Then he said, "Fortunately, you didn't need a radical, only a modified. Also, I looked at you, and I said you are a very active woman, and I did a different cut." He held the bedsheet against his chest and said, "If you want to go sleeveless, you can go low-cut, and you'll be beautiful." I said, "Look, doctor, I'm not worried about the low-cut. I'm a turtleneck girl, so you didn't have to worry about that. I'm not out for looks, I'm here for health reasons. What do you think? I walk around in evening gowns? I'm down-to-earth."

That wasn't very nice of me. I could see it in his eyes, and I knew it was not me talking. It was the *wounded* me. I said, "I'm sorry, I know you did a beautiful job. I'm grateful and really glad to be alive. I'm happy the glands aren't affected, and I don't have to have any treatments." He smiled and took my hand, and I felt he understood everything—how it is, I mean, after you wake up with it gone.

I understand that for most women the hardest day is the third one, when they've recovered from the shock of the operation and have to summon the courage to look at themselves. I never had a really hard day at the hospital, but I used to cry at night, for two or three weeks after I came home. It was like I was in mourning, because really a part of me was dead. That's how you feel.

A year later, I was visiting in Berlin, and I was undressing when my little niece said, "Oh, Auntie Chris, you have only one breast. What happened to the other?" I said, "Don't worry about the other. It went to heaven." *(Laughs.)* She said okay, so that little girl intuitively knew more than the other grown-ups.

My father was a doctor, and I'm curious medically. I immediately wanted to know what it looked like. The first time they changed bandages, I said, "Let me look." My tongue was in my cheek, but I wanted to see. Dr. Ashikari was there, and I really couldn't believe he did such a fabulous job. A good surgeon knows how to cut, but a great one knows how to cut so it will heal with the least harm. That's what he did and why he's so special. I could see myself in an evening gown, and then I realized why I had gone to the trouble to tell him I was a turtleneck girl. I didn't believe I could ever be anything else.

As soon as you can get up and walk, they send you up to a special room where they pick up the pieces and start to make you whole again. There's a social worker and a physical therapist with certain exercises to help you regain use of your arms. Every day we went up there, like walking wounded, with pillows under our arms. It was very moving for me to see all of us there—young girls and old ones, black and white, every sort of woman—all with one breast or maybe two breasts gone, sitting there, each with her own story, talking about what she hoped for and what she feared most when she went home.

We also had a volunteer lady who came to tell us about her mastectomy, from the Reach for Recovery group—women who have been through it and volunteer their time to help others. Our lady was truly enormous. *(Laughs.)* Honestly, with the one she had left she could have supplied the whole floor. She had a prosthesis in place of the missing breast, and I asked her where she got it. She said, "Do me a favor. Feel me and say which one it is." I said, "Well, I usually don't go around squeezing other women's breasts, but let me feel." I couldn't tell the difference, and I asked, "In your estimation, what is the best kind?" She said, "Invest a little more money," and she gave me the name.

So I went out and bought this prosthesis. It's been five years, and it's like new. I bump into people, they apologize. They don't know what's happened to me. Nobody knows the difference, and I feel very comfortable. I don't think I want a reconstruction. I was thinking about it for a while, but it doesn't matter to Peter. Maybe I will, maybe I won't. But it's not that important.

PETER: *(Interjects)* Obviously, if she felt she wanted it very much because it made her a whole woman again—if that's the right term—I would not stand in the way. In discussing it between us, I expressed my feelings, and she said, "If it doesn't bother you, it doesn't bother me." That was it. It may change in a few years' time. It's still a possibility. But she's as attractive to me today as she was before it happened.

CHRISTA: I'm getting my distance. I feel very happy to be alive. I expected the first days in the office, after the mastectomy, to be terrible because I felt everybody knew, and they would look. But because of my positive attitude, I was laughing about it, and it went all right. I have to tell you a funny story. One day as I was leaving the house, I became very conscious about my breasts being straight. I had on a very thin dress, and I was already out on the road, when I had this phobia. It was a new problem for me, because before this I naturally never worried about whether they were straight or not. You don't think about those things. I said, "Peter, are they straight?" He says, "Wait a second," and runs down into the basement then comes up with the level. *(Laughs.)* He lays it across them and says, "Now will you believe they're straight?" I said, "Yes, Peter, I believe," and that cured me.

PETER: Shortly after her mastectomy, we went into group therapy for couples who have experienced it. I was shocked at the reactions of some men when their women openly expressed concern about what effect this would have on their sex lives. You could see the men were turned off. For them, this was no longer the woman they had married. She was not a whole woman anymore. She was a sort of freak. I couldn't understand this. We discussed it frequently, and for me there are two aspects in loving someone. There's the physical part, and there's the human being, the whole person. The whole person should be predominant over any physical part. If somebody is disfigured, in the face or body, a love for the whole person should overcome whatever has happened to the physical part. We've been very open about this, and Christa has never been ashamed to appear naked before me, as I understand some women are made to feel by their men after a mastectomy.

CHRISTA: He kept me feeling like a woman, like someone he wanted and loved. More than anything else, I think that held me together when I told Dr. Ashikari about the pain in my groin, and he sent me to see Dr. Jones.‡

I walked to Dr. Jones's office to get an appointment and had to wait. I was ready to leave when he came out, a good-looking young man who looks like a light-skinned Indian but is black, and he greeted me in German. I thought, "Oh, this is my kind of fellow." I told him about the pain, and he examined me and said, "Did you have breakfast?" I said yes. He said, "I feel something, I want you to come back with an empty stomach, and I'll reexamine you." I came back, and he said, "I feel the ovaries enlarged, but I want to know why they've enlarged. I would like you to first take some tests. Then come into the hospital, and I will examine you under anesthesia because you couldn't possibly stand it otherwise."

He gave me five tests for cancer of the ovaries—all negative. I said, "So I don't have to come in for examination under anesthesia?" Dr. Jones said, "Yes, we have to do that, too. I'm not convinced yet." I thought here was a supercautious man, but I checked in, they opened me up, and they found cancer of both ovaries—one larger than the other. So they had to do a hysterectomy, I mean four hours of it.

When I came out, they broke the news. It was cancer but not related to my breast. It had not spread through my body. Thank God, Dr. Jones was so thorough—unlike the other doctors I had seen. He said in another six months it would have gone too far. He thought he got everything, but because of the blood flow, he decided to put me on chemotherapy. He was putting me into a control group with other patients, supervised by Dr. Ochoa.* It was to be two years of chemo, and after that they would go in again and see if I was cancer-free or what the story was. Did I agree? I remember I got out of bed and kissed Dr. Jones's hand. "Doctor, do you mean I'm going to be alive two years from now? Fabulous!"

I thought, "Whatever you say, I'll do it." I started taking chemo drugs in tablet form and kept asking Dr. Ochoa, "Aren't there any side effects?" He said, "Everyone reacts differently." Well, I had no side effects. I felt good. I never had a cold while everyone else in my office did, and I had more energy than ever before.

After two years, they opened me up and went in. The first to tell me the good news was Dr. Ochoa. "I've got good news, the first tests are negative." I said, "How wonderful!" He said, "Yes, we are kind of pleased, too,

---

‡ Walter B. Jones, M.D., associate attending surgeon, Gynecology Service, Department of Surgery, Memorial Hospital.

* Manuel Ochoa, Jr., M.D., attending physician, Solid Tumor Service, Department of Medicine, Memorial Hospital.

but we have to wait for the wash." That was the last test. On Friday, Dr. Jones came in, and looking into his face, I knew it was good. He came over and gave me a peck on the cheek and said, "You know, you're a grand old lady. The wash test is negative. As far as we are concerned, you are clinically cured." *(Pauses, overcome with emotion.)* I still don't believe it happened to me. I looked at him by my bed, this man who had saved my life, and I thought of his humility, his saying, "I don't know, we have to double-check and make sure."

PETER: After this second time around, people were astounded at Christa's mental attitude, her outlook on life. They couldn't believe she had been afflicted twice with this deadly disease. Even in my family, my mother and her friends could not accept the seriousness of it because of Christa's cheerfulness.

CHRISTA: Cancer scares people so much they unconsciously back away when they learn you've had it—as though it were contagious. If you have open-heart surgery, they don't say, "That fellow's going to die." But if you say you've had a cancer operation, especially if you've had two or three of them, they'll shuffle backward, convinced you're a goner, and maybe they'll catch it from you if you sneeze. If you say, "I'm fine, my doctor says I'm *clinically* cured, which is more than just being cured," they still can't believe it. But you can overcome that, too. At the office, my coworkers felt like I did at first—that cancer is a death sentence for anybody who gets it. Then, as I began to feel comfortable and very positive, my coworkers felt the same way, and they accepted it, too. If you just give people a chance, they are very generous with their feelings.

PETER: It's a funny thing. I always wanted to play it on the safe side, always wanted to make sure we have enough money when we retired, buying insurance, annuities, and so forth. When this happened to Chris, all of a sudden I became very aware that life is unpredictable. You never know from day to day. You can plan for life at 65, but also you might never get there. So now I have adopted a different attitude. We are going to enjoy life now—not tomorrow. If we want to do things, we do them without worrying, because the material things will somehow or other take care of themselves.

CHRISTA: I'm really not a crusader. I can't go around and tell people there is no such thing as a personal contract with God, or a contract to live to be 90, or that you might get cancer, and tomorrow you are dead. Yet I know this now. You have to learn to live with your chances and go ahead. It's not easy, but if you are honest, it becomes easy. Then you can laugh at it, and you can hope, too, because that gives you a hold on life.

It's been five years since I had my two cancer operations. I was so charged up to see the eighties. Now that they are here, I'm charged up again, hoping to be able to see myself with white hair and what I'm going to be like as a little old lady.

Every Wednesday, she goes to Memorial Hospital to tell her story and give counsel to women emerging from breast surgery. She is a volunteer in the Reach for Recovery program, composed of women who have experienced mastectomies.

I was a widow when I had my surgery. I had two teenaged daughters who were away at school, I lived in New York by myself, and I was completely unprepared for it. I came in for a biopsy, with no thought of a mastectomy. I was so dumb I didn't even know what a mastectomy was. I had never heard of it.

We are seated in a bare room on the eighteenth floor of Memorial where shortly some postmastectomy patients will gather to receive instruction in physical therapy and personal counseling. We have met beforehand to talk privately about intensely personal problems encountered by Rosalie Stahl after her mastectomy.

She is 55, with the trim figure of a woman in her forties. She has high, pale cheekbones, sea-gray eyes, gray-white hair, and she wears a smartly tailored purple suit with a beige silk blouse. It is not possible to detect visually which of her two breasts is formed artificially by a prosthesis.

"I was a textile fashion designer in New York until I got married. Then we moved to California. My husband was in industrial development. It's not housing—you build factories and warehouses. After he died, I chose to come back to New York and brought my children with me. The business in California continues to operate. I go back and forth."

One day, I felt a lump, but didn't give it much thought. I'd had them before, especially during my period. It persisted, however, and my doctor insisted I come to Memorial for a biopsy. I thought, "I'll go in and be out tomorrow, so I won't tell anybody. Why upset the children? Or my mother out in California?" When I got here, Dr. Urban* told me, "If this was malignant, we should operate immediately." I agreed, but I never really believed it could happen.

After the operation, I woke up briefly in the recovery room, not really knowing anything, but aware that something dreadful had happened to me. They have you so drugged and bandaged, you don't know what you're

---

* Jerome A. Urban, M.D., attending surgeon, and acting chief of Breast Service, Department of Surgery, Memorial Hospital.

feeling, but in the back of my head, something was going on. When I finally came out of the anesthesia in my room, I saw my daughter, who was supposed to be at school in Boston, and that did it. Somebody had called her, so I must be in serious condition.

The next morning, my older daughter, Robin, was at my bedside. She had flown in from California, and I thought, "They are here because they think I'm dying, and I *know* I'm dying." But I couldn't find the words, I couldn't talk. And they were petrified, unable to talk to me. It was awful, just like a deathwatch—but they did try. They'd say, "Well, hi, Mom," and I'd open my eyes, but then I'd fall asleep again. I slept most of my stay there. It was my way of protecting myself—by sleeping, blocking it out. The nurses got me up and sat me in a room with other patients who were talking, but I never opened my mouth.

I can talk about the whole thing now. In fact, I have helped hundreds of women who are like I was—unable to say or do anything. I was in some nightmare and didn't want to wake up because then I would have to face reality—and worse. So I clung to this semiconscious state, and my daughters came every day for a week.

When I finally was sent home, we were all in my room. I cannot tell you what provoked this, but one of them said, "Oh, Mom, I was so afraid you were going to die." I said, "You were afraid? I was *sure* I was going to die." With that, we all began to cry. It was like verbal vomiting. I mean all of us. It just poured out. How much we loved each other. How much they wanted me to live and how much I wanted to live to see what their lives were going to be like. It was a purging. We opened up, and that was good. About three days later, they each packed up and went back to their various schools, and there I was—alone.

I could have called my mother to come and take care of me, but I didn't want her. Now I tell myself, "You idiot, wouldn't it have been marvelous to have someone there helping to pamper you for a while?" But I couldn't handle it at the time, and now it's just too late. I cannot tell my mother at 86 that I didn't trust her eight years ago. But I have a feeling that she knows anyway and is smart enough not to put me on the spot. Mothers know. They have a way of knowing. She looks at me strangely sometimes, when I'm staying with her and close the door to get undressed, which is not normal between a mother and daughter. She will say to me, "Have you been for a checkup lately?" I'll say, "What do you mean Mom?" She'll say, "Don't you go to the doctor regularly?" Then I tell her, "Sure I do." I know what she's asking, but I cannot bring myself to talk about it now. So that's part of it.

I also found that I could not look at my body. It's necessary to go to the doctor quite frequently after surgery. For the first five weeks, you go about every five days, and he removes a couple of stitches and just observes. The first time I went, Robin went with me. And before I knew what was happening, she was with me in the examining room. I asked her to leave, and she said, "No. I want to stay here." Robin is very sensitive, we were good friends, and she was doing teacher training for brain-damaged and retarded children. So she had a lot of understanding, and she stood there.

I wanted to protect her from seeing this mutilated, deformed body that was now her mother. But she would not leave, and, of course, I looked at her face, at her expression, at her eyes. I expected to see some flicker of revulsion, but there was nothing. I said, "Robin, cut it out. You don't have to be a martyr." She said, "Listen, Mom, you're my mother. You're a whole person, not a pair of boobs." Of course, I cried, and that was the beginning of my being able to look.

But it didn't change me, like a miracle, right then. For a long time, I would bathe, and find I had a washcloth on my chest. I didn't do it on purpose, but there it was. Subconsciously, I was protecting myself from seeing it. I cried an awful lot. Every time I passed a mirror, I wondered: Why did this happen to me? What did I do that was wrong for my body? Or wrong for God? Maybe He was punishing me? I always had a good figure, and I thought, "Oh God, my life is over. Who's going to want me now?"

I was involved with a man at the time who desperately tried to reassure me, but I could not hear it, could not accept it. I was convinced he was just being kind to me. It took me a long time to realize that he really loved me, that he was involved with a whole person who had a personality and a character, a sense of humor and an intellect, and who wasn't just a pair of boobs.

I finally had to go into therapy. Or maybe I just fell into it. My daughter Robin got involved with something in California that I found too difficult to handle. So I went to a psychiatrist to help me cope with her—only to discover that I had really gone for myself. After about four sessions, I finally said, "Oh, incidentally, I had a mastectomy last year." The psychiatrist almost fell off the chair, because I had avoided it so desperately. Even then, I didn't want to discuss it, but we finally got into it—how mixed up I was. Just imagine it. I, who now tell all the patients how important exercise is—I, who had always been involved in swimming, tennis, and dancing—I had stopped doing exercises, almost deliberately. As a result, it was difficult for me to move my arm. I finally had to go to the Rusk Clinic because I had done everything to make it harder for myself.

The relationship with the man I was involved with at the time of my surgery ended some years later. It had nothing to do with my mastectomy. Then I met another man, and we saw each other rather frequently, but there was no physical contact between us. Finally, he said, "Listen, Rosalie, we have to talk. There is something wrong with what's happening here." I pretended not to understand because I didn't know how I was going to handle it. But he insisted. He lived out of town, and he said, "I'm coming in on Tuesday, and we will talk about this."

Well, I was a wreck. Finally, he came, and as soon as he opened the door, I tried to make light conversation. "No way," he said, and he pulled me into the living room, sat me down, and said, "Okay, now what's wrong? What's wrong with me?" Meaning himself. It was such a shock to me that he could have thought there was something wrong with *him.* It never occurred to me because I was so involved with my own problem. I said, "Well, there's this thing that is wrong with *me."* "What?" "Well, I had this illness." "What?" "Well, I had an operation." "All right, Rosalie, *what?"* I said, "I had a mastectomy." "Well, so what? What has that got to do with me?" I just could not fathom his thinking. Here he was saying it was okay, that he understood and he still wanted me. It was the greatest thing that could have happened. That a new person could accept me with this flaw. Now I handle it very easily. I say, "My body has been altered." That's it.

You were probably quite shy and nervous the first time you went to bed with him?

My God, I was miserable.

Did you insist on it being in the dark?

In the dark, and I wore a bra. I could not think of exposing my whole body. Of course, he finally said, "Take that damn thing off." I feel nauseous now, just talking about it. But I did, and it was fine.

Along with the denial of exercise and all the other things that masked your identity, did you initially also deny yourself full pleasure in making love?

Oh yes. There was a long time when I hated it.

Did you finally begin to enjoy it when you were still with that first man?

Yes, I think it finally came when I realized that Joe really loved me.

So the acceptance of yourself as a whole person allowed you to start accepting his love and, with it, also the enjoyment of love?

Yes, until that happened, until I felt comfortable with myself, I was shoving everything away from me. Like a lot of these women you are about to see coming into this room. They will say, "I'm not going to look at it. I'll look at it when I get ready, when I get home." They are creating a special world for themselves. They are out of sync with normal time and reality, until they can look at it and accept it. But listen, it's difficult for anyone, no matter who. When I hear a woman in a group saying, "I'm fine, I've accepted it, it's great," I know she's covering up, and there's going to come a time when she has to face it, and she will not be so positive about her reaction.

In five years of counseling here, you have talked with hundreds of women. What are they most concerned with? Is it perhaps their fear of loss of sex, of how to deal with their husbands or lovers, of how to dress in order to conceal their mutilation?

How they dress is a superficial thing. That's their way of avoiding the real problem. Their husbands or lovers can be a problem, but that varies and depends upon each partner, especially if the woman is made to feel secure. No, I think the main concern is, "Will this recur? Am I going to die?" Because it's hard to say the word "cancer" and that's part of it. To get them to verbalize it, to say, "I had a mastectomy because I had cancer." More than sex or going to bed with someone, or how you dress it up, the biggest problem is to be well and alive and *feel* it. You can't be haunted by concern that cancer will come back. You get a headache and wonder—is it going to be cancer of the brain? Is the pain in your neck cancer of the spine? I went through that until I realized that I was driving myself insane. I had had headaches before, and I took a Bufferin for a tension point in my neck, or I did my exercises. Finally, I realized that my body was behaving normally and these minor ailments had nothing to do with cancer. That was the beginning of my final adjustment—to not relate every ache and pain to a recurrence.

Do you find that beautiful women have a harder time after breast amputation than others?

I think you are only beautiful if you think you are, and how you look is quite a separate thing. There are a lot of women who have enormous egos, who are not beautiful, but they *feel* beautiful—and so they attract men.

Those women accept the fact that their bodies have been changed. They are just happy to be alive—and sensitive to the real problem. No, I don't think you can say who takes it harder—the beautiful or the ordinary. It's hard on everybody, because every woman has an image of herself and also has her own dreams and her own special fears.

All of us have the same problem. We must realize that we are a whole person, though we lack one or two breasts, that we have nothing to hide, and that we have to be honest with ourselves and our families. We have to share. That's what living is all about, isn't it? I had been coming here for a year, talking to these women, before I suddenly realized this. It happened right here, in this hospital.

I am a very uptight-thinking lady in some areas. I mean I'm not a toucher of strangers. One day, on the floor of the old building, I met a woman whose face and neck had been cut away—a horrendous sight. I was waiting at the elevator, and she came up to me and asked me a question. She was obviously very distressed, and I found that I had put my arm around her—this stranger, who normally I would not have been able to look at. Yet I touched her, and I put my arm around her, and I answered her question, and I talked to her in an intimate way.

When I got into the elevator, it suddenly dawned on me what I had done, and I was thrilled and frightened. I had such a variety of reactions that I could do what I had done, and finally I said, "Well, Rosalie, if you can do that, if you can touch that woman, you've made it." It made me feel great. That's when I began to realize why I was coming here every week. It was the sharing of myself, of whatever I have that might be worth a little bit to somebody else.

At this point, our talk was interrupted by the arrival of seven postsurgical mastectomy patients—gathering in a group session for physical therapy and counseling, led by social worker Sona Euster-Fisher.

Over the years, thousands of women have come in small groups to a room on the eighteenth floor of Memorial Hospital for physical therapy and personal counsel to speed their recovery from breast amputation. Amid tears and laughter, they variously discuss sex, self-identity, their husbands, their hopes and fears. It is, as Christa Freund puts it, "where they pick up the pieces and start to make you whole again."

The seven women, wearing personal dressing gowns, enter the therapy room with a pillow under the arm on the side which has suffered surgery. Those holding two pillows have lost both breasts. The gowns vary, indicating somewhat the women and the character of their homes. Those emerging from recent surgery walk slowly, with the dazed look of a bird that has been stunned by a blow. As they are seated in a circle, a social worker* briskly places a name tag on each one.

A large, one-way mirror separates one side of the room from a smaller observation chamber, used by teachers and students. It allows an observer to study the women and hear their comments through a one-way audio system, without being seen or heard. The patients are advised beforehand of those present in the observation chamber.

A dark-haired young woman, in her early twenties with lovely features, sits next to the glass. Her hair falls freely onto a deep red robe, and with a pillow under her right arm, she begins to rock back and forth like someone in a neurological ward. Pausing, she speaks to the woman next to her: "I'm Marjorie." The other woman, a honey-blond who had once been a great beauty, says, "I'm Giulietta." She looks down at the younger girl with the air of one long used to personal triumphs. To their right sits another blond with a ponytail, wearing a green robe embroidered with palm trees. She speaks with a French accent. Next in the circle is a tall, elegant black woman with fine features, thick lips, her hair in a tight bun, her body arched as though seated on a throne while surveying the small circle of women through large-framed, sequined glasses. Beside her sits a woman in a pink robe, dark hair cut short, framing a round face with eyes like daisies. Next is an old woman with white hair, wearing a white quilt robe. The last one is a dark Italian madonna in a blue robe.

---

* Sona Euster-Fisher, M.S.S.W., formerly Department of Social Work, Memorial Sloan-Kettering Cancer Center.

Marjorie leans forward until her lips touch the glass partition. They are now only a few inches from ours, and her eyes seem to stare through the mirror into our own. "I want to go back to my room," she murmurs, her lips moving on the glass.

The session begins with the physiotherapist explaining there are two types of postmastectomy pain. First, there is pain from the surgical incision which manifests itself in three ways: diagonal, horizontal, and transversal. She warns: "If you feel any type of *incisional* pain, don't move further." The second type is *referred* pain, which can be felt in the shoulder, arm-pits, arms, back, and in the opposite breast. That pain can be described as "furry, sharp, sticky, or a numbness in the elbow." It may last a month or even a year.

In the first exercise, the women stand up and individually face a perfo-rated stick on the wall. They lift their "good" arm as high as it can reach and then place a peg in the stick. The arm is then lowered and both hands, placed against the wall alongside the stick, begin to finger-crawl upward. The "bad" arm keeps pace with the "good" one until, feeling pain, it falls behind. After a pause, both hands once again seek to crawl together to-ward the top peg.

Marjorie tries and gives up, grasping her pillow again. Giulietta takes deep breath as her hands begin to crawl upward, the fingers delicate, w manicured—pausing finally as they reach shoulder level. Her lips m wordlessly as she attempts to go higher, but the pain is too much, an allows her hands to slowly crawl back down again. Exhausted, she forward, her cheek pressed against the wall. Her lips continue to wordlessly, and her eyes close. Then she bravely shoves away, hands start upward again, the delicate fingers trembling, her lips t pain.

The black woman with long legs and arms seems to have Like a basketball champ, she outreaches everyone. The others unison, force their hands to crawl the wall as though feebly se from a prison cell.

Others exercises follow. Hands are clasped atop the h down behind the neck. In another, bending over with the g on the back of a chair, the bad arm is swung crosswise, circles. Finally, using a rope over a high hook, the goo raising the bad one upward.

Exercises over, the social worker introduces Rosalie in the Reach for Recovery program, composed of w mastectomies. "Mrs. Stahl had a breast removed ei now describe her experience and answer any questio eyes converge on Rosalie Stahl's beige blouse and the two identical breast mounds.

SOCIAL WORKER: Rosalie, perhaps you can tell them how it affected you at first.

MRS. STAHL: At first, I felt very depressed until I realized this wasn't getting me anywhere. It wasn't accomplishing anything. In fact, it was making it worse. So each day, I tried to do a little more. If I couldn't do it, I would wait, and a few days later I would be able to do it.

MARJORIE: The reaction of others and how they looked at you—was that hard?

MRS. STAHL: If you act naturally, they actually feel relief. Most everyone wants to accept you, without problems.

BLACK WOMAN: Not my mother. She'll insist that I tell her I'm dying. If I say I'm all right, she'll feel like I don't love her. *(General laughter.)* She'll insist on doing the shopping, because I do worry about that—some ⸱ep in the supermarket knocking into me, bumping my arm.

⸱S. STAHL: I found that in supermarkets I became physically ill from ⸱conditioning. My thermostat was broken. *(Women smile.)* I just ⸱olerate it and felt a lot of extra pain. If I went out into the warm ⸱found it helped. After that, I always carried a sweater. I think ⸱ was when I went to be fitted for a prosthesis. I was just ⸱e breast and thought, "Here I'm going to be made whole ⸱ came home, it was like I'd been in an accident. It was ⸱ot the fault of the sales people. It was just me. I ⸱lo something about myself.

⸱, when they showed us the various types of pros- ⸱d it was gone. Until then, I don't know what I ⸱e false breasts, I knew I had lost my own, and ⸱e. I had always hoped, but at that moment ⸱lly hit me—I couldn't handle it, and I

⸱*):* It's just the idea that you have ⸱ body which normally has been ⸱at's not you. I don't know i⸱

⸱ of you se⸱

Marjorie leans forward until her lips touch the glass partition. They are now only a few inches from ours, and her eyes seem to stare through the mirror into our own. "I want to go back to my room," she murmurs, her lips moving on the glass.

The session begins with the physiotherapist explaining there are two types of postmastectomy pain. First, there is pain from the surgical incision which manifests itself in three ways: diagonal, horizontal, and transversal. She warns: "If you feel any type of *incisional* pain, don't move further." The second type is *referred* pain, which can be felt in the shoulder, armpits, arms, back, and in the opposite breast. That pain can be described as "furry, sharp, sticky, or a numbness in the elbow." It may last a month or even a year.

In the first exercise, the women stand up and individually face a perforated stick on the wall. They lift their "good" arm as high as it can reach and then place a peg in the stick. The arm is then lowered and both hands, placed against the wall alongside the stick, begin to finger-crawl upward. The "bad" arm keeps pace with the "good" one until, feeling pain, it falls behind. After a pause, both hands once again seek to crawl together toward the top peg.

Marjorie tries and gives up, grasping her pillow again. Giulietta takes a deep breath as her hands begin to crawl upward, the fingers delicate, well manicured—pausing finally as they reach shoulder level. Her lips move wordlessly as she attempts to go higher, but the pain is too much, and she allows her hands to slowly crawl back down again. Exhausted, she leans forward, her cheek pressed against the wall. Her lips continue to move wordlessly, and her eyes close. Then she bravely shoves away, and her hands start upward again, the delicate fingers trembling, her lips tight with pain.

The black woman with long legs and arms seems to have no trouble. Like a basketball champ, she outreaches everyone. The others, in scraggly unison, force their hands to crawl the wall as though feebly seeking escape from a prison cell.

Others exercises follow. Hands are clasped atop the head, then slide down behind the neck. In another, bending over with the good arm resting on the back of a chair, the bad arm is swung crosswise, then in opposite circles. Finally, using a rope over a high hook, the good arm pulls down, raising the bad one upward.

Exercises over, the social worker introduces Rosalie Stahl as a volunteer in the Reach for Recovery program, composed of women who have had mastectomies. "Mrs. Stahl had a breast removed eight years ago and will now describe her experience and answer any questions." For a moment, all eyes converge on Rosalie Stahl's beige blouse and the two identical breast mounds.

SOCIAL WORKER: Rosalie, perhaps you can tell them how it affected you at first.

MRS. STAHL: At first, I felt very depressed until I realized this wasn't getting me anywhere. It wasn't accomplishing anything. In fact, it was making it worse. So each day, I tried to do a little more. If I couldn't do it, I would wait, and a few days later I would be able to do it.

MARJORIE: The reaction of others and how they looked at you—was that hard?

MRS. STAHL: If you act naturally, they actually feel relief. Most everyone wants to accept you, without problems.

BLACK WOMAN: Not my mother. She'll insist that I tell her I'm dying. If I say I'm all right, she'll feel like I don't love her. (General laughter.) She'll insist on doing the shopping, because I do worry about that—some creep in the supermarket knocking into me, bumping my arm.

MRS. STAHL: I found that in supermarkets I became physically ill from the air conditioning. My thermostat was broken. (Women smile.) I just couldn't tolerate it and felt a lot of extra pain. If I went out into the warm sunshine, I found it helped. After that, I always carried a sweater. I think my worst day was when I went to be fitted for a prosthesis. I was just getting used to one breast and thought, "Here I'm going to be made whole again." But when I came home, it was like I'd been in an accident. It was very traumatic and not the fault of the sales people. It was just me. I realized then I had to do something about myself.

GIULIETTA: Yesterday, when they showed us the various types of prosthesis, I suddenly realized it was gone. Until then, I don't know what I thought. But when I saw the false breasts, I knew I had lost my own, and it hit me—my sexuality was gone. I had always hoped, but at that moment I lost my hope, my sexuality. It really hit me—I couldn't handle it, and I got hysterical. (Unable to continue.)

OLDER WOMAN (with German accent): It's just the idea that you have to add something else to your own natural body which normally has been all yours. Now you're adding something that's not you. I don't know if I'm expressing it right. . . .

SOCIAL WORKER: Oh, it's quite clear. The two of you seem to be reacting in a normal way.

GREEN ROBE: I think it's that women are always supposed to have a bosom—you know, out here—and now it won't be there anymore, until you get a prosthesis. I don't know what it's going to be like when I get home . . . but so far I don't feel I've lost any sexuality. It's just that it's always been there, and you're supposed to look pretty good in sweaters, and now it's missing.

BLACK WOMAN: That's the problem—when you go home. I was prepared before I got here. I did all the crying and despairing, and I went through surgery very well until yesterday morning. Then I sort of lost hold of that grip on myself. And now, going home has got me worried.

MARJORIE: We were talking about that yesterday morning before my operation, but it hasn't done anything to me yet. Maybe that's because it just happened to me? It's like reading a story about someone else.

GIULIETTA: Not with me. It's happening to me so much I can hardly stand it. I want to run, and I can't. I don't believe it. I'm *in* the story. I keep telling myself it's going to get better, but I don't feel it yet. *(Voices murmur agreement.)*

GREEN ROBE: I understand her *(nodding to Marjorie)*. After the operation you don't feel it. Then, when you're feeling better, it hits you. Yesterday, when we went through these exercises, a switch was pulled. It hit me that it was finally done, and now I have to face life as it comes each day . . .

OLDER WOMAN: Did you cry?

GREEN ROBE: No, because I finally said to myself, "What happens today, happens today. What happens tomorrow, will happen tomorrow."

OLDER WOMAN: I didn't think I could cry, but I did. It just sort of all came together. First, the woman in the room next to me was feeling terrible, and I told myself I had to help her, then I could help myself. I thought, "We have to all stick it out together." Then I went back to my room, and the doctor gave me his report, and it was good. After that, I got another bouquet of flowers, and I had a phone call. Then, all of a sudden, on the phone, I let go. *(General sound of understanding from other women.)* I cried, and I said, "I guess that's good."

MARJORIE: How'd you feel after you cried?

OLDER WOMAN: I think I had to have that, although I'm supposed to be strong. I was always strong, and my husband had said, "Don't worry, you'll make it because you're strong."

SOCIAL WORKER: I have to make a comment here. You said it's bad to cry, or something like that, and also you're supposed to be strong. There's an awful lot of value judgment in those statements. I think it's important to realize that people react in the way that relieves them. Also, not crying doesn't necessarily mean you're strong, nor does crying mean you're weak.

PINK ROBE: It means you're human.

BLACK WOMAN: But what happens when we go home? Not that I expect to wear a size forty-two when I'm really a thirty-six! *(General laughter, including her own.)*

SOCIAL WORKER: You should receive temporary ones to go home with.

MRS. STAHL: It's hard right now for any of you to have any sense of what it's going to be like on a day-to-day basis without a breast or without two breasts. For me, it was like being on a different planet. I knew I had a mastectomy, and that it couldn't grow back. *(General murmur and smiles.)* But as long as I kept the gauze pad on, I could imagine all sorts of things. The man I was with was one of the those who can't stand a scar of any kind, can't tolerate illness in himself or anyone else. But you know what? He changed my dressing because I refused to look. It *had* to be changed because I could take showers, and there's nothing like wearing a wet gauze pad! *(Laughter.)* So *he* looked long before I did. I looked at him while he looked at me, I was really cheating! *(Laughter.)*

GIULIETTA: When you get back home, the first night you go to bed with your husband, what do you do?

MRS. STAHL: It can be hard or not, depending on you and your husband, but mostly it depends on you. I was not very good. In fact, I was terribly confused and obstructive for a long time, until I began to realize that I was a whole person, and not just a pair of boobs.

SOCIAL WORKER: *(To Giulietta)* This may sound silly, and I don't mean it to be. What do you think you want to do the first night?

GIULIETTA: I don't want him to look at me.

SOCIAL WORKER: You don't?

GIULIETTA : No. *(She sobs, and Marjorie extends a Kleenex.)*

SOCIAL WORKER *(quickly):* I understand how you feel. It's quite normal. But perhaps your husband will want to see it and show you that he loves you just the same.

GIULIETTA: I said I'm not showing it. He came to me here in the hospital and said, "Let's look at it," and I said, "No." He said, "I want to look." I said, "I'm not looking, and if I'm not ready for it, then I'm certainly not ready for you to see it."

BLUE ROBE: I understand that. My doctor came this morning to say good-bye because he was going on vacation. He said, "Look at your scar." I said, "No, I'm not ready yet." He said, "When will you be ready?" and I said, "I hope, with some help from the nurses, that it'll be *before* I go home, so I won't need somebody to hold me up when the time comes. But I want to do it one step at a time." He said, "Do it now." I said, "No, it has to come from inside me . . ." and I started to cry.

SOCIAL WORKER: There's a lot of reality in what you're saying. One step at a time.

BLACK WOMAN: I already took the steps. I wondered what I was going to do when I got home and the bandage came off. Then my husband came here and wanted to see it, saying, "Let me, so I won't be shocked when you get home." So I let him see it.

PINK ROBE: My husband says he wants me whether there's something missing or not.

SOCIAL WORKER: Can we go back to looking at ourselves? What was your first reaction, those of you who have looked?

GREEN ROBE: I can't look, even if I want to. I mean, in my room here the bathroom mirror is so high, and I'm so short. *(General laughter.)* In the shower, they take the bandages off, and I do look—but I'm looking down. My operation was such that I do have nipples, but they're not in the right places. I'm going to have reconstruction so I have flaps here, pockets there. God knows what it's going to be like when I get home and look at all of it in a full-length mirror.

SOCIAL WORKER: What do you expect will be the difference at home when you can look at it straight on?

GREEN ROBE: I guess I'll be looking mostly at the nipples because now they're up higher—not that I'm going to stand there all day looking at them! *(General laughter.)*

GIULIETTA: I told them before the operation that I must have reconstruction. So I must have flaps or whatever, too.

SOCIAL WORKER: But you haven't looked yet?

GIULIETTA: I don't know why I can't look. I just can't. So many years being used to a body, then having it so different. Maybe it's because I still think I am what I was. It's America, and unfortunately it's the body beautiful, and now I'm just . . . *(Voice breaks again.)*

GREEN ROBE: I don't feel that way. I feel like I've been given a second chance. If you have to give up a breast in order to live, that's not the worst thing that can happen. We haven't lost an arm. Or a leg. We've got our eyesight. We can hear. We can speak. We're still able. I'm grateful to God. Once I've got the prosthesis and put on my bra, my friends may know—but nobody else. I'm not gonna put up a sign, saying, "One Breast Missing." *(Laughter.)*

SOCIAL WORKER: I think we can say you all gave one or two breasts to save your lives, but that doesn't mean it's pleasant or comfortable. Everyone adapts in a personal way.

PINK ROBE: I told my husband when I left, "Now you're going to have one for the price of two—half a loaf is better than none!" He got hysterical. *(Laughter.)* Then I'd cover myself and say, "How do I look without it?"

GREEN ROBE: I did that, too! *(More laughter.)* My husband and I were standing in front of the mirror, and I took a towel and said, "How's it look?" He said, "Great! What's special about you is how you keep changing. It's never boring." *(Murmurs of approval.)* I loved him for that because he was saying, "You're going to face it, and I'm facing it with you."

BLACK WOMAN: *(To Mrs. Stahl)* Can I ask a question? How'd your husband take it?

MRS. STAHL: He helped me to accept what had happened to me—to accept me as I am. To realize there is nothing wrong with having one breast, having a scar on one side, and a scar is not necessarily ugly. He *likes* it—on me! About four years ago, we were in a motel, and he said, "You know, your body hasn't changed at all in all these years we've been together." And he meant it. He really meant it. *(Pause.)* But you know, as he gets older, his eyes are getting weaker. *(Uproarious laughter.)*

SOCIAL WORKER: I think we can all agree you are fortunate to have men who love and understand and accept. But unfortunately, it's not always that way. Often women have to overcome sexual and social problems that arise, and that can only be done by having a respect for yourself as a whole person. I believe you all feel that instinctively.

PINK ROBE: I worked in a cytopathology lab for years, and when this happened to me, I said, "Well, now it's your turn. You're on the other end of the microscope." But after seeing all sorts of operations for twenty years, I knew mine was far less than many others. It really is. I'm saying this with all my heart. Also, women have a great deal of strength, much more than men have—and I don't say this just because we're a bunch of women sitting here in this room. As vain as we women think we are, men are much more vain. And women have a much greater fighting instinct. I've had women friends who've had mastectomies. They've asked the same questions as we are now, and, believe me, they've done wonderfully. *(Mixed voices of approval, with scattered applause.)*

SOCIAL WORKER: That's a very good point to consider in closing. Also, as Mrs. Stahl has demonstrated to us, a great deal now depends upon how you feel about yourself. If you feel whole as a person, you'll be accepted as one. If you feel you are just as beautiful a woman as before, then people will tend to accept you that way. It's up to you, and it's never easy. Nothing worthwhile is ever easy. But it's your life, it is worthwhile, and you will find that it is easier to overcome this each day you face it.†

---

† Further comments from Mrs. Stahl, carried in the preceding interview, have been deleted here, along with additional counsel from the social worker, Sona Euster-Fisher.

In some cases of bone metastasis, it can be overwhelmingly frightening when five nurses try to lift a patient in bed and have an arm or a leg break while they are doing it. These are highly skilled, gentle people, and they come out devastated. It does something to you deep inside. It puts you in touch with your finality, with the fact that you are flesh and blood. You are not immortal.

She's 33 and blond, has a soft laugh and light blue eyes that sparkle when she smiles. The only indication that Sister Rosemary is a nun, and not just one more pretty staff member wearing a white jacket, is the "Sr." on her name tag, and a silver ring with a Greek Cross on her left hand.

We have met in the coffee shop at Memorial to talk about the inevitable risk of becoming emotionally involved with cancer patients and, on occasion, feeling a love for them.

She is a supervisor on a thirty-five-member staff in the Department of Social Work, and she also teaches in the department's institute for postgraduate social workers. "We bring them here from all over the country to help improve their skills in the care of the cancer patient, the family, and the staff. My subject is stress, staff stress. I've been working to develop a greater understanding of what causes this stress."

I believe we have the highest medical standards here at Memorial—at least, from my perspective. But if we're going to talk about maintaining high quality, especially in a human situation, I believe we should understand what people have to go through to get it.

This place, like any other hospital or research center, is staffed with human beings who, like everyone else, have their own problems. Inevitably, this is intensified by the work we do, by the nature of the disease we are fighting. Staff members working directly with patients—doctors, nurses, social workers—are especially subject to stress from this. It can drain them emotionally and leave them vulnerable to experiences that can evoke deeply personal fears and feelings. For instance, uncontrolled bleeding can bring out profound fears—not only in the patient but the staff as well.

I'll never forget a man who had a tumor around his carotid artery—here, in the neck. This man could die if his artery blew out, because then he would bleed to death. I never quite understood what that meant, but some nurses were very anxious, and the house staff was also tense about it.

The man was so frightened. He had this tumor growing in his neck, and he could feel it. I could understand it intellectually, but not too well emotionally. Then, as the tumor grew and began to bleed a little bit, I could see his fear growing with it. He was so panicked, he refused to leave Memorial to go to a terminal-care facility. He wanted to stay with people he knew. The doctors wrote all sorts of orders to justify him staying here because we knew the transfer would be too destructive—it would devastate him. In my stress groups for nurses and doctors, they began to talk about finding it harder and harder to go into this man's room when he rang. I respected their feelings, but I couldn't quite understand why.

Then one day, I heard a nurse, a young nurse calling from his room. My office was near the room, and I ran to it. *(Pauses.)* I've never seen anything like it in my life. His tumor hadn't blown the artery, but it was bleeding profusely. The nurse had nothing to stop the blood other than her hands and her body. She was holding him close in her arms with a towel, trying to stop the bleeding. At the same time, she was calling for help because she couldn't reach the buzzer. I yelled for help, too, and grabbed other things to help her stop the flow. I have never seen anything so devastating. It's the fear of total loss of control of life, the greatest vulnerability human beings can experience. His life's blood was flowing out, and there seemed to be really little anyone could do but apply pressure. The anxiety in my chest was so great, I could hardly breathe. He didn't die that time, but he did shortly afterward from further bleeding.

Later that year, I did see a carotid blowout. It came out with such force that it was hitting the wall. It was most difficult to witness. I could hardly breathe, and I felt my heart beating as I looked at it—at the overwhelming vulnerability of human life. They managed to put pressure on it and bind it off. There are precautions for this, but you don't always know when it's going to happen, and you have only a short time to do something before it's too late.

There are other areas of staff vulnerability. For instance, a patient may remind you of someone you've loved and evoke a traumatic experience buried in your past. You suffer a close identification which can immobilize or limit you—leaving you even more vulnerable. Or you can be needy, just needy, having troubles in your personal life. You come in here, and some patient, for whom you have a close feeling, might be dying or experiencing an unexpected complication, which is too much to handle. And you identify again. You can just become flooded with emotion.

Besides all that, there's the nature of the disease and the fact that we're all bound in a common struggle against it. We have one enemy, we think and work against it, and there's no letup from it. You often find the house staff, interns and residents, social workers and nurses, saying this is an unreal situation. But, in fact, it's so real that it's frightening. It is focusing on one point in the human experience to the extent that it seems almost inhuman, but it's really not. You know that old Indian story—what does an elephant look like? A group of blind people are placed around an elephant. Each one touches and describes what he feels. So the elephant is a big snake, or a tree trunk, or a heavy rope, and so on.

What we are confronted with here is not an inhuman situation, but rather a close-up on one part of a person's life, one particle of a person's total experience, blown up to an overwhelming proportion by people who are trying to save them, people going to the limit of their energy, their mental and psychic capabilities totally focused on one point of a human body, one part of a single life.

Do you see the interweaving of all the services and disciplines—doctors, clergy, social worker, volunteers—as a sort of extended family for the patient?

I think it often is, except that here, in life terms, it is more total. Here you are dealing with life and death, with a perspective of tasks needed to help people survive, and priorities for these tasks and the staff members responsible for them—the physician, nurse, pharmacist, social worker, whatever. So we have to work against our medical family falling into common social stresses—of excluding some members, of rivalry and conflict, of the usual struggles you see in a normal family situation. Priorities are always a source of potential conflict. When you deal with someone dying at home, everyone wants to be important to that person. That's always a latent danger here, or in any hospital, where you have many professionals striving to help the patient.

Everybody wants to help. So you find the clergy saying, "We're helping the patient deal with this," and the nurses saying, "We're helping the patient deal with this," and the social workers and psychiatrists saying, "We're helping the patient deal with this." Everyone wants to save the patient, but there can really be no "first" at all. There has to be a sharing of different disciplines. Each one has its own specific moment to be important, its specific contribution toward the total effort.

The patient needs everybody in the effort, each one working to help him, his family, his life-sustaining social links—all of it re-creating the human experience again for both patient and family. This means you do not allow the patient to be an island in the middle of loss and sickness and debilitation. You do not let the experience of illness be called inhuman. You try to humanize it. To not leave someone on a riverbank because they are no longer functional. To keep integrating them into the flow of life and to help them to stay there.

I see the clergy, social workers, psychiatrists—that is, the support professions, in addition to everyone else—as bridges to people's lives. I don't see one stopping, followed by the other. They are parallel, bringing into play the long perspective of someone's life, beyond the hospital. They help re-create and support that life. No one has it all in hand. For instance, the spiritual dimension of someone cannot be the only truth in someone else's life. I've really come to that. The clergy does not have it all. The medical field does not have it. The social workers do not have it. Everyone is another link in the total, integrated life of the patient.

So we're all about the same thing in the broadness of the truth. Each of us crosses over a bridge from his own field. The clergy bring the integration of the spiritual dimension. The mental health professionals come with the psychosocial, the psychological, the interpersonal, and intrapsychic aspect of people's lives. They are separate, yet inseparable, in the sense that they're all going to the same place in the patient's total life experience.

Yet you can't really say that everybody here feels close to everybody else. There is rivalry, friction, even hatred. It's only human and to be expected.

First, let me say that when I first came here, I wasn't quite confident of my professional skills. I'm still learning, but then I was just beginning. When I walked into a room, I wasn't sure that I would know what to do or how to respond. I felt that I had to have the answers. I looked around and thought, "I really don't belong here, with these gifted professionals." I was intimidated by their separate, individual skills, but this has since evolved into a rather strong affection for them, especially after seeing their dedication to their work.

Yet there is, as you suggest, a conscious level at which some people cannot acknowledge belief in another, whatever the other might be—God, Buddha, the wholeness, whatever. On the other hand, there's also a deeper level for most of the people here which prevails over that, over all that constantly hinders us, over all that corrupts and hurts, over all the needs to control, to conquer, to possess. What finally counts, the true measure of what is here, comes from this deeper level of giving together without any counting of self.

People will write countless articles, explaining why we work in a situation like this, in a cancer hospital—articles that never refer to this central truth. They'll talk about competitiveness and achieving all sorts of objective realities. They'll talk about us having our needs met—the obvious needs, and the unconscious needs to be loved, to be wanted, to be needed, to be singularly helpful.

But what they should talk about is the fusion of ourselves without counting—or even being aware it is happening. For when it comes to the moment that really counts, you look at the people here, at how they work, and you find it all coming together—you find someone who gives rather than someone who takes. They are taking while they are giving, of course, but the giving usually wins out.

I no longer get annoyed with the human frailties, the demands and competitiveness, because ultimately when push comes to shove, these people give of themselves from this deeper commitment. Perhaps I should say it's a higher level because here they are selfless and often even heroic in their personal sacrifice. It occurs all the time in this place, almost as though it is to be expected and is to be received without recognition or acknowledgment. It's just part of the reality of this hospital—and most of us who work here.

TWO

LOVE

The heart has its reasons, which reason does not know. We feel it in a thousand things. I say that the heart naturally loves the Universal Being, and also itself naturally, according as it gives itself to them; and it hardens itself against one or the other at its will.

Blaise Pascal
Pensées

Nature has arranged that it is impossible for man to feel "right" in any straightforward way [because of] two motives or urges that seem to be part of creature consciousness and that point in two opposite directions. On the one hand, the creature is impelled by a powerful desire to identify with the cosmic process, to merge himself with the rest of nature (Agape). On the other hand, he wants to be unique, to stand out as something different (Eros).

Ernest Becker
The Denial of Death

Not only in this section, but elsewhere throughout the book, we encounter episodes and acts of love possessing a singular strength and beauty. In various ways, they seem to emerge as part of any cancer experience.

Many who survived believe that love was crucial for them, both in turning back the disease, and in leading them to an altered state of being where they are more open to life, with a greater awareness and a heightened sense of joy in day-to-day living.

These are climactic experiences, yet they often occur when least expected by the patient or the family—descending suddenly, like a shaft of sunlight pouring into a town hall or a church, touching the shoulders, the hair, the cheeks, and hands, wrapping each figure in a light which seems to invest them with a special grace.

So, too, in these stories the mantle of love envelops the patient and those gathered nearby, suffusing them in a reflected light. It also appears to endure beyond its time, to be more visible than previous loves, to be more capable of returning in moments of need—flooding the whole being with a feeling of love that is purged of all doubt or fear by the devastation of the illness. In this way, love enters with an unquestioned identity, it is accepted entirely, it has an enveloping wholeness.

We witness its effect in many ways. At the bedside, tiny miracles flourish. An extended hand wipes away a lifetime of misgivings. An embrace, a whispered word brings down barriers of guilt and hate. Proud spirits kneel humbly, feeling a sudden release of self and a shock of recognition. Fannie

Krevsky, in washing feces from her husband's pants, says, "I finally know about pity and love. I don't care what happens. I'm willing to undergo it."

On other occasions, it occurs more slowly, as though love was seeded to flower in separate moments of need or despair. A college dean's dockside appointment with his wife becomes a beacon fixing his course through dark days—serving also to illuminate progressively the profundity of their love. A husband, in doubt about his wife's survival, plants small trees around the home, which his wife accepts as proof that he believes she will live to see them grow—using this to help her climb to recovery.

For others, there is the presence of two or more loves with the need to give priority to one—followed by a sudden awakening to the immensity of the primal love. A woman refuses to allow her pregnancy to be terminated, thereby risking the spread of her cancer—causing her husband to realize that his love for his wife outweighs the risks of the unborn child, even though it will be the last baby they can ever have. Another woman, grieving over her dying brother, neglects her husband who is undergoing radiation for throat cancer until she finds him in a bar one day, talking to strangers—discovering then that she could never love anyone as much as this one man.

At other times, the love appears to be so vast that it can only be grasped through prayer, or only approached by going through one or more persons. For Pascal, it is the love of the Universal Being, when not loving oneself as the heart dictates. For Becker, it is to identify with the cosmic process, to merge with nature—when not obeying an opposing desire to be unique, creative, and separate from all others.

Some of these survivors, with the agility of bilocating saints, exist within both states of love at the same time. John Alexion, sustained by a love for his wife, also dwells within the prayers of Vincentian priests. Estelle Marsicano, held aloft by her husband's love and what she perceives as his faith in her, is also transported by the laying on of a bishop's hands, feeling then the warmth of God passing through her.

Others describe their transcendent passage from the self-love of Eros to the universal love of Agape as a natural and inevitable event. James Brown, after having his leg amputated, attempts to help a little boy facing the same fate: "I was going along without my girl, with nobody real close. Then, before I know what's happening this little boy is with me. It's like you can't go very far, all alone by yourself, without caring for somebody else—like it's more natural to care for each other than anything else."

We also see this type of care and love coming from the nurses, the social workers, the volunteers, the doctors and staff at Memorial Hospital. It is part of the give-and-take between the patients and those caring for them,

essential as breathing in the hospital's life. It is irrepressible, and it will out
—no matter how one seeks to restrict or confine its force.

For a nurse, Patricia Mazzola, it was beautifully manifested when her
brother, as a patient, became "everyone's brother." Nurse Dorothy Dona-
hue sees it as an inevitable part of having "a series of extended families."
For Nurse Sabina Cunningham, it is the sort of loving that goes on all the
time: "The whole person, a body's innocence is being violated. We're caring for that, we're loving that part of them."

Even when one nurse, Maureen Roden, goes beyond the limit—going
into Eros with a physical love for her patient, Bruce—she seems to have
made of him an apotheosis of all her patients in the past as well as those to
come. Upon seeing him for the last time, she says, "I had the strange
feeling that I had known this man long before I ever met him—and that I
would meet him again somewhere."

I'm a DES daughter. I know it, but there's a lot of women who don't know it, and they should be aware of what might happen to them, especially if they want to have a baby. Before it was banned, they estimate that three million women took this drug to help their pregnancies.†

It didn't do much harm to the mothers, but it played hell with their children, who are abnormally prone to cancer of the vagina, cervix—you name it. Some of the males have low sperm counts and abnormal semen and sperm forms. Poor things, that must be a living nightmare for them.

They have records for only about four hundred women who've gotten cancer from this, but there are undoubtedly many hundreds more which haven't been reported because they want to keep it a secret or because they don't know their cancer was caused by DES. Many mothers are so guilt-ridden they can't talk about it, or they don't know or don't remember if they took the drug. But it's important for every young woman or girl born before 1971 to know about it because this form of cancer, clear cell adeno-carcinoma, is curable if diagnosed early, even though it usually entails surgery that leaves you incapable of having children. That's why I held onto my pregnancy and wanted to have my baby even when they told me I had cancer of the vagina.

She's 30—dark hair to the shoulder, dark brown eyes, a large woman with an attractive body and sensitive features, wearing a purple tunic. "I've been overweight ever since this happened, but I'll lose it when I go back to work." We are sitting in wicker chairs on the front porch of the Kramer bungalow in Tarrytown, New York. It's been a hot Sunday, and the first evening breeze is bringing some relief. Nathan Kramer, Lois' husband, comes out onto the porch with drinks, then sits down to join us. Tall and lean, with a dark mustache, he is manager of a plumbing supply firm.

---

* Identity of patient and husband have been altered.

† DES (diethylstilbestrol) is a synthetic hormone that mimics the action of estrogen, the female sex hormone. From 1943 to 1970, it was prescribed during pregnancy to avert threatened miscarriage, but was eventually banned in 1971, when it was discovered that the daughters of women who had taken DES became highly susceptible to cervical cancer. With some DES-related cancers occurring in women up to 29 years of age, the buried menace of this drug will not be gone until the year 2000—if then. It is still sold (with FDA approval) for use as a "morning after" contraception pill. Despite warnings to use only in emergency situations, it is popular on college campuses. DES has also been linked to development of cancer of the breast and endometrium, or lining of the uterus.

I had a miscarriage and went to see the doctor—my mother's gynecologist. He knew I'd been exposed to DES, but the idiot told me not to worry about it. "Jewish girls don't get cancer," he said. It's supposed to be less likely because Jewish men are circumcised, but that's bullshit because now all men are circumcised—or most of them, anyway.

I knew better, but I believed him anyway, because it was easier to believe and not worry about it. Then I conceived again, and when I was three months pregnant, we switched over to a community health program under Blue Cross. So I had a new gynecologist—a Dr. Brown. He looked at my cervix and said, "You're a DES-exposed daughter." I said, "I know that . . . what about it?" He said he didn't like the look of it and sent me to a specialist at a Long Island hospital.

This was another prima donna—the lugubrious type. He took one look and told my husband, "She has cancer. I'll do a biopsy, but I'm sure she has it anyway." Nice guy, right? You need that kind like you need Hitler.

NATHAN: *(Interjects)* I remember him coming on very heavy, saying, "Your wife has cancer"—like it was her fault, like she was guilty of breaking the law. I thought, "Why does he do this to us? Does he enjoy it? We need help, we need encouragement, or at least nothing negative!" I asked him about the baby, and he said, "If it's between your wife and the baby, which is more important?" I asked if that meant I'd have to choose between one or the other, and he said, "If she has cancer, you don't have a choice. Either we operate, or you risk losing them both."

LOIS: No doubt about it. If the cancer had appeared then, at three months, I'd have lost my baby. It's happened to other DES girls who were pregnant when the cancer appeared. They aborted the baby and operated on the mother to save her life. But luckily, my cancer did not appear then. The report came back that I merely had cervix edema, or swelling, which is common in ninety percent of girls who have been exposed to DES. So Dr. Brown decided to watch it with regular Pap tests through the whole pregnancy.‡

Then, in the sixth month, the test came back showing something was wrong—and that was it. I knew I was in trouble. He sent me to Columbia Presbyterian, to a specialist, who wanted to investigate it further with another biopsy. I said, "No way. I'm pregnant, I've been cut enough. They

---

‡ The Pap test can detect established cancer of the cervix, but its great value is diagnosing precancerous conditions, which can be treated before developing into cancer. In a simple, painless procedure, cervix and vaginal fluids are examined for abnormal cell changes. The test is considered essential for all women, including teenagers, at least once a year—especially if there's been cancer in the family. Since first proposed by the late Dr. George N. Papanicolaou in 1950, it has saved an estimated half million lives.

did that to me in my third month, nothing showed, and you're not doing it again."

I was a lunatic at that point, in my sixth month. I knew a biopsy was necessary, but I wasn't listening to them then until my gynecologist promised he would not terminate my pregnancy, no matter what the test showed. So they took a biopsy, and we began the nightmare of waiting for the results. It had been hell the first time, because I knew I'd lose my baby if it came back positive. This time, I was even more tense because I knew the surgeons would want to operate right away, and I wasn't going to let them take my baby, no matter what the results were. Well, they told my husband first.

NATHAN: Yes, I was working in the supply warehouse when the doctor called and asked me to see him. I left work, and on the way there, I knew it was bad news because if it was good, he would have said so.

He tells me the biopsy is malignant, and Lois has cancer of the vagina. Just like that—bang! I'm stunned, like I've been hit by a truck, and he says to me, "I know we promised Lois we would not terminate her pregnancy, but it's my duty to tell you, the husband, that the safest route for your wife is to operate now. Otherwise, this cancer will have three more months to grow. It's not fast-moving, and it's in one place, but we have no way of knowing that it'll stay there. If it spreads, you risk losing your wife and the baby. If you act now, at least she will be saved. There's a high survival rate with this type of cancer when attacked at this stage." I said something like, "But she'll lose this child and never be able to have another one," and he said, "That's why she'll want to hang on, no matter what happens. But you have to also consider how much you want to risk losing your wife. That's why I called you in first. I know what she wants, but you have to also know the risks and what you want."

I walked out of there with a terrible headache. I get them in stress situations, and, to be honest with you, I don't always remember things correctly when I get like that. I had a coffee, and it didn't help, so I had a beer and tried to think about what to do. For the doctors, it was a clear-cut decision—abort the baby and save the mother. They had nothing to lose and everything to gain. I had a lot to lose—either my baby, or maybe my wife *and* the baby. But especially my wife. You always say to yourself, "Gee, I really love her." It isn't until something like this happens that you realize how much you can love someone, just when you might lose them. So I thought, "I want to keep my wife. She wants to keep the baby. So maybe I want her more than she wants her own self? If she wants to risk her life for an unknown baby, do I want to risk her that much? If I let her do it, and she dies, I'll have nobody to blame except myself for not putting my foot down and saying, 'No, you can't do it, I won't let you risk it.'"

It was a terrible decision to make. You become like a judge, and you wonder, "What right do I have to make such a decision? How can I say which is good and which is not?"

LOIS: *(Interrupts)* Except you weren't having the baby, I was. And it wasn't your total decision. It was ours.

NATHAN: Right, but first I was holding it all in my head. I learned it on a Thursday and didn't tell you until Saturday night, all the time wondering, "How do I handle this, how do I tell her without making a mistake? I felt very emotional, almost like I was breaking down, wondering how I was going to tell her about it. . . .

LOIS: *(Interrupts)* We were giving my parents an anniversary party that Saturday, a family get-together with some of their friends. We'd been planning it for a long time.

NATHAN: I didn't want to burden her with the news until after everybody'd gone. Then I sat her down and said there was something I had to tell her—and she knew what it was. We both cried then. It was very emotional.

They had met on a blind date, arranged by Nathan's aunt, who was a matchmaker. Lois recalls, "She said she had a nephew back from college who would like to meet a nice tall Jewish girl. My father said, 'I have a daughter.' He had never done that before, but he couldn't say no to this aunt." Nathan recalls, "My aunt said, 'Call this girl. Your eyes will pop out of your head.' Well, I'm not the most dynamic person when it comes to calling blind dates. I was very nervous, I was shy, but I called her up, and we talked for about an hour. Lois later said that I mumbled, she didn't understand a word I said or who I was, but when I asked if I could come over, she said okay." Lois recalls, "It was raining, pouring, and I figured we'd stay in my house. I didn't put on makeup, just blue jeans and a turtleneck. We sat on the green couch, and it was so romantic." (Laughs.) "My father and Nathan talked about football the whole night." Nathan: "What else could I do? Also your little sister was there with her friend, snickering at me, giving me the third degree. I was a setup, I was a pigeon." Lois: "My parents loved him and said he was a nice boy. I said, 'He was very nice. I didn't get a chance to say two words to him.'" Nathan: "But, boy, did she make up for it later, right up to the final wire." (Laughs.) "At a friend's wedding—you know how you get romantic at those things?—I sort of threw it out, for conversation, saying, 'I'd kinda like to be a June groom in maybe two years or so.' She said, 'You got it all wrong, or you've got me wrong. June comes once a year—this year or never.' And that was it."

LOIS: When Nathan told me I had cancer and the doctor thought it was safer to abort the baby, I sat there, holding myself, saying, "No way, I want to keep this child, and we aren't going to tell anybody about the problem." I knew our parents would go crazy and drive us crazy—especially my mother because she would feel guilty and dump her guilt on me. She'd already done it when I had my miscarriage, because DES girls are prone to that, too. I told her, "Ma, listen. There's three million women who took that lousy DES. The doctors passed it out like aspirin. So it's not your fault. If I'd been in your place, I'd have taken it, too—so stop worrying about it." Nathan's mother was the same. She's a good woman and means well. But when I had my miscarriage, she went around crying all the time, like it was her worst problem, when it was really my problem, not hers.

No, we had three months before us, and we had to cope with this, without the whole family walking around moaning and crying over us—or our friends looking sad when they saw us. No, no way.

"But first I had to find a supersurgeon. My doctor told me I would have to have a radical hysterectomy-vaginectomy and cesarean section. I didn't know what 'radical' meant, I didn't really think they were going to remove my vagina and rebuild it. I was in a fog and didn't listen. But I remember him saying, 'This is not normal surgery. It's not just walking in for a hysterectomy. You have to find a very special, highly skilled surgeon because I don't even know if this has ever been done before—that is, all this surgery at one time.'

"He gave me a list of names, including Dr. Herbst in Chicago—one of the doctors who proved the dangers of DES in women, and who keeps a registry of all cases that are reported.* He and his doctors were fabulous with me when I phoned them. They answered lots of questions I'd been too dumb or too afraid to ask, like what was going to happen to my sex life. They told me, 'The surgeon will reconstruct your vagina, your sex life will come back, and you will enjoy it.' Anybody with DES trouble should call them in Chicago. They'll answer a lot of questions that girls are afraid to ask.

"When I told them that I was going to see John Lewis at Memorial, they

---

* Arthur L. Herbst, M.D., professor and chairman, Department of Obstetrics and Gynecology, Chicago Lying-In Hospital. Drs. Herbst, Howard Ulfelder, and David C. Poskanzer published the first negative findings on DES in the April 1971 issue of the *New England Journal of Medicine*—thirty years after the drug was first used in the United States.

said he was one of the best surgeons in the world for this—and I couldn't do better."†

As soon as I met Dr. Lewis, I felt at ease. He knew we were scared, and he calmed us down—he has a father-type image. He told me I could be treated two ways—by surgery or by radiation—but he felt surgery would be more effective, and also radiation would probably destroy my sex life. So I said I wanted surgery.

After that, I began to live with this for three months, waiting for it to happen. I went to work every day, and that was okay. I'm an executive secretary in a computer company. I didn't let anybody know my trouble, and I was doing fine—making decisions and dealing with people. So I could turn it off by day. But I was really shook up at night. We couldn't have intercourse for fear of stimulating the cancer growth, so there was no sex, not even in other ways because I was afraid to have an orgasm for the same reason. So I'd lie there all tensed up, trying not to think about it, but feeling it anyway—feeling my baby growing and wondering if the cancer was growing, too, if maybe it was going to invade the womb and take hold of my baby, you know, a sort of a race against time, and I'd think "My little baby can't run anywhere, he's trapped in there, maybe he doesn't even have a chance." Then I'd get the shakes, because the poor little thing . . . *(Stops, unable to continue.)‡*

NATHAN: All of a sudden, she would be crying. It would be late at night, with those thoughts coming onto her, and she couldn't help herself. There's an expression people say, if you live with a person long enough, you start to look like them. Well, you get to *feel* like them, too. So I felt, "It's bad for her, it's bad for me." She has the cancer, and I don't, but I'm holding onto her, trying to take the sorrow away from her, letting it come into me. So we suffer together. Her dilemma is my dilemma, and we work it out together because it becomes one problem.

Lois laughs. "We had to do a lot of lying, too—especially to my parents. They've always been very overprotective. I mean, when I decided to go to Europe with my friends—I was 19 and had my own money to go—my mother's first reaction was 'What are you going to do if you get sick in

---

† John L. Lewis, Jr., M.D., chief attending surgeon, Gynecology Service, Memorial Hospital.

‡ There was no concern that the mother's cancer would pass to her child. The myth and fear that cancer is "contagious" is, unfortunately, widespread, even among highly educated persons.

*Europe? How can you take care of yourself, if I'm not there?' She's like
that. She also calls me at nine o'clock in the morning every single day, even
now she does it, and that's the way it is. So when I had to go to the city or to
the hospital, I had to lie through my teeth. She'd ask me, 'Where were you
at nine o'clock in the morning?' The lies were getting harder, so I told her I
was going to the Lamaze natural childbirth classes. Then she'd ask me what
they did at Lamaze, and I'd make it up for her, and she never knew."*

About two weeks before the operation, my amniocentesis report indicated
I was close to borderline, that the baby was about ready.* Dr. Lewis had
to be in Chicago for three days, and he wanted to do the operation before
he left. My husband asked him, "If you were not leaving, would you do it
now?" He said he wouldn't, so Nathan said, "Well, we'll take our chances
and wait for you to come back."

Before leaving, Dr. Lewis put me in Memorial to be ready for when I
came to term. You should've been there. *(Laughs.)* They'd never seen
anything like it, before or since. Memorial is not designed for delivering
babies, it's a cancer research/teaching hospital. This was one of their first
—scheduled—births. There'd been another one before me, unexpected,
from a woman who came in for something else and was so enormous they
didn't know she was pregnant until she suddenly delivered a baby on
them.

The nurses were all excited—a baby's going to be born! *(Laughs.)* I had
a fetal monitor, and they were constantly in my room, watching it and
listening to the baby's heart. It was such a novelty for them to be able to
hear a baby's heartbeat. They'd heard it in training, but many hadn't
heard it since then. They were all over me, mothering me, and *(laughs)* I
guess I really needed it because I began to feel less afraid and that my baby
was finally safe.

It was due on May twelfth, the day of Dr. Lewis' return, but everything
was ready if it happened sooner.† Since there were no facilities for babies

---

* Amniocentesis is the study of amniotic fluid surrounding the fetus during pregnancy—
mainly to determine prenatal and developmental abnormalities, as well as the lung maturity of the unborn child, and the sex, if parents wish to know.

† Before leaving, Dr. Lewis left detailed instructions on the procedures to be followed in
event of labor before his return. Besides a brief capsuling of patient's previous history,
recent blood count, urinalysis, and other factors, he carefully specified instruments to be
used and cautioned that postoperative intensive care should reckon with "major fluid shifts
that occur at the time of termination of pregnancy." Details for pediatric care of the baby
included a list of doctors on call from the N-5 nursery unit at New York Hospital, phone
numbers, call schedule for six days prior to due date, plus his numbers in Chicago. If birth

at Memorial, Dr. Lewis worked out a plan for a pediatric team to be there from New York Hospital, which is just across the street. There's a tunnel connecting the two hospitals. For his radiation, the Shah of Iran was brought to Memorial through this tunnel. Now my baby was going to be rushed the other way, from Memorial to New York Hospital, in a transport incubator. It was a very sophisticated procedure and to make sure there were no hang-ups, they'd done a few dry runs, going from the operating room to the sterile quarters across the street. So everything was in order, except my water broke the day before Dr. Lewis was due back.

NATHAN: *(Interrupts)* She phoned me and woke me up at four A.M., yelling, "My water broke! It's going to happen!" I'm still in a fog, and I said: "You better call the nurse right away or tell somebody else."

LOIS: I said, "Shmuck, wake up! Everybody already knows. Come to the hospital. They're going to operate!" Then, Dr. Lewis called me from Chicago—poor man, it was still the middle of the night for him, too—and he said, "Don't worry, everything is under control. You'll be in the best hands possible. Dr. Jones is the backup man. You couldn't find a better surgeon for this anywhere."‡

Dr. Lewis had already introduced me to Dr. Jones. He's a black man, although his skin is so light you don't realize it at first. A very handsome man. Everybody on the floor had said, "There's no way Dr. Jones is ever going to touch you, because this is a big case, and Dr. Lewis is going to do it." So now it was like a movie, and suddenly Dr. Jones is the star. Well, I was lucky because I had the best of two worlds. Dr. Jones is not only a fine surgeon, he's also a marvelous, understanding human being.

They took me down and operated right away, at six-thirty in the morning. . . .

NATHAN: *(Interjecting)* I jumped into the car and headed for the city, real excited because my wife is going to have the baby, and this is zero hour. It was early, thick fog all the way, and I'm driving like a maniac. When I think about it now, I shudder because I must've been crazy. I kept saying, "You're going to be a father when you drive home." And I'm saying, "Everything's going to be all right, yes it is, you bet it is, hip-hip-hooray!" *(Laughs.)*

When I got there, Lois is already in surgery. It's about seven—before the hospital gets going for outsiders. Nobody knows anything. I'm walking

---

was to occur before his return, he specified that Dr. Walter B. Jones, among other assistants, be called in.

‡ Walter B. Jones, M.D., associate attending surgeon, Gynecology Service, Department of Surgery, Memorial Hospital.

around the lobby and start down a corridor looking for the operating room area when a security guard stops me, saying, "You can't walk around here." I said, "My wife's just had a baby." He smiles, "That's great, mister. But you got the wrong hospital, it's across the street." "No," I said, "It's here somewhere." "Not here," he says, "nobody comes here for babies, just for cancer." His eyes narrowed like he thought I was crazy, but then an orderly came by, and the guard says, "This man's tryin' to tell me his wife's havin' a baby here." The orderly said, "She's already had it. Congratulations. It's a girl." He also said my wife was still being operated on, and it'd take several hours—but the baby was now in the tunnel, en route across the street.

I ran to the phone and called Lois' father—my father has passed away —and I'm afraid I was yelling at him, "Hey, Pops! It's a girl!" They'd expected it to happen the next day. . . .

LOIS: *(Interrupts)* They were all going to come in, the whole family. Can you imagine it? Gathering around, looking at me like I was going to die. *(Laughs.)* There must've been a God watching over me. He saw it coming and spared me.

NATHAN: I was in the clouds. You know what they say about a new father? It's true. Your feet never touch the ground. For hours you walk around with your head in the clouds. You become a kid again. I went over to New York Hospital, and they have a facility there which is amazing, one floor specifically designed for premature babies, marginal babies, those who are underweight, sick, exceptional. . . .

LOIS: *(Interrupts)* Ours was exceptional.

NATHAN: Okay, exceptional. Anyway, I go in there, and she's in an incubator, and everything looks all right. They said, "Would you like to hold her?" I said sure, so they took her out, and I sat in this old wooden rocking chair, and it was so amazing. The hospital is all stainless steel and glass, all sanitary and white. It was like science fiction, being in a space-ship and in the middle of this spaceship was a wooden rocking chair. I felt like I was in a *Star Trek* or *Space Odyssey* movie, set in the future after mankind had been wiped out—yet, by a miracle, I'm confronted with a specimen of past men. I'm holding my child in my arms, and she is going to start the future race of man again—the tiniest little thing, all wrinkled up, but so cute, and she looked exactly like me.

LOIS: *(Laughs)* Which means this next race of men will be just as blind as the last one, because the baby looked exactly like me.

NATHAN: Anyway, Lois was on the operating table ten hours. Her father came, and we walked the streets, waiting for it to be over. I don't remember a thing we said or did, except we stopped for some Häagen-

Dazs ice cream. Finally they told us it was all over, and they'd gotten everything out. Dr. Jones had done a brilliant job.*

LOIS: We named the baby Rebecca, and she went home at four days. That's when I saw her for the first time. They brought her to the lobby of Memorial, and I came down to hold her. They wouldn't allow her up in the hospital because she'd been in a sterile ward until now and needed to build up her defenses. So I came down. It was Sunday, and Dr. Jones and Dr. Lewis came all the way into town to be with us. The hospital was bubbling, the baby's picture was everywhere, and even the visitors in the lobby crowded around to look at Rebecca. It was like a party for a home-coming—only she was going home, I wasn't.

Dr. Lewis was ready to do a second operation right away, to rebuild my vagina, but Dr. Jones came to my room one afternoon, and he saw how much I wanted to go home to my baby. If I stayed for reconstruction, it would mean another two weeks in the hospital. He spoke to Dr. Lewis, who agreed to let me go. So Dr. Jones brought me a mold—you have to wear a mold at first so the vagina doesn't grow back together and close up. He taught me how to use it and said, "If you can get this mold in and out by yourself, we'll let you go home."

So I did that and came back six months later for reconstruction surgery. They took a graft from my leg and made me a new vagina. There were no complications, and I went home, but I was really scared about having sex the first time. Thank God, I had a husband to do it with. Some DES girls don't have husbands, and it's harder if you don't have sex on a regular basis. Now it's like before. I have all the feelings, and I don't think any-body would know the difference. Nathan says it's just the same. We can't have any more babies, of course, but we have Rebecca, and she's all we've always wanted.

It happened seven years ago now, but whenever I go back to Memorial for a checkup, the nurses, the social workers, the guards, everybody who was there then, they all smile when they see me and say, "She's the lady who had a baby here"—as though something wonderful happened that day, and they like to remember it. So do we. Like Nathan said, it was the beginning of a new world for us.

---

* Following the cesarean section to deliver the baby, the procedure consisted of a radical hysterectomy, a vaginectomy, and a pelvic lymphadenectomy—or removal of nearby lymph glands capable of harboring undetected cancer cells. Tissue specimens were ex-amined at each step of the operation with some samples conserved for further study and others sent to Dr. Herbst in Chicago for his DES research and registry.

He planted the trees for me, all of them small. He said it would be fun to watch them grow into big trees. It was his way of telling me that he knew I would live. That helped, I know it did. I'd go out and look at the little trees, I'd touch them and feel stronger. That's how I knew I would live—my husband and these little trees. Also, maybe God—and Dr. Fortner.

We are in the backyard of the Marsicano suburban home at Bay Shore, Long Island. Estelle touches the trees—maple and spruce—her short, delicate hands on slender limbs, cupping the green leaves. She's 40, with dark hair, chestnut brown eyes, a round face, a perky nose, and a tender, lingering smile.

We pass in front of the house, across a neat lawn with a flagpole and an American flag flapping in the April wind. "My husband fought in Vietnam. He was in the Marines, with helicopters. Then he got a job at PanAm and started at the bottom, washing airplanes. He'd go out on the wings with a mop and wash them. Then, you know, he took a home course in electrical work for about a year, and he passed a lot of tests until he had two or three licenses, and now he's an electrical specialist for 747's. He makes sure they fly, but I kid him a lot. I ask him, 'Did you work on that 747? Then I'm not flying on it!'" (Laughs.)

A blue Corvette pulls up, and Anthony Marsicano gets out. He wears light blue jeans with a red checkered sports shirt, and he strolls casually up the walk under the flag—a lean man with a trim, dark beard. He shakes hands without a word, his dark brown eyes steady on the visitor until, finally nodding with a half smile, he asks, "How about a cup of coffee?"

We go into the kitchen, and at the table Estelle says, "I don't know how to start." Tony, as her husband is called, says, "Start at the beginning. Tell him how they almost killed you."

Well, I began to feel not so well. I was always tired, and I had a pain up here. *(Points to right upper abdomen.)* So I went to this doctor we'd found when we moved out here from Brooklyn, and he said it was just a nervous colon. Then I got the flu, and since this doctor was away, I went to another one, a younger doctor, who said, "You know, your liver seems large."

When my doctor came back, I told him about it, but he said it was nonsense. Then he said, "I have a large liver, too, if you want to feel mine." He claimed my trouble came from a nervous indigestion, and he put me on tranquilizers. The pain wouldn't go away, and he started giving me painkillers. Then I started to have dizzy spells, until I finally went to him, very upset, and he sent me to this surgeon at Meadow Brook Hospital.* *(Turns to Tony.)* I guess we shouldn't say their names?

TONY: No, they'll sue us. But they should have their licenses revoked. They're a social menace—both of them.

ESTELLE: Well, it was out of the frying pan into the fire. This surgeon saw me in his office, and a week later in the mail, I get a letter with the whole procedure of an exploratory operation he's going to do on me. *(Laughs dryly.)* Can you imagine it? No tests, no exams—just open me up and look?

TONY: We had no idea of cancer at the time, and this sudden plunging for an exploratory upset us. Fortunately, we have a very close friend, Anne, who's a registered nurse. She told us to get another doctor, since the surgeon was knife-happy and our own doctor had Estelle popping pills for a year without getting to the bottom of it. Finally we said, "Why don't we go see the doctor we had in Brooklyn, old Dr. Baskin?" He used to be our family doctor. So he put Estelle in Maimonides Hospital for two weeks to do nothing but tests. Finally he said, "From what we can gather so far, your wife either has a cyst or a tumor in her liver. The next thing to do is an exploratory. We can do it here, but if there's a tumor, she's going to need the best surgeon in the field. I suggest Dr. Fortner at Memorial."† I said, "Oh my God!" My head was spinning, and I had to tell Estelle. I wanted to make it easy for her, so I said, "Look, they think you have a cyst or maybe a tumor, but it's probably just a cyst."

ESTELLE: *(Interrupts)* I told them, "It's not a cryst, it's cancer, I know it." But Tony and Dr. Baskin said, "Don't be silly. You can't know until Dr. Fortner examines you." Well, at Memorial they put me through more tests, then they did an exploratory operation and found I had *two* tumors in my liver. Dr. Fortner said it was only a primary—that is, the cancer had started in the liver but hadn't gone anywhere else. He said this was a good sign. It meant we had a better chance, but at that point nothing seemed good to us.‡

---

* Name altered.

† Joseph G. Fortner, M.D., chief attending surgeon, Gastric and Mixed Tumor Service, Memorial Hospital.

‡ The exploratory was done to determine the extent of the cancer and whether or not it was possible to do a resection, or surgical separation of the diseased area. As much as 80 percent of the liver may be removed; the remaining section begins to enlarge immediately and, within a month, has usually regenerated itself. Estelle Marsicano did not have sufficient cancer-free area to allow for such procedure. Dr. Fortner, one of the world's most experienced surgeons in this field, has also pioneered new surgical techniques in surgery of the colon and pancreas.

TONY: *(Interjects)* It was either a liver transplant or chemotherapy, and Dr. Fortner finally decided to take the chemo route. The survival rate at that time wasn't very high going either way. Fortner wasn't giving any odds, but one of his assistants leveled with me. He said, "Your wife might live a year and a half—if she's lucky."

I didn't tell Estelle. I never lied to her, but I did hold back some things, and, believe me, this one really bottomed me. I thought, "My God, what's the use of going through the hell of chemotherapy—only to die at the end?"

When I went to Dr. Fortner with this, he became very upset. "Nobody should have said that. Nobody can give you any figures. She might live less than that—or a lot longer, which is what we are trying for." We were in his office, and I must have looked pretty beat because he calmed down and tried to help me. "Look at it this way," he said. "You're lucky. This cancer probably started a year ago when your wife first went to her doctor. It could have spread elsewhere, but it hasn't because it's slow-moving. Maybe we still have time to stop it. I don't know, but I think we have a chance. We often succeed with a certain type of patient, and I think your wife is one of them." "What type?" I asked, and he said, "People who don't give up, who fight back, seem to do better."

I believed him. Dr. Fortner is a great surgeon and a man to trust. But that's all we could do. Nothing was certain, and even he had admitted my wife might not live a year and a half. He was going to use a new procedure on Estelle, and he'd had some success with it—but I couldn't shake the feeling that the percentages just weren't with us. My father had died of brain cancer, and I kept thinking about him.

When they took Estelle into the operating room, I went to church—St. Catherine's, across the street from the hospital. I sat through Mass, then stayed on—asking for her health, and for some sign to help me believe that she would live, and also to help me carry on. We have two children—two boys who were then only 5 and 2. When I returned, Dr. Fortner said the operation had gone all right, and he allowed me to see Estelle in the recovery room.

ESTELLE: *(Interrupts)* They fixed me up with a little box, like a camera case, that I wore with a belt. It had a small pump that fed drops of chemo medicine through a little tube that went right into my liver.* It kept going

---

* The unit pumped three chemical agents (actinomycin-D, methotrexate, and 5-fluoroura- cil in a saline solution) into the liver via a catheter tied into the hepatic artery. The procedure has since been modified, eliminating box and pump. Using the same hepatic catheter, injections are made once a week. With the opening temporarily closed, patients lead normal lives—including such sports as tennis and swimming.

all the time, day and night, even in bed—for three months. In church or at night you could hear it humming away, and sometimes it was a real nuisance. If I was making the bed and leaned over too far, or sometimes making love, it'd pop loose, and the medicine would start spilling out. *(Laughs.)* I'd just plug it back in and go on with whatever I was doing. I said it was Dr. Fortner's magic box, and it was going to knock all the cancer bugs out of the ball park. *(Laughs.)*

TONY: Estelle was just like Dr. Fortner thought she'd be—tough-willed, with a lot of inner strength. She was always saying, "I'm gonna beat this thing, it's not gonna get me." But I couldn't forget my father's death, or that other doctor saying, my wife would be lucky to live a year and a half. But for her sake, I never showed it. I'd say, "This is really doing you a lot of good" and "You're going to win this, I know it." But inside myself, I didn't know it at all. She was losing weight, she didn't look good, and I had this growing fear that we were really getting nowhere.

We were going to plant a lot of trees, but after I learned how serious her illness was, how little time she might have left, I began to think, "What's the use? If she doesn't make it, I'll probably move away." Then I realized this was a ridiculous attitude, and I decided to plant the trees as if nothing was wrong. On my day off, I'd plant a few of them and say to her, "We're going to see these trees get nice and big together." Maybe I was trying to convince myself, too—because each time I said something like that it made me feel better.

ESTELLE: *(Interrupts)* Do you think that's part of love? I mean, what happens when you love someone? Because it's really strange how I got strength from him when he says he didn't have any. He kept all the bad news, the doubts and the fears, to himself—protecting me. I was scared, too, but I kept believing him. When he said, "You'll make it, I know you will," I held onto that for dear life, like I kept holding onto those little trees, watching the new leaves coming out. Also, Anne would take me to her church, St. Peter's-by-the-Sea, for healing services, where they have a laying on of hands. One day, Bishop Bardsley of Coventry placed his hands on my head, and I felt a sort of tingling warmth going through me, even after we left. I think that helped, too.

Anyway, I had to go into New York, to Memorial, every Monday to have them put more chemo into the box—and also for a checkup. Toward the end of the third month, the doctor is measuring my liver, and he says, "This can't be." Then he checked his chart and measured me again. The look on his face said everything, and my heart was going like crazy. "It's fantastic," he says, "her liver is going down, it's going back to normal." I wanted to hug him—Dr. Carrillo from Venezuela. Little did I know that this was only the beginning, that the worst was still to come. . . .

TONY: *(Interrupts)* There was a long way to go, but that was the turning point for me. I felt now we had a chance, at least. Fortner said we'd halted the cancer in her liver, but the next thing we had to do was wipe it out, and make sure it didn't flake off to other parts of her body.

ESTELLE: They took away the box that was going only to my liver, and began to give me intravenous injections that went through my whole body. It made me very, very sick. I used to go for treatments on Monday, and every week it was hell. I would start to throw up every fifteen minutes after we got home. They gave me sleeping pills to help me get home, but sometimes if we were late and got caught in the traffic, I'd begin to do it in the car.

My friend Anne, who's a registered nurse, would come over every Monday night to help me because I would throw up so severely. I had times when I was spitting blood and sometimes the medicine was so strong my mind would kind of—I don't know—hallucinate. I could tell when it started going through my head because I'd begin to shake all over, and I'd have this stare, this funny look in my eyes. Anne would know, she could see it, and I'd be saying, "I feel like my mind is going." I really had to fight in order to hold on. I would just stare at one little flower on the wall, just concentrate on it so this wouldn't get me. After a while, they cut the chemo in half so it wouldn't be so hard on me.

Tony was wonderful. While Anne was in with me, he took care of the children. Before dinner he'd walk into the dining room with a towel and play chef to them like it was a fancy restaurant.

TONY: *(Interrupts)* You had to do something for them. When we came home on Monday, Estelle would go right to bed and start throwing up. It tore my heart out to see her suffering so much and not be able to do anything about it. The kids would hear it, too—a really frightening sound. At the time, they didn't know she had cancer—so I'd say, "Mommy doesn't feel good. She took some medicine, and it makes her sick, but it's going to make her better soon."

For dinner, I'd set the table for them with napkins, some flowers, and write out a little menu. Then I'd ask them if they wanted cocktails, and I'd fill a martini glass with grape and orange juice, or something like that, while I had a real martini with them. Then I'd say, "Sir, would you like another?" and we'd have a second round. They'd get a big kick out of it. There'd be one thing on the menu, hamburgers or something, and they'd say, "We want hamburgers!" Then I'd let them go downstairs to watch TV until it was time for bed.

After they were in bed, I'd go downstairs while Anne was still with my wife. I'd lay on the couch to get some sleep until four or five o'clock when Anne would go home. Then I'd take over until I had to go to work.

ESTELLE: Sometimes it would continue into Tuesday. I'd have heaving spasms and visions like some drug addict—you know what it was for? For a giant root beer ice cream soda! *(Laughs.)* Anne would return in the morning and give me a little ginger ale. She'd say, "That's all, just sip it." I was dying, I was parched, my tongue was hanging out. I felt I was in a desert. She'd also give me little chips of ice that I thought were the most wonderful things in the world.

By Wednesday, I would be all right again, a little weak, but able to take care of the house—also I was a den mother for some Cub Scouts. The rest of the week would go fine until Sunday evening when I knew I had to go in the next day for another round of chemo. In the winter, I'd pray for snow, so it'd be impossible to drive into town. A couple of times it really did snow. Anne would peek out her window and say, "Oh no, she did it again. God made it snow 'cause Estelle was praying for another reprieve."

Then, going in on Monday morning—Tony got his days off switched to Sunday and Monday—I'd start to salivate. I could smell it and taste it even before I got there, like those cheap hair sprays they used in the beauty school where I worked for years. You'd breathe it all day, then at night. Even on weekends, you could taste it in your mouth.

"The doctors told me, 'The more sick you get, the better it's working.' But it didn't work that way for a lot of people. There was a little group of us who used to sit and talk before we went in for blood tests, before we got the chemo. Some of them weren't doing so well. Their depression was so great because no matter how much treatment they were getting, they had this feeling that they were not going to get better. So I'd tell them to have faith, to hold on. I'd say, 'Someday we'll say hello and talk about our grandchildren.' I used to try and kid around with them like that, to maybe help a little.

"Then maybe you'd come in one day and see one or two of them turning yellow, and the next time they are no longer there. You know what's happened to them, and it's so tremendous for the others who are left, so overwhelming. . . ." (Breaks up.) *"Let me get control. . . . It's like a kind of family, you know. You go in there together, and you get to know each other, you grow to love them almost. . . ."* (Breaks again.) *"You see, I knew I would. I knew this would happen when I got to this part."* (Tony gestures for her to skip it, but she shakes her head.) *"No, this is the most important part. This is where it begins to happen, when you know whether you are going to live or die. Your doctor doesn't tell you. You learn it there, from*

them. You can see it in their eyes, the way they look at you, wondering why you're making it and they are not—why are they going to die?

"After a while, you have to psych yourself up to walk in there because it's really—this is just plain old corny—but it's like you're living in hell. You see them turning yellow, then disappearing, and it's like you're living in two worlds. This one, where people are in hell, is the real one. The other one, your family, your children out there on the Island with those little trees, it's a fantasy, far away, not real.

"Then you know that you're becoming like them, going their way, and you have to fight it off. You have to hold on and not let it get you, not get lost. It's hard because you can't help but feel close to them, to the others with you. I've never said this before, but you even begin to feel especially close to those who are disfigured, the ones with a leg or arm off, and there was one man with a side of his face gone. I'd look into his eyes, they were soft blue like the sky, and I know this sounds impossible, but I felt he was happy. You see their horror, but you also see they are being helped, and you see these moments of happiness. It's incredible how much you can lose, how disfigured you can become but still laugh, still hold onto life. Look at that Kennedy boy. He skis, he's become a lawyer. So you begin to cope because you know there are worse things in life than losing an arm or a leg. That's how it seemed when I'd get depressed and sometimes when I'd think maybe I wouldn't see any green this spring. Then I'd say, "Oh yes, I will." And I'd be so happy to see the birds, even the slightest little bug. You look at it, and you feel its life, its tiny little life, and you feel happy for it, too, that you haven't killed it. . . ." (Breaks up again.)

TONY: *(Interrupts)* So that's how it was. They started stretching her treatments out to every two weeks, then once a month. Actually, she was on chemotherapy for about three years, and now she's been off it for about seven years. They say she's cured. That's pretty much the way it went.

ESTELLE: There were others who made it, too. Kathleen, a beautiful black girl, had eighty percent of her liver cut away, and she's doing fine. We used to joke a lot, and we thought this laughing and feeling good for each other might delay the medicine making us sick. There was also Helen, a young girl from Florida who had a large part of her liver cut away. I just got a letter from her with a photo where she's wearing a bikini. She looks great, and she has daisies painted over her belly scars. *(Laughs.)* She says it drives the boys crazy. They all want to come and pick flowers in her garden. *(Laughs.)* My hairdresser says he'll do it for me, paint some daisies over my scars, but Tony's too jealous.

TONY: *(Interrupts)* No way! For that, it's got to be me—or nobody! *(Both laugh.)*

I loved running. It was my whole life, you know. I'd go to school, go to work, but track was everything. I ran the hundred yards and cross-country, and I always used to place second or third. I was only 17, and the coach was counting on me. So when they told me I might never run again, man, I just didn't want to live no more.

He's 21, a light-hued black with a handsome, sensitive face, a close-cropped Afro, the soft, brown, trusting eyes of a child, and the lean body of a runner. He wears tight blue jeans and, at first glance, the only way to distinguish the artificial leg is the larger instep of the right running shoe.

We are in his bedroom in the Brown family apartment in Brooklyn. The room is decorated with bright posters of a leopard, a dragon, a blue pirate ship, and an orange-blue Superman. Records and disco equipment are stashed to one side. "Yeah, I play the clubs around Brooklyn," he says, explaining he also works as a TV attendant at the Brooklyn Jewish Hospital, and is a liberal arts major at Brooklyn College. "They got me running, man, even the way I am now." Slaps hand and shakes head as though still amazed at what happened.

First, I had this bike accident in June when I hit a car at the front. It bruised my knee and sent me spinning up into the air, but somehow I came down on my feet next to the curb. I guess the trauma and everything, you know, the force inflicted on my knee, was the beginning of it—how the cancer started to move.

So the ambulance came, and I went off to the emergency ward. There I met a lawyer who wanted to take the man's insurance company to court so I can get some money for the injury. I was in the right, you know, because I had the light, and he was edging out before the light changed. This lawyer, he set me up to go to a medical center, and the doctor there said I had water on the knee. He went to inject a needle in me to draw out the water, and he drew blood. So he used a heat lamp on it to try and dissolve the water. But that didn't work, either, and I went home. So then I received a letter from this lawyer, saying they'd paid for the medical expenses—but whether the case was won or lost, I don't know.

The next week, I went roller skating and banged my knee against an iron pole, in the same spot. The pain was so terrific, you know, it felt like my leg is gonna saw off right in front of me. I was talking to a couple of friends and told them I can't hang out no more. I had to go home because my knee was bothering me so bad.

I laid off it a week, and the pain went away. So I went to practicing on the leg that was hurt—running in high school track. The pain stayed away for two weeks, and I went roller skating again, but my friend, by accident, he kicked me in the same spot. This time the pain was so real I almost passed out. I must have skated only two times around the ring and couldn't make it no more, so I went home.

I had the pain for about four days, and then it was graduation day. It hurt every time I walked, but I went anyway. I was doing well there, my work was beautiful. Nothing went wrong in high school, I was so innocent. I wanted to go to college out of state, to study law and run track.

After graduation was over, I brought back my gown and hat since they expected them all back. Then I went to the track coach to get my trophies, but I couldn't wait around no more, the pain was downing me so much.

"The pain didn't leave me, so I told my mother to take me to Brooklyn Jewish Hospital. I didn't want to go; I was scared of hospitals, except at Brooklyn Jewish I had friends since I was working there as a TV attendant, you know, putting sets in rooms for the patients.

"They gave me a whole series of tests, and they told me to perform a couple of exercises. I performed them well, and they just can't see what's wrong with me. Then they saw like a spot in my knee above the tibia area and didn't know what it was. The bone doctor came over and said they would have to do a biopsy on me. Right then, you know, I started to shake and get scared a little bit.

"I went down to surgery and had a biopsy done, and then I must have waited around a week before the results came in. The results were . . ." (Pauses, unable to say it.) *"I couldn't bear the results, man. When he told me there was a malignant tumor, I couldn't believe I had cancer. When I knew that, how I might never run again, man, I just wanted to die. I just didn't care no more. Life was gone for me.*

"My doctor knew I was taking it rather hard, and he told me he was going to get me the best care, so I would have to go to Memorial Hospital. I asked him, 'You think that can fix me so that I can run again?' And he said he didn't know but Memorial was the best, and the big bone man there was Dr. Lane.* I asked, 'Can I have one day off to see my family before I go there?'—and he gave me two days to see my family and my girlfriend."

---

* Joseph M. Lane, M.D., attending surgeon, chief, Orthopedic Service, Department of Surgery, Memorial Hospital.

When I got to Memorial, I had butterflies, and I was scared. I never was sick. I went seventeen years without sickness or a stay in a hospital, and for something severe like this to occur, you know, just shocked me.

Then I met Dr. Lane, and he lifted my spirits; he was beautiful to me. He showed me the real meaning to life, how I had to stick with this, and how I can get over it. He told me, "You did very well. I don't know how you decided to come to this hospital, but you've caught it at the right stage." From the way he came across to me, it gave me so much faith that I said, "I can handle whatever it takes. Whatever comes, I can handle it."

Okay, so I got settled into the hospital, and that week I went through a whole series of tests. When it was over, Dr. Lane came in and said I got osteogenic sarcoma—cancer of the bone.† I asked if maybe I could have a bone replacement so I wouldn't lose my leg, and he said he'd do what was possible.‡ But first I had to do a chemotherapy treatment to shrink the size of the tumor. When it was over, he would see what was possible for me.

"Anita was the chemotherapist, and she was telling me that I'm going to be in for the roughest year of my life because the medication is very powerful and will do things to me I wouldn't normally expect. She told me I would lose my hair, I would get nauseated a lot, and there would be periods where I won't do what the doctors say. I would mentally start to crack, and say, 'I've had it, I'm not taking any more treatment.' She was talking like that as a friend, getting me ready for it, but when she told me this, you know, I was scared.*

"My girlfriend came over to visit me a couple of times, and right then me and my girlfriend broke up because she couldn't go through what I was experiencing. She couldn't handle it, and on top of that, she had other problems. So I lost my girlfriend when I needed her most, right when I was going through a really rough time. But I had so many other friends from where I worked at the Jewish Hospital who treated me with the utmost

---

† The use of -oma at the end of a medical term means "tumor" while the rest of the word refers to the kind of tissue in which it is growing: sarcoma, tumor of the connective tissue, bone, cartilage, or muscle; carcinoma, tumor of the epithelial tissue (tissue that lines body cavities); lymphoma, tumor of the lymph cells; and so on.

‡ With increasing frequency, surgeons are able to substitute diseased portions of bones or joints with prosthesis replacements made of metal or synthetic materials.

* Anita Nirenberg, R.N., administered drugs as instructed by Gerald Rosen, M.D., associate chairman, Solid Tumors, Department of Pediatrics, Memorial Hospital.

respect. They gave me gifts to keep me happy, and many people prayed for me and my family."

Anita, she set me up for the first treatment, and I was worried about my hair. I said, "Once that goes, man, I don't know. I'm gonna lose something inside. I'm not gonna be the same no more." *(Laughs.)* So be it, and that first injection started to do just that after about four days. When I saw my hair falling out, man, I just about passed out because I was really shocked. I was telling my sister, "Braid my hair for the last time, braid it up real good." *(Shakes head sadly.)* She braided it up, man, and then everything just fell out, and I said, "Oh no!"

This was just the beginning. It shocked me, and my mind was really confused because there was gonna be twenty-two of these treatments. So Anita, she had a group of patients come to talk to me. One patient, I think his name was Jimmy, had been going there for two years and was on his last treatment. He told me, "James, in the beginning, it's real tough. Martin Luther King said he climbed to the mountaintops, and it's like that, climbing to the mountaintops, when you're fighting cancer. You're gonna have your ups and downs, and moments when you're gonna call it quits." Then he said, "You gotta stick it out, man, because there's only one ball game here, and it's your own life. You got no choice. You gotta play to win if you want to stay on this earth."

Talking that way, he really got deep into me, you know, he scared me. But then I thought about what Dr. Lane told me, and I said, "I can handle this; I can take these treatments without a hassle." I didn't know what it was gonna be like, I mean how hard it would be.

Every Tuesday morning, I went to get the treatments. I would have my blood exam, then get the weight done, and after that I'd join a long line with other patients waiting to be hooked on the medicine. I would be there all day. They won't let you go until your urine is clear, because after the medicine is flowing through your body, it's like killing everything in your body, it's like making it weep. A lot of patients don't go to sleep when they've taken this medicine, but I'd get sleepy, and they'd say, "Look at you. That's good, that's beautiful, you're sleeping through it."

I was so weak when I left the hospital, I'd be throwing up sometimes coming through the front door, throwing up a long trail to the cab. When I got home, I liked shuttin' myself off, you know, from the family and everything. I'd turn to this room and close the door. It used to be me and my mother, and she'd come through every four hours to give me the pills, except I had a lot of complications from the medicine. It affected me psychologically, you know, in the mind. That's why, just like they warned me, it got so I couldn't take no more.

My mother would come to give me the pills, and in the beginning, she watched me take them. Then, when she saw it going right, she didn't wait around no more, especially at midnight. *(Laughs.)* You see that loud-speaker over there? It's got a hole in it, so I'd throw them in there. Or I had this basin, because I was spitting up mucous, and I'd throw them in there to dissolve. But I wasn't slick about it, because she caught me at it. *(Laughs.)* She got really upset, "James, why aren't you taking these pills? These are for your own good." I told her, "You're not goin' through what I'm goin' through, and I can't take no more." She said, "You want to die?" —and right there, she got me thinking I don't want to die.

I knew I had to stop faking it, and I said, "If I'm gonna beat this, I have to think stronger." So I got it in my mind that I'm almost finished. I wasn't even halfway through, but each time I took the pills, I said, "I'm near the end," and didn't think about all the other treatments to come. That's how I managed it, but if my mother hadn't stuck with me, I don't think I would have made it. The main thing is to have loving people beside you that cares, because if you don't have that, man, there's no way you can make it.

"I was asking if there was anything to help me cope with this pain and one patient, who seemed to be making it all right, said, 'Have you ever tried marijuana?' I never smoked, but I told my mother that I had to try this to relieve the pain, so I tried it, at home, and it helped a lot. I met up with all the patients on the seventeenth floor where they have the chemotherapy. A lot of swell people, man, and they were also smoking on their own, to help them cope with it, to get off the pain. While I was smoking, I took the treatment like a flash. It eliminated any problem with two of the big medi-cines, but there was one of them the marijuana didn't have no effect on— vincristine."

I was on my eighth treatment, and Anita said, "It's time for your surgery, we'll finish the rest of the treatments later." It was the first week in December, and I was talking to myself, saying, "Man, this is the final moment. You have three nights—three nights of your last days on earth!" There was this other girl, a nurse helper, I met at the hospital. She's Patricia Brown, just 20 years old, and we used to call each other Mr. and Mrs. Brown. *(Sighs, shakes head.)* I got very fond of this girl. Then during those last three days she came to me, you know, and she stayed with me. She was the most beautiful person I've ever seen.

On the night before surgery, Dr. Lane came into my room to tell me the results of the final tests. He said the chemo had shrunk the tumor so small you could hardly see it. I said, "If it's that small, is surgery necessary?" He said, "Yes, we still have to cut it out, otherwise the little spot will grow back again." I said, "Ah! I thought I had a chance there."

I was still hoping to have a bone replacement, not an amputation, but he said the tests showed the tumor was all around a main nerve in the leg. If they had to sever that while taking out the tumor, my leg would be paralyzed, you know, and I'd be dragging it around for the rest of my life. Right there, everything I hoped for, the whole idea of a bone replacement, was dwindling away slowly.

So he gave me the options. If I insisted, he was gonna try for bone replacement, even though there was not much chance for it to work. He said I'd have to wear a brace for a long time, I'd be in the hospital a lot more, and there'd be more pain. The way he was explaining it, my best option was the amputation. I asked, "Where would you do it?" He showed me here (points to midthigh), and my heart was breaking because I never thought it'd be so high up. I said, "But the cancer is right near the knee," and he explained, "You have to cut out more than what is being seen, just in case it might come back again."

I thought about these possibilities, and I told him I wanted the amputation. Dr. Lane stayed with me in my room for about an hour, talking to me, keeping my spirits up. He said, "You know what I want you to do? Become president of the Chase Manhattan Bank, and all the money you make, I want you to donate it to the cancer works here." I said, "Sure, man, you got a deal." (Laughs.) If it hadn't been for him, I would never have made it that night. Dr. Lane is the most beautiful man, person I've ever met. Also before this, in the morning, he'd sent me Dr. Sculco, who was going to do the operation.† He is a very nice doctor, just like Dr. Lane, where the patient comes first all the time.

My life was different before I experienced all this. I had never met so many wonderful people before. They give you so much confidence, you just know they're gonna do you right. So when Dr. Lane said Dr. Sculco would fix me up real good, I said, "Wow! He's gonna fix me up!" I'm on cloud nine, you know, and that's the attitude I walked in, from there on.

The anesthesiologist, she came, and I had a whole room full of guests. She said, "Are you James Brown?" I said, "Yes, ma'am." She said, "How're you doin', baby?" She comes out like this, you know, and I say, "Oh wow! What've you been doin' these past months in the hospital?" Actually, she's a wonderful woman, and she told me various things to expect, and she asked me if I had any long illnesses or did I smoke or

---

† Thomas P. Sculco, M.D., assistant attending surgeon, Orthopedic Service, Department of Surgery, Memorial Hospital.

anything. I told her everything is fine, I haven't been smoking, and I'm ready to go through the anesthesia with no problems.

So after she left, a male nurse came. "Are you Mr. Brown?" I said, "Yes." He said, "I'm here to shave your leg." I said, "Okay, man, come on and do the job." So like me and him, we started talking. He was a young guy like me, going to college, and he said, "How did all this occur?" I told him I used to run track and was heavy into it. He said, "That's a very sad story, brother. For this to happen to you makes me very sad." He'd been shaving my leg, just breezing along, but then he started shaving it real slow, taking extra care like he didn't want to hurt it no more, giving it all respect like it was gonna stay with me. I was feeling him caring so much for me. Like I said, it's having the caring and loving around you that helps you make it.

In the morning, the nurse came by to give me the injection to make me drowsy. I said, "Come on, baby, let's get the show on the road!" I turned around and—wham!—she stuck it into me. I was in a happy mood that day, saying "Come on, let's get it over with." It was like a sensation going through my body. I'm awaiting the call, you know, to come down to surgery and have it done.

I'm looking down the hall, waiting for the guy with the stretcher to come along. He must have come around nine o'clock, after I had the injection. My ma, my sister, my grandmother, my cousins from Queens was all there. My grandmother, she gets on this tremendous crying spree, and I couldn't stand for anybody to start crying around me. I said, "If you're gonna cry, you better go because I'm in good spirits, and if I see you crying, I'm gonna feel the same way, you know. I want you to have the same strength that I have under me. I'm going into surgery, and my mind's at ease at this moment, and I want your mind at ease."

Finally the attendant that rolled the stretcher came to get me. He would usually bring the stretcher to just beside the bed, and you would slip right onto it. What I did, I hopped out of bed onto the stretcher and said, "Come on, man, let's get the engines going, let's get on down to the operation room." So I hopped on there, and I was upside down, you know, looking back at my family as I was going down the hall. I looked at them, all bunched up like a photograph, and a sad feeling came over me . . . *(pauses)* but I had to keep it in, I didn't want them to notice.

I had this feeling that I won't be seeing my leg no more, and I was talking to my leg, kind of meditating to myself. I said, "Well, old buddy, you came into the world with me *(pauses)*, and you won't be around that much longer. It's going to be kind of hard *(pauses)* to get over the loss of you, you know. You've been with me for seventeen years, you've brought me my desire, my hopes, my dreams but things happen for a purpose—it's a thing we have to accept."

"On my way down to the operation room, I said a last good-bye to my family—my cousin who's a kind of jittery guy. He makes sure like nothing, nobody does things to me. He says, 'James, do you want me to come into the operation room with you?' I said, 'No, man, stay here and wait till I come out.' " (Laughs.) *"As we rolled onto the elevator, there's people in there, and he says, 'Would you mind to move aside, my cousin's comin' in.' He's like one riding his Cadillac. 'I want you all to get out of the way, just make room.' He had me laughing, you know, as I was approaching the operation, and I said good-bye."*

They rolled me into a waiting room place next to the operation rooms, and I was waiting there, alongside an older patient and he had a few words, like "You goin' in now?" I was drowsy, man, and the world's gettin' ready to leave me at that point. He said, "What're you goin' in for?" I said, "I'm goin' in for the amputation." He said, "Yeah," and I said, "What're you goin' in for?" He said, "I'm goin' in for the same thing." He looked around 60 or in his late fifties.

Then they came to wheel me into the operation room, and I was looking around with amazement. I was shocked, and I said, "Wow, are they gonna use all this stuff on me?" Nobody was in the room yet except the sisters, who were setting everything up.‡ I said, "Where's the chisel, where's the saw, the electric blender and all the rest?" *(Laughs.)*

They transferred me from the stretcher onto the table. Then, who walks in but the same anesthesiologist, and she says, "So we meet again. How you doin', babe?" I'm all happy and everything, getting ready to fold up, and I said, "Oh yeah, go on, do your trick on me, put me on a cloud." She had this needle, and I felt it. "Ah! That's very good. I'm glad . . . I'm glad it's happening to me." So right then, I floated off, and I didn't see the doctors or surgeons come in because I was real gone.*

The next time I woke up, I was in the recovery room with some nurse bending over me, and I was very sleepy. Then I woke up again in my room, just one eye opening up, and who was standing there but my girl-friend, Patricia. She's from the islands, from Puerto Rico, and has the

---

‡ They were operating room nurses, a highly specialized and exacting part of the nursing profession. See Pat Mazzola, p. 547.

* Dr. Lane was there at that moment. Memorial policy requires the attending surgeon to be on hand when the patient is put to sleep.

most beautiful smile and face. She gave me a kiss and then I looked down and didn't see my leg, just the flat bed cover, and I said, "Well, I guess they did it."

I was falling asleep but Patricia was kissing me again, and I felt wet from her tears. That woke me up real fast, and I said, "What's the matter?" "Nothing," she said, and I said, "So why you crying?" "I love you," she said, "I never loved anybody like this before." I tell you, man . . . *(Pauses.)* It was so beautiful. She really cared about me.

"After a couple weeks, Dr. Lane sent a rehabilitation team to help me learn how to walk with a prosthesis, you know, the artificial leg. They were two instructors from Rusk Institute, and they said, 'We're going to start you walking now so you'll know how to use your prosthesis when it's ready.' They had a pipe-shaped leg with a foot on it, and they hooked it onto the cast around my stump. I practiced walking on it an hour a day—slowly, gradually pressing my foot on the ground. It had a device on it, so if I applied too much weight, a beep sound would spring out. I was making a lot of mistakes at first, but after a couple weeks I was doing fine."

Then Dr. Lane sent me home from the hospital, so for a few weeks I had to go to Rusk for the final fitting of the prosthesis and to learn how to walk up ramps and other obstacles. I was still getting around on crutches, so my girlfriend Patricia would come by every morning to take me into town, on her way to school.

She'd left Memorial to go to a Catholic college in Yonkers, and me and her were very close, as close as two people can get. I wanted her as my personal girl, and she stuck with it. No matter what happened, if we had a problem or a quarrel or if everything seemed real low, she would be the first one to call and make things up. That was so beautiful. She'd say, "Forget about it, honey, let's just start again. These days are bad times, and you can forget about our errors." I would say, "Wow!" But I was also thinking, "What's up with this girl? She keeps comin' back, treatin' me nice, no matter what." I was getting this complex about my missing leg, wondering what she was going to think when I got the prosthesis, you know, how we'd be able to make it, like when she wanted to go dancing or to the beach or things like that.

One day I had to take a paper to Rusk, and she had only one class, so we drove into town and then up to her school. There was this coffee shop and I'm going to wait there for her. I was moving on my crutches toward a table, and this couple went right by me and took the table. The guy, he's paying me no heed, like he don't know what he's done. But the girl she stands up, very upset, and tells him, "You took this table away from a cripple."

I thought, "Wow! Are they talking about me?" It was the first time anybody called me that, and it was a kind of jolt because I was thinking of myself as a man without a leg, not a cripple, because that sounds more like you're broken everywhere, not just in the leg.

Patricia, she comes back with some friends and wants to have a coffee but I want to go. So she goes for the car, and on the way home, we have this talk. I said, "Why are you treating me so nice?" She said, "Why shouldn't I?" So I said, "How come you like a man with no leg?" She says, "Because I love the man, the legs don't matter." I said, "How you know that?" She said, "What you feel, I feel—if you're not happy, I'm not happy. That's how I know." Then I said what was bothering me. "How do I know you're not treating me nice, and just staying with me 'cause you think I'm a charity case?"

She stared at me, I mean she looked at me real sad and said, "How could you say that?" She began to cry and said, "Everything was going so good, why did you come out and say such a hurting episode?" She was crying and sobbing like her heart was falling into pieces, and right away I felt her hurt, I felt her pain in me.

I apologized and said I was all mixed up, but after that it was never the same again. That night she called my mother, crying on the phone, and my mother said, "James, why are you driving this girl away?" I said I wasn't doing anything of the sort, and don't pay it no heed because it was nothing. But something had broke, and nothing could put it back together again. Even when we tried, it was not the same anymore. Then one day she went and enlisted in the Army Air Corps and went off to Alabama. I really loved that girl and I . . . *(Sighs, shakes head.)* I just drove her away worrying about that leg, for no reason at all.

When I got the new leg, the prosthesis, I started walking straight like everyone else, and I also started to get straightened out in the head. I was doing the last part of my chemotherapy when I came in—I mean, I just walked in there, man, with my new prosthesis. Anita and my friends on the seventeenth floor, they were cheering and applauding like this was some kind of hero. Right there, I felt better, and then Anita, she had me as a spokesman for some new patients with problems. I felt kind of shy, but also rather good that they could rely on me to talk to other patients.

I thought back to the first time that patient had talked to me and set me straight. So I approached it the same way, but I came out rather softly, you know. One of them was this 9-year-old boy who was giving his mother a hard time about taking the pills. So I came around and said, "Man, what's happening? Why don't you come on and take the pills?" He was stubborn, man, really stubborn for a 9-year-old boy. So I pressured him. "Come on, man, you know you can do it. If I can do it, you can do it." I was trying my damnedest, looking at him and looking back at myself when I first began, and I wondered, "Where does a 9-year-old get all this strength to say no?" I thought about how desperate I was once and how much terror must be inside his little heart, and I pleaded with him. "Please take the pills, man, don't put all this aggravation on your mother." But nothing worked, I couldn't reach him, so they forced the pills down him.

I stayed around until it was over, and I said, "You didn't have to go through this, you could have just downed the pills, and you can even have them crushed to make it easy." Then I said, "What would you rather have? The doctor wants you to tell me." So he told me he'd rather have them crushed, and at home because it was more painful away from home. A couple of treatments later, he started to really get the hang of it, and we became friends. His name was Eddie. I asked him, "You ride skateboards?" He said, "Yeah." He was sitting on my bed, thinking about a bone replacement because if he could get that, he could ride skateboards again.

So I told him, "There might be a possibility you will lose your leg." He looked at me with a kind of sad look, but then I demonstrated to him how I walked with my prosthesis, and I told him how I could ride bikes again. I was trying to get his mind on a clear basis, to not get mixed up like I was. I wanted him to know that if he lost his leg, he could function normally again. So I told him, "When you finish everything, you're gonna be out there riding skateboards, riding bikes, and everything." Then I said, "Stay cool, don't give your mother a hard time with the treatments, and I'll be seeing you every day."

The next thing you know, he is hugging me like I was his big brother or daddy, saying *(pause)* if me and him hang out together like I promised, he was going to surprise everybody and get well real fast. Then he said, "When I get well, if you need something, I'll go on my bike and get it for you." *(Breaks up, unable to continue.)* This is very touching to me.

You see, he was believing me, and right there me and him was like one person almost, so close. I was going along without my girl, with nobody real close. Then, before I know what's happening, this little boy is with me. It's like you can't go very far, all alone by yourself, without caring for somebody else, you know—like it's more natural to care for each other than anything else, especially the handicaps.

I never used to pay no mind to handicaps or anything. But now, I'm one

of those people, one of those individuals, I'm a statistic. Only there's
millions of us out there, living inside that statistic, you know, walking
without legs, making it without arms. I look at those people . . . *(pause)*
I just feel for those people because, like we got parts of us that's missing,
but what's left is more one piece, more concentrated in caring and loving.
So we're like everyone else, you know, only more so because of this.

I'm married almost forty years, and the first time I ever saw my wife really break down was when they told me I had cancer. She said something like "I don't want to live without you." I said, "Now, Grace, you don't mean that." She said, "Yes, I do. My life would be nothing without you." I was overcome, and I put my arms around her, and I said, "You know, honey, in the Navy I faced danger many times and came back, you've always seen me come back, right?" She nodded, and I said, "So I'll come back this time. You get your pretty little self down to the dock, and you'll see me coming in again." I guess we sort of held onto each other, and then she said, "All right, John, I'll be there waiting for you. I'll get myself all pretty, just for you, and it'll be like always, when you come back." And that's how we attacked this, right through to the end.

He's a big man, over six feet tall, weighing 190 pounds. "I work out three times a week and try to watch my weight. You have to in this job." He's dean of the College of Business Administration at St. John's University in Jamaica, Queens—one of the three largest collegiate business schools in the New York area. A Navy veteran from World War II and the Vietnam War, he is now a captain in the Supply Corps of the Naval Reserve. Occasionally, the salty phrases of a sailor resound on the polished desk of the business dean.

Seven years ago, I started to experience difficulty in voiding, which is the medical expression for urinating. I figured it was to be expected at my age, but gradually it increased. Then one day I was driving north from a business conference in Hollywood, Florida. I remember I had to stop every hour or so to get out of the damn car and go to the side of the road. Besides that, it was becoming painful.

As soon as I got home, I went to our family doctor, who is also a personal friend. He said, "I'm going to send you to a urologist who's young but very expert. Most physicians consider him the best in Queens."

"I'm not one to neglect my health. I was already getting the best in medical checkups—one a year from my doctor, plus a second one from the Navy, as a senior officer in the naval reserve. Each one included a digital examination of the prostate.

"Let me say this right now to anybody, any male of middle age: 'For God's sake, if you belly up to the urinal, and you have trouble taking a pee, get your ass over to the doctor and have your prostate checked out. Even if you don't have trouble, even if you think you're all right, but you're over 40,

*go anyway for a checkup at least once a year.' That's because prostate cancer, when it starts, often produces no symptoms, no urinary difficulties or warnings. But in the digital exam, the doctor probes through the rectum with a gloved finger, and most often he can feel hard lumps or growths that indicate possible cancer. If it's caught in time, you should have no trouble. If not, it can spread and get out of control. It's very common, and every male faces it, as women do breast cancer."**

The urologist, Dr. Lowell Kane, examined me and found no hard lumps. But the gland was swollen, and he concluded that a transurethral resection was necessary. A TUR, as it's called, is relatively simple and can be done without making incisions into the body. Also, it's done under a spinal or general anesthesia, so it's painless. A special instrument, a resectoscope, is inserted through the penis up to the prostate gland. You can see through it and manipulate an electrically charged wire loop to cut away the obstructing tissue growth, which then flows back out through the same instrument. It's really remarkable, and the best damn thing ever for the male prostate.

They did it for me at Hillcrest Hospital. I was out of bed in a couple of days and planning to go home, when one afternoon Dr. Kane came into my room. Grace, my wife, was there with me. She's a registered nurse—retired now, but she still holds her license as an R.N. Dr. Kane said, "I'd like to see you both outside." I was in a semiprivate room, since it was only minor surgery, so I assumed it was just a matter of being alone. But in the corridor, I saw the strain on his face, and then he gave me the bad news. "I have to tell you," he said, "that the results of the pathology of your excised tissues indicate there are cancer cells in your prostate." *(Pauses.)*

I'm stunned and so is my wife, but he tries to relieve us by saying my chances for recovery are very good. "When you catch this at an early stage," he says, "the survival rate is very high." I ask him my alternatives,

---

* Close to one half of all men past 50 develop some swelling (hypertrophy) of the prostate gland, located below the bladder and surrounding the urethra, the tube that carries urine from the bladder to the penis. This can result in urination difficulties—frequent and urgent need to urinate, difficulty in starting, slowing of stream, dribbling, and incomplete voiding of bladder which can result in bladder infection. About 10 percent of all men prior to 80 require surgical help. The swelling is usually benign but must be closely watched, since early prostate cancer can develop without warning. As a result, only 10 percent of these cancers are discovered before spreading—lessening chances for a cure. It accounts for 18 percent of all forms of cancer in the American male, exceeded only by lung cancer, at 22 percent. Thus, from the age of 35, every man should have an annual digital rectal examination.

and he says, "There's only one surgeon in this city that I would recommend—Dr. Willet Whitmore at Memorial Hospital.† I wouldn't bother with anyone else."

I asked how much cutting they would have to do if the prostate had to be removed, or whatever. He said that would depend entirely on what Dr. Whitmore determined. He actually meant just that, but we assumed he might be shielding us from further bad news. He's a very decent man, Dr. Kane. I was taking it stoically, but my wife was in shock, and he put his arm around her and told her not to worry because the odds were in my favor. She held on like a real pro, but after he left she began to cry.

"Being in a position with some business and university contacts, I then proceeded to find out how soon Dr. Whitmore could take me, only to learn there was a long list, an international list, and I'd have to wait several months.

"At that point, my closest and dearest friend, Milton Felson, insisted I get another opinion while waiting to see Whitmore. So I went to the chief urologist of a major hospital in New York. The name of this hospital and this doctor, I do not care to divulge. He was old enough to remember my father, Dr. Alexander J. Alexion, who was a prominent New York urologist.

"This elderly doctor proceeded to lay a bomb on me. The only procedure he would consider was surgical castration and a radical removal of the prostate, to get rid of any male hormones that might stimulate further cancer growth. I thought, 'Jesus, that's why Dr. Kane wouldn't talk about it and bucked it over to Whitmore. They're going to turn me into a six-foot eunuch.' " (Laughs bitterly.)

I called our family doctor to ask him about it, and he came over to the house. He's Dr. Walter Kaufman, a most unusual character. He's a Jew who escaped with his family from Hitler's Germany—a tremendous guy. We were among his first patients in Queens and became close personal friends. I asked him if he thought radical surgery, including castration, was going to be necessary. He said he didn't think so because this was usually done only in extreme cases, and I was still in an early stage. Then he said, very casually but matter-of-factly, "John, I know you pretty well after all these years. Let me tell you something. If they discover the cancer has spread throughout your body, don't let them cut you up. Just let it go at that."

That startled me because I hadn't really thought of it spreading any-

---

† Willet F. Whitmore, Jr., M.D., attending surgeon, chief of Urology Service, Department of Surgery, Memorial Hospital.

where beyond the prostate. Except for the urinating problem, I felt in great shape. I asked him, "You think it might have spread?" He said he didn't think so. There were no signs of it, anyway. So I said, "Then why did you say what you did? Is there a chance it's spread, and we don't know it?" He said something like, "You never know everything about this disease. That's the problem always. You never can tell. But if you get ready for all possibilities, you're in better shape for whatever happens."

"So that's where it was. One doctor said he would castrate me, and the other said I should consider the possibility of having disseminated cancer with no hope of recovery, but Grace would have none of it. She kept talking about our date on the dock, how I'd promised to come back to her and how she was going to be there waiting for me." (Smiles.) *"Looking back now, I realize that date with her was the best thing I had. It kept me on course through those dark days. She was not about to lose any part of me. That counted a lot, but I also believe I had God's help through prayer with my family, my friends, and the Vincentian priests at St. John's."*

Then Dr. Whitmore had good news. After a series of tests in the hospital, he said he did not believe that the radical procedure of castration and prostate removal was indicated for me—which only shows how you can get yourself mutilated for nothing if you don't get to the right doctor.

He has a very pleasant manner, and he's also very sympathetic and reassuring. He said, "Apparently you are in the early stages of this, and you should know it is very common to the middle-aged and elderly male." Also, the probabilities of getting cancer of the prostate increases with the age, so that a male of 50 years has about a 20 percent chance of having it, a male at 70 about 40 percent, and so on.

He also pointed out that many males with cancer of the prostate don't die of it for two reasons: It's often slow-growing, and other causes of death may prevail in men past fifty years of age.

So that was it, and he gave me a crapshooter's choice of alternatives. I could leave it alone and take the chance that it would remain relatively localized for the rest of my natural life. I could also submit myself to some form of radiation. Or I could undergo a special procedure for people in the early stages of the disease. It's called the I-125, which I later learned was developed by Whitmore and his associates. Radioactive iodine enclosed in small titanium capsules is inserted into the prostate, where they usually destroy the cancer cells. At the same time, it does not destroy or impair the delicate mechanism of a man's erection, nor limit his ability to ejaculate.

I asked Dr. Whitmore his opinion on what was best for me, and he said,

"The procedure is still new and experimental, but judging from our limited experience, the preliminary results appear favorable with patients in your particular condition. Also, you're relatively youthful, in good physical shape, so I think you should have no trouble." I asked if he thought the cancer might have spread, and he said, "We see no evidence of that." I didn't particularly relish the possibility of having to wear a bag for urine, and I asked him, "What if it's gone to my bladder?" He smiled and shook his head to reassure me. "The odds are in your favor. I'd bet on you." I said, "That's funny, Doc, I was betting on you." *(Laughs.)*

After Dr. Whitmore left, I remembered my doctor warning me not to let them cut me up if the cancer had spread. Of course, a lot depended on how much cutting and what your life would be like afterwards. Jesus Christ, look at what happened to John Wayne, that poor son of a bitch. They took this out, that out, until they finally took out his whole stomach. I'm only saying that at some point you have to make a decision on whether the quality of life is worth staying alive. I already knew about that from my own family.

"My dad, as I mentioned before, was a very fine physician in his day. He married late in life, when he was 45, so by the time I reached maturity, he didn't have long to go. Just the same, I avoided facing this, the loss of my father, until one day in 1944, when I came off active duty to see my parents. I was 28, so my dad was then 73. I went first to see my mom because I knew he was in his office, taking care of patients.

"My mother was very upset. She said, 'Your father has had a series of strokes. He recovers, but then it happens again. His colleagues have banded together. . . .' The doctors in those days were a very clubby lot and closed rank for one another. My mother explained, 'They prescribed the latest medication and diet for him, but he'll have none of it. Go and talk to him.'

"I went to see my father in his office. He was a very proud man, very austere, and I was shocked to find he had the wasting-away look that Franklin Roosevelt had in the end. With great delicacy, I began to reproach him for not taking his medicine, and he started to tell me to bug off. But then he relaxed and said, 'Let me put it this way, John. I've been a physician for most of my life, and I know what's wrong with me. I know exactly how much time is left. If I were to take this bland diet, take these medications and lose weight, I would prolong my life for eighteen months, give or take a month. But if I don't and I continue to live the way I am, I've only got about nine months to live.' Then he said, 'Now, I'll admit to you that perhaps I've given your mother some difficult times. . . .' This was true, and it was the only time in his life I heard him admit it. He had a very demanding personality, he wanted everything his way. Then he said, 'I've

reached the point in life where I really enjoy a pony of cognac at night, one cigar a day, and a fine gourmet meal. If I were to give up these things, my personality would definitely change, and during those additional nine months your mother would be living in some kind of hell because I'd be really upset over all of this.'

"He shook his head and said, 'It's not worth it, John. I'd rather accept only nine more months and live as I've always lived, knowing the inevitable is always there and accepting it, working every day, doing my job as a physician, and let it go at that."

"That's what happened up to the last day. It was on a Sunday. He went to church and came home. My brother was working in a Navy research lab in Washington, and I was off on Navy duty. Dad always liked to go to our rooms, the 'boys' rooms as he called them, to take an afternoon nap. He went up there after a nice Sunday dinner, laid down, and in his sleep he went off." (Pauses.)

I thought a lot about my father before they took me down to the operating room. If the cancer had spread and there was no chance for me, I'd be in the same boat that took him away. I knew I had to get ready, so that when the bos'n's pipe sounds up there for me, I'd set the sea anchor detail, and get the ship under way. Except there was no sign the cancer had spread— at least Whitmore didn't think so. That was the big difference between my father and myself.

I was in the operating room for about four hours. When I came out of the anesthesia in the recovery room, I felt relaxed and in fine shape, except I thought I was in San Juan, Puerto Rico. There's a hotel there with a roof garden restaurant that has little tree toads that make a musical peeping sound. Still half under the anesthesia and hearing the peep-peep of the heart monitors in the recovery room, I thought I was back in San Juan, on that roof garden, drinking a daiquiri with Grace. It's weird how easily you can lose a concept of time. Anyhow, I was transferred to my room, and when Dr. Whitmore came to see me, he said he'd won the bet. The cancer apparently hadn't spread to the bladder or anywhere else. That Whitmore is really a beautiful man.

Three months after I was discharged from the hospital, he wanted me back for a postop exam. I went into one of his rooms, and he started to examine me. After a bit, he began to frown and shake his head like something was wrong. Then he started to look at his earlier notes on my case. Apparently, cancer enlarges and hardens the prostate, even when it's been knocked out. Whitmore was astounded to find no residual swelling, no hardness, no nothing. The prostate had been reduced to totally normal.

He kept shaking his head, and he said, "This is hard to believe, this is terrific." In his opinion, it was largely due to my mental attitude of positive thinking. He said, "You know, John, I'm convinced that the mental attitude of the patient plays a large role in the recovery process and, in some cases, might even make the difference between life and death."

I said, "In this case, someone else also played a large role. She's a marvelous woman who believes in promises."

You're very vulnerable in this work—all of us. Sometimes it happens to the nurses, doctors, or other staff members, including us, the social workers. You spend your days getting to know someone. You are with them as they delve deeply into their lives. You learn about their hopes, their fears, their way of looking at the world. All the while, they are fighting for their lives, and there are moments of truth that bring you quite close.

We are still in the coffee shop at Memorial. Sister Rosemary—a social worker specializing in stress as experienced by members of the hospital staff, as well as patients and their families—previously described the inevitable risk of emotional involvement with the cancer patient.

She now turns to a higher form of human involvement: the interdependency of all the various disciplines of medicine and personal care as they are brought to bear on the patient. For her, this defines the true, inner reality of the hospital and its staff.

My religious and spiritual beliefs are the background of my life, but my social work training gives me my skills. For me, there is no dichotomy in this. What makes it hard is to be with someone you know who is in crisis. You try to help people deal with deep fear. And in the presence of such personal suffering, you can feel quite vulnerable.

It doesn't happen very often—in fact, very seldom. But it happens, and you can expect it to happen to anybody who works closely, caring for someone. I'll never forget a young man who had leukemia—Peter. I did a psychosocial evaluation on him when he was first diagnosed. Then we shared a great deal, through two years of life. He got married during that time. I went to his wedding—somewhat rashly, but I went anyway. Basically, I'm saying "rashly" because I had other patients on the floor, and I had to invest just as much energy in them.

One day he came in, and he's doing very well. He was strong with a big, thick red head of hair. "Would you like to come to my apartment for dinner one evening? We'd like to have you." I said, "You know, I really can't do that." He asked, "Why?" And I said, "Well, you know I really have to be available to you and everyone else who are patients here." He said, "So when I finish chemo in a year and a half, and I'm cured, will you come as a friend?"

I knew it was unlikely that he would be cured. And I cared deeply for him. It was hard to know this and listen to his dreams, which would probably never be realized. I wanted to say, "Don't do this to me!" even though he was unaware of the stress he put me under.

A short time later, he appeared at my door and was in tears. "I'm out of remission*—if something happens to me, I want to die on this floor." I said that all of us on the staff would not leave him alone. We would be there whenever he needed us. Well, he was admitted and began to sink very fast. About three weeks after his admission, I had to go away for a couple of days. When I came back, one of the nurses said, "Where have you been? Peter bled into his head last night." I went to his room and found him without response. I spoke his name, but he could no longer speak to me. Three days later, he died.

Peter was very dear to all of us. For a couple of days, I found it very difficult to work with other young leukemia patients. I kept a distance. This kind of loss demands time to integrate yourself, both personally and professionally. There is a part of you that does not want to reengage again and confront such a painful experience—but gradually that subsides.

Besides working with patients, she is a supervisor in her department of social work and her seminars on staff stress are attended by postgraduate social workers from all over the United States. Among the 1,500 nuns in her order —Sisters of Charity of New Jersey, founded by Elizabeth Ann Seton—are eight other social workers. She lives with two other sisters in an apartment in Jersey City, New Jersey, which makes it a long day for Sister Rosemary. "I get up at five thirty, say prayers, have breakfast, and take a bus and subway to get there. I also attend daily Mass across the street at St. Catherine's, unless there is some real emergency."

Of course you're emotionally involved with patients all the time. We're only human, after all, and we wouldn't do this work unless we cared about people, about human beings. There's a difference between being open, in order to hear what someone really thinks and feels, and meeting your own emotional needs. For instance, if I was to really worry about a patient liking me, wanting him or her to like me, and wanting to be part of his or her family, I would limit my ability to determine what he or she really needs. If I were overly involved, the necessary objectivity and distance which allows people to express and deal with their anger and frustration would be missing. The other thing is that you can become so involved with people you can love them almost in a selfish way. You are using them, rather than being there for them.

---

* "In remission" means that the disease is in abatement, permanently or temporarily. "Out of remission" means that the symptoms have returned.

Are you aware of this when it is happening to you?

Gradually you find you are staying longer with people. You are more personally upset or anxious about their situation. You become more tired, often with feelings of inadequacy and helplessness about being unable to change their medical condition. You can lose your effectiveness in both professional and personal caring. The staff soon becomes aware of it, at different levels and at different times. When it happens, we try to help each other.

You speak of caring for people. Perhaps it can be a higher form of love?

Oh no. I'd say love is a greater form of caring, though I often think the word "love" is used very loosely today. It can mean you withhold on your needs in order to care for others. That kind of love you usually get here. And sometimes because of this love, patients are able to get angry with you, because they know you're not going to run away. They know you are going to come back into the room, and that can be as much a love and caring as the softer, more gratifying kind.

When I say "love" it means for me the highest potential of the human being. It incorporates understanding and deep caring, as well as liking and being willing to set yourself aside for the better of the other person. You could say it's being a good professional. That's not a cold term because if you really are good, and if you really care, then that is love in a very true and real way.

So a higher form of love is giving up your identity for someone else?

Not your identity, but maybe some of your own needs. There are other places to get your needs met, and all of us seek to get our needs met. That's clear. But in working with cancer patients and their families, it's not up to them to meet our needs. If we use them for that purpose, we lose the maximum of our potential—and we lose our true, professional purpose for being there.

PATRICIA ANN MAZZOLA, R.N.

Chairman, Division of Nursing, MSKCC

I don't think you can stay here without getting emotionally involved with the patients. It is a beautiful part of working here. You can really enjoy it, but you also have to know how to handle it. The problem with some of our nurses is that they don't know when to step back, they can't drop the responsibility when they walk out the front door. Particularly the new graduates, who tend to become overly involved and lose their perspective. But they get a lot of support from their peers, and we now have a psychiatric nurse clinician, along with a social worker, to help them deal with the problem. Even so, we have lost nurses who admit that the emotional involvement is just too much for them and they cannot handle it.

She's 40, an attractive figure, dark hair, brown eyes, and a face with the soft hue of Mediterranean women. One detects on it the imprint of thousands of hours spent in Memorial's intensive care units, struggling with patients between life and death. When she smiles, however, all this seems to fade—the eyes alone remaining constant and vulnerable.

We've met in her office at Memorial, from which she now directs the hospital's 713 nurses. She wears a white lab coat over a smartly tailored light brown linen suit. She speaks with easy yet careful, clinical detachment, broken occasionally by a laugh and personal candor.

It's very natural, this involvement. You always have families waiting outside the unit, and often it's a touch and go situation for a long time. So you relate to this, to the patient and their loved ones.

With some patients, I can become involved and have no problem, but with others I just have to stay back. You know when it's beginning to happen to you, when you're going too far. It's when you start spending extra hours with the patient, or taking thoughts of that person home with you.

The chances of that happening to you increase in proportion to the time spent with the patient. The longer you care for them, taking care of their physical and emotional needs, the closer you become. It's highest in the medical and pediatric units, less in the recovery unit where you see a patient for a relatively short time. Some nurses prefer that, working in an emergency situation without the risk of overexposure or involvement with the long-term patient. I don't know if I would have survived in this hospital, working in a medical unit, because I might not have been able to step back enough in such an extended situation. Maybe I would have, I just don't know.

"I've been here sixteen years, most of it in the intensive care units. I came first as a staff nurse in the Recovery Room, then became head nurse, and after that was a clinical instructor in the three intensive care units—Special Care Unit, Coronary Care, and Recovery. I had an interlude setting up the Nursing Recruitment Department, then I went down to the operating rooms as director of OR Nursing. So it was another emergency area—we have fifteen operating rooms going all day long.

Even there, in the operating room, you can get highly involved with the patients. You see it especially with the surgeons when the operation fails or falls short of what was expected. Some of them find it almost too difficult to talk to the family afterward, to say, "There's nothing more I can do."

I'm thinking of one surgeon in particular who becomes quite upset, as if each patient was a member of his own family. It's the same with them as it is with the nurses or the social workers or anyone else who works here. You have to have a psychic barrier that causes you to step back before you go too far. It's not easy when you first come here. You've dedicated your life to curing the patient, and you find sometimes you just can't do it. Sometimes you can only palliate and ease the decline. But your goal is always more than that—to defeat the disease and send the patient home free of it.

It happened to me when I worked in the OR. My brother was admitted with the diagnosis of cancer of the kidney. He was only 39, and I'd tried to get him to Memorial earlier, but he wanted to be operated on by his own physician at home near his family in Tennessee. The operation was not successful, and he eventually came to Memorial, wanting to take any chance he had in order to live.

Despite the odds, Whitmore said he would do everything possible to save my brother. A consultant surgeon was also called in, and he spoke with my brother the night before. He said, "I might be involved in the surgery, and if it becomes extensive, we may have to go on the pump."* He was a very decent and kind man, this surgeon, and my brother immediately felt close to him.

The next morning they brought my brother—his name was Paul—down to the OR,† and I went in to stay with him until he went to sleep. The night before, he had been in one of his moods, saying, "This is it, we'll either make it or break it. If they can't get it all, I want to die on the

---

* Pump: Heart-lung machine.

† Operating room.

table." I had said, "You're not going to die on my OR table. There is no way." That morning in the OR bed-holding area, he was in a different mood—getting ready to fight it, no matter what happened. Before going to the OR, he took my hand and smiled as if he wanted to give me courage. "Don't worry, Pat," he said, "I'm not going to die on your table—no way. I have too much to live for, too much to do." *(Pauses, sighs.)*

Whitmore operated on him for about seven hours, trying to free up the tumor. He couldn't. It was just too far gone in every direction. It was originally diagnosed too late, and nothing else could be done.

But the struggle to save Paul went on and on. After the operation, everyone became involved, and there was such an air of hope, of not giving up. . . . *(Pauses.)* Like he was everybody's brother. Everyone wanted to do what they could in their own way—chemotherapy, radiation, immunotherapy.

He was also putting up a good fight, saying, "I want to live, I've got to live, I have five children." Then he said, "I'll do whatever they want me to do if it will give me some chance, and maybe I might just be that rare one to survive this."

He did—for a while. He went through things that I don't know if I could have taken—the radiation and the chemotherapy that made him so sick. But he was determined to live up to his last possible day, and because of this, he did live several months longer than expected. But once he had settled everything—taken care of his children, his business, when this was all finished—he began to deteriorate. And that was it.

I learned a lot about myself from that experience and about the others who tried so hard to save Paul. It was as if he was everyone's brother, and not because he was related to me. He was a young man who should not have died, given early diagnosis and proper treatment, and everyone felt it emotionally. The consultant surgeon could not go back and sit down with him after the operation. He said, "I just can't handle it—it's too much." Of course, Paul, like other patients, asked "Why is he avoiding me? Why isn't he coming back to see me?"

I think it's helpful to reveal what happens to all of us, including the surgeons. Why shouldn't people know about this? We're only human beings, we want especially to succeed, to not lose a human life. When it happens, it's very hard to take. It's always like the first time, and we always feel this deep emotional commitment. We couldn't stay here if we didn't.

Sure, it's happened to me. I can't come up with numbers, how many times, but it's happened that I loved someone in my care, and it probably will again.

Her patients are invariably women, ages 15 to 85, on the gynecological or tenth floor of Memorial. She has gray-blue eyes, dark hair, a lovely smile, and is 35. We are having coffee in her glass-partitioned, head nurse station.

You know, you can't help it, you can't help feeling this way with some of them. *(Smiles.)* They are in and out of here, sometimes for a couple of years, and there are some personalities that are just magnetic. You need to know them, they need to know you, also their families. It's an incredible situation, you know, as opposed to a general hospital where it's not the same thing.

When I interview, I tell a new employee that not everyone can work at Memorial. It's not easy to work here. There are a lot of stressful situations, whether it's the complexity of care, which can be very frustrating, or whether it's the emotional drain of constant intimacy with our patients. Many of them survive, but you see a lot of deaths at Memorial, too.

You have to work with that, which is another thing I try to tell a new staff member. Nurses always have an idealistic thought about themselves —that we are here to cure someone, to take care of them, make them well or better and send them back into the community. But if we're not able to do that to everybody, we are always able to comfort them in some way, to find out how to relieve pain, to give them a sense of being able to hold onto their image of themselves.

You have a patient with five bags on the abdomen, intravenous lines going into them, tubes coming out the nose, another from the bladder, and in the leg another intravenous line, with a machine over them, monitoring their life signs—all of this, and suddenly you realize you're forgetting things that are creature comforts. I mean the extra pillow under the arm, the back rubs that sometimes get overlooked, the cream on the elbows— things that everyone loves and makes them feel like they are being cared for, you know, as a person, not just a receptacle for a lot of tubes.

We find that staff meetings are very helpful in talking our feelings out. You just sit with a cup of coffee and shoot the breeze about something that's really upsetting you, some patient that's ornery or self-centered or wants attention all day long. Or someone you care a lot about, someone you feel very deeply about, maybe too much. *(Pauses.)* Maybe you love them and don't know it or want to admit it. You've been caring for them for a couple of years, on and off, and now they are going to die even though you're offering them whatever you have to offer.

"We had a patient here for sixteen weeks. And you know what? She was dying for sixteen weeks. She didn't want to die. She was fighting it off, and it was very tough because everyone loved her so very, very much, and we all liked to take care of her. Such a marvelous spirit, so beautiful and always wanting to lift up our spirits." (Laughs softly.) *"Rosa Martinez. Everyone wanted to help her, but they couldn't find a way to help her die easier because she was fighting it so. She wanted another year. She was grasping for that extra time, and it was hard on the staff to face that every day, hoping that maybe the following day she would be a little more relaxed, wouldn't be as agitated and anxious and hyper, asking questions like 'Do you think I'll ever get out of here?' while everyone knew she would never get out, no matter how much we loved her and wanted her to make it. But you can't turn around and say, 'No, you'll never get out of here.' You have to sort of work around it, without lying to her. You fudge it, to give some hope, always some little hope.*

"When you care so much, when the patient is loved by so many of us, it's especially hard—even for those who've been here a long time. It's something you just have to face. You sort of get yourself together and start thinking about how you're going to help this person."

I try and spend a lot of time with patients even though I'm manager of the unit, so to speak. I want to know what the data are really saying about them, and you can only get that by talking with them. Also, I want to relieve them of some of their pressures, using the expertise I've acquired over the years. So it's sort of like having a series of extended families. And everyday that they're here, or the longer you know them, another page turns, and you find out something else.

We continue to look after many patients, even after they go home. They've been here sometimes four weeks, maybe six or eight weeks. They came in a whole person—as they think of themselves, anyway—and they leave with maybe a colostomy, or a conduit, which is a diversion of the urine, or maybe a very large wound defect that needs to be cared for until it's totally healed. Before they leave, we do what we can to help them retain that concept of still being a whole person, even though their body is not the same.

We teach them a lot, and we hope they will be able to take care of themselves. But in order to insure that, we send out visiting nurse referrals on many patients to ensure a continuity of care. The referral goes to a visiting nurse service located close to where the patient lives. Then they go in and follow through on what has happened, what needs to be done at home, and they send us reports on how the patient is doing. *(Pulls out card index file.)* Here, this patient, Maria, lives over on a Hundred Eighty-ninth Street. We sent a referral to the West Manhattan Center, and here's a report on how she's doing with her recovery. I also encourage the nursing staff to call the patients and ask how they're doing. When we contact them, I write down whoever talked to them, the date, that the patient is now able to take care of her colostomy, that her skin seems to be doing well, and that we've reminded her of her next appointment with the doctor. So they know we are continuing to care for them.

Here's another one, Viola. *(Lifts out card.)* We called her two months ago, then she called us on Christmas Day. Last month, she was in to see her doctor and came up to see us. She's doing well and in great shape. It's very rewarding for the staff to see this happen. When they return like that, it goes through the floor like an electric charge. Everyone feels it. You're flooded with a quiet sense of joy, that you can win at this, that the caring and loving do matter.

It's happened to me several times, this feeling of love for a patient. It's happened to practically everyone I know. I was with one patient very recently. He was a young fella, and I couldn't stop thinking about him every five minutes. I couldn't pass the door without going in or doing something for him. I didn't know one of the other nurses felt the same way, until the day he went home, and she cried. Then I started. It was hard not to feel that way, because he was going home to die. We won't see him again.

She's nearly 40, blond, blue eyes, with a tall, willowy figure and long, delicate hands. Her voice is low and modulated by a rich Irish brogue. We are in the nurses' lounge on the eighth floor for thoracic surgery patients at Memorial Hospital.

His mother called me one day, you know, to kind of thank me for what we had done for him, the reassurance we had given her. She said he was doing very well, but apparently he had some bleeding. I thought, "Oh God, now it's going to begin for him." Then I checked myself. You have to do that. You have to say to yourself, "No, that's enough. I'm not letting this happen to me again." Yet sometimes it happens anyway. It might sound strange, but often you are not aware of it, even though there are signals or warnings. Others can see it, though, and we tell each other to be careful when we see it starting in on them.

I think it tears up the patient more when you get too involved. At the same time, there's a certain close involvement you can't escape. It comes with the job. If you take care of someone for two weeks, or even one whole week, seven days in a row, you can't avoid being involved with them and the family, or whoever is close to them. In many ways, you become even closer than the family because you're there when the family isn't. You're with them, in the center of the major crisis of their life, bathing them, touching them, making them comfortable. Also, there's something else most people don't realize. Often the patient suddenly finds his family is no longer so close to him. He sees they are afraid. They are apprehensive about taking him home with them.

This really bogs you down. Whenever they see you, they ask the same questions all over again. "How can I cope with it?" They love the patient, or at least they think they do. But they are terrified of being unable to handle it. They see this sick person—whether they're going to die or not—coming home and changing their life around, or making life impossible for someone else in the family who won't be able to cope with it.

Also, these cancer patients demand closer, more personal care than others do. If you disappear for a week's vacation, or if we are short of staff, they're immediately aware of it and become very demanding. They start checking on you, to see how long it will take you to come when they put on the call light. That's an amazing thing in this hospital. In other hospitals, patients just wait. But here, it's "Nobody's checked my dressing or my tube." They can really panic. All of a sudden one of them is yelling for you to come urgently. You walk into the room and find they are angry because they were told they were to have a test done or were supposed to go to the OR—but it hasn't happened. "Why haven't I gone downstairs for my test?" Or, "Why didn't I go to the OR at ten o'clock?" Things like that, and they get really angry. If you speak softly, their tone of voice gradually comes down. If they scream at you, or you hear them screaming, you might run to the door, but once you get to the room, you walk very quietly and talk very softly. That way, they cool off and almost always are apologetic.

You have to understand them, I mean why they are like that. It's the nature of the disease that causes them to act that way. They feel the pressure of it possibly growing, of it taking over their body. In other hospitals the patient can usually assume that whatever he has will each day be diminishing or slowly mending. But here, there's that pressure on them, or within them, and they want you close by to help them with it.

So you know why they are looking for you the minute you come on duty, how much it means to visit with them. Maybe it's only to fix something they've been waiting for you to do, because they feel closer to you than someone else. And when you do it, it shows that you care especially for them. It gives them a sense of being lifted up, of still being able to hold onto themselves.

That's why you can't blame them when they start pushing the call button to see how fast you come to them. I don't know if I can explain it, it's so difficult, but if you look at these people, this cancer, the problem isn't only whether they are going to die or not. The problem is somewhere else, in the nature of being afflicted in the first place. It's a whole person, a body's biological innocence is being violated. We're caring for that, we're loving that part of them. You know what I mean? I think it's this that brings you closer to the patient here than it would elsewhere. So you have this unusual involvement to begin with, and sometimes it gets deeper, more complex than it should. Because the more vulnerable they are, the closer you come to them. And it isn't always just a week or a month. We have some of them coming back here, in and out, for several years. So this feeling, the involvement builds up also because of that.

*Besides the inevitable psychological involvement with cancer patients, the
physical and medical bonding between patient and nurse has increased with
the growing responsibility of nurses in the care of patients. "We start our
own IV's and change pleur-evacs* where a few years ago we didn't do that
kind of stuff. If a patient has a temperature, you automatically draw blood
to check his blood count before it is affected by antibiotic treatment. You
have to know when to act before a doctor comes—and when not to act.
There's a lot of paperwork and other controls, and it often comes at you all
at one time. Some days we have forty-two patients, and, especially on a
surgical floor, you find most of them going down to surgery in the same
period. Then you have them coming back up again with an overflow of
postsurgical needs and problems."*

Also, I think it's very important to greet the patient when they reach the
floor, especially in a cancer hospital, because you're interested in what's
going to happen to them, and how they feel about it. I find it's very
important to take them to their room, to spend a few minutes talking with
them, maybe getting them something to drink, asking them if there's anything bothering them, if there's anything special they want. All that sort of
stuff helps. You can see the tension easing. That's when you begin with
them, noting from day to day the subtle changes in their spirit or their
general condition. We write it all down on the patient's chart because
we're with them all day or all night while the doctor sees them for maybe
ten minutes, twice a day. Some doctors don't bother to even read what we
write. Then you have to go and tell them, and even then sometimes they
don't listen to you—but not often.

*Back home in Ireland, and later in England, she had worked hard, often on
twelve-hour shifts, but without such involvement and responsibility for the
patient. She left behind two brothers and five sisters. "We were a very close
family, and I was the only one that traveled to the U.S. The others stayed
on, or went to England. They thought I was crazy, coming here, but I got
the opportunity and took it.*

*"When I arrived here, sixteen years ago, I also thought maybe I was crazy
because it was so different, and work in a cancer hospital was so difficult.
Not the work as much as it being mentally exhausting and the tension. But
I guess after a while you can get used to anything. I did, even before I
noticed it. And now I wouldn't go anywhere else. I feel like I belong here
somehow, but I can't explain it."*

---

* Containers for collecting fluid and air after a chest operation.

Despite her personal beauty, Ina, as her friends call her, has never married. "I have male friends, I enjoy life, but sometimes I think with women you either have to get married, be a nurse, or become a nun. Those three things. And for me, it's being a nurse. Maybe it will change some day, but I don't know. You never know in life, do you?"

He's 32 and resembles a young Ernest Hemingway—tall, large hands, broad shoulders, dark piercing eyes, and the thick mustache. We are in the glassed office cubicle of the head nurse, on the sixteenth floor of Memorial Hospital.

When you become too involved, too close to a patient, you go over the top. You enter into them, into their feelings, their fears, their terror. You become part of their own processes working against them. You end up unable to help them as you should. Sometimes you can pull yourself back, but it's difficult because it's so mixed up with your total belief in the worth of caring for people. These are not scientific models. These are people, and people can draw you close, very close, when they are in need and fighting for life.

Yes, but if you penetrate into their sense of fear or terror, why wouldn't you have a more encompassing view of their feelings, as well as your own—and so be able to help them more, with greater understanding?

What happens, in such an involvement, is that you close down your focus, instead of allowing it to remain open. Your interest in the patient should be solely in terms of the patient, in trying to understand what is going on with them. But when their process of terror, or whatever you want to call the fear, enters into your own life, it becomes *your* terror. Then you start thinking about it in terms of yourself. You see this happen frequently with young nurses. They have a patient that has a lump on the breast. One or two weeks later, when they get very close to the patient, they start feeling around their bodies to see if they have a lump.

Yet most nurses admit that an occasional overinvolvement is inevitable, and sometimes there's even a feeling of love for a patient.

Of course, and not until it happens do they feel their full potential or the depth of their commitment. Also, not until they go too far do they know where the line is, how it can happen, and how to check themselves.

You've fought in Vietnam. Would you compare this to the need to experience fear in order to be brave?

Yes, because then you discover that freedom from fear is bullshit—merely an illusion. You think you're going to escape fear, but a soldier finds that he doesn't escape it. He just has to learn to live with it and deal with it as he can. That's how it is here, in not becoming involved with patients. You try not to get yourself into that position, because like the soldier, you want to avoid the conflict in yourself, or anywhere else. The true hero isn't out to start any war. *(Laughs.)* He isn't out to prove himself.

But it's never easy. As a nurse, you're in a position that breaks down all barriers. You take off the patient's clothes, and they lose their protective identity. It just happens. Then you get to know them as they are. You are taking care of them, after their operation or receiving chemotherapy or whatever. You touch them, you help them wash, you help them in other private ways—and all the barriers they've lived with all their life are suddenly erased. Sometimes you can't help it. You come very close to them, and if you lose them, it can be very hard on you. But it can be wonderful, too, when they make it, and you feel a part of their personal victory.

I was in a real hurry when he came in. I knew he was a leukemic with fever, but all I could think about was how this meant more work, more antibiotics to hang. I told myself, "Here we go again. It's two o'clock, they're going to order medicines, and I'm going to be running around and never get out of here."

But there was something about him that I liked, just a look about him. We started talking and laughing. He was really uptight about being there, and I was going, "Oh, c'mon, it's no big deal." I didn't know he was out of remission—that is, his leukemia had returned after earlier treatment seemed to have stopped it. That's very serious. Once you relapse, you usually die, because most leukemics are resistant to chemo treatment the second time around.

She's 23, with black hair and blue eyes, and when she smiles, she looks like Judy Garland. We are in a quiet corner of an Italian restaurant near Memorial. It's her lunch hour, and she is wearing her white uniform with the hospital name tag: M. Roden, R.N., Dept. Nursing.

We just started laughing, and I liked talking to him, and gradually I'd find more and more excuses to go into his room. After he was on the floor a week, I went to New Orleans, to the Mardi Gras. I thought about him while I was there, and I told my roommate about it. She began to worry, and said, "Forget the patients, don't get involved with patients." I said, "I know, I just like him. He's nice. I don't feel anything more for him."

She's been a registered nurse for almost two years. "But I worked as a nurse's aide and a practical nurse at college. You have to play the ropes to get where you want to go. To get a good job, you have to have some background experience, besides being a new grad. So at first I was an aide. Then after I passed medical-surgical nursing in my junior year, I was eligible to take the boards to be licensed as a practical nurse. So I got that, my LPN, and then in the final semester at Niagara University you have to specialize in one area. I chose oncology and worked at Roswell Park Memorial Institute. It's a cancer-research hospital in Buffalo, like Memorial Sloan-Kettering.

"I did a semester there on practically the same type of floor I'm working on now—lymphoma, leukemic, acute medicine, leftovers, whatever you want to call these patients. When they don't fit on one floor, they're on my floor. I had worked in a nursing home, so I was used to people dying and the sickness and the sadness that goes with it."

When I came back from New Orleans, I worked evenings, the three to eleven-thirty shift. You really get to know patients in a different way working that shift. During the daytime, it's more rushed. Get this one washed, get that one to a test, or whatever. After a long day of that, the patients are more exhausted, and often sicker because of their chemo treatment during the day.

That's when I really got to know Bruce. What'd he look like? Well, he was Greek, about five-nine, with black hair and a beard and brown almond-shaped eyes. His eyes were really what first attracted me to him. They were beautiful.

Then I found out he was an artist, and he showed me slides of his paintings. In his last year at college, at Cornell in Iowa, he did like a hundred-fifty paintings. Since he was in remission from leukemia, he didn't know if he would survive or how much time he had. So in his last year, he painted night and day. He wanted to put down as much as he could of himself while he had the chance. All of his paintings were very sad, I thought.

Then I got the flu and was out for a week—just when he got very, very sick and had an out-of-body experience. With some chemotherapy, all your counts get wiped out, and you become highly vulnerable to infection. He got it and almost died. They gave him amphotericin B, which is a very strong antibiotic.

One night when he was quite sick and his pressure was extremely low, he fell asleep and suddenly felt he was going through a long, dark passage. He saw his body leaving him, and just then one of our nurses was walking by, and he began to scream for her, "Roxanne! Roxanne!" She came running because they were all afraid he was going to die. As she entered the room, he kind of came out of it, and he saw his body slowly sink back into him. It was like he died and somehow came back to life. Then he lay there, waiting for me to come to him. He knew I was sick, but he also felt that I was going to come, anyway. What's really weird about this is that he was right.

I had this terrible flu with fever, but somehow I knew what was happening to him. I thought he was going to die, and I sent my roommate, Janine, down to the floor to see how he was doing. She came home and said, "Bruce is really sick." It was what I'd suspected, but I asked, "What do you mean?" She says, "I think he's going to die," and I said, "If he dies, I hope he dies before I get back there."

Only when I said that, did I realize how much he meant to me. We were close, but I never knew it was that close. I didn't want him to die. I wanted to go to him and do what I could. I got up and went to Health

Service, because I'd been really sick, to see if maybe I could come back to work. They said I had to wait, but I got permission to go up to the floor.

It was Bruce's birthday, and I looked into his room and said, "Hi, I can't come in because I'm still sick." He asks, "When are you coming back?" I said, "Soon. How are you?" "Not too good," he said, but then he goes, "I've been waiting for you, but you don't have to come in. Just stand there so I can look at you. That's all I need."

It was enough to drive you crazy. Later, we wondered about it, if maybe wanting me so much kept him from dying. Most people who have that experience of going down a dark corridor say there's a feeling of contentment with a light at the far end and a nice sense of floating away. I've talked to them about it, those that came back. But Bruce was different. He didn't like it. He knew he was dying, and he didn't want to go. He saw me, but then I was gone, and he was frightened. He never expected to love a woman again, and he thought maybe this turned him back from dying.

On the following Monday, I came back to work, and from then on we were inseparable. I took care of him practically every day until he was released. No matter where he was, I somehow maneuvered it so that I could have the group of patients that included him.

I didn't care what anyone had to say. People would ask, "Why are you always in that room, whispering and everything?" I didn't care. To hell with them. And after work, I would stay there. We'd watch TV, look at slides of his paintings, talk. The nurses would be coming in, the supervisor kicked me out of the hospital one night. The hell with her. The next night, I'd go back and stay there. I just didn't care.

I never neglected my duties to other patients. And believe me, there are times when you don't want to do a damn thing for some of them. The cranks, the mean ones, those who are always testing you to see how fast you can get there—and it's never fast enough. So you say, "I'm not going into that room again." You keep busy with other things, intending to let it slide into the next shift. But then you go in, anyway. You go into their room, and you always feel better afterward—after doing what you don't want to do. You know, the biggest reward is not the paycheck. It's there, with the patient. If I just move them or comb their hair or give them a heating pad or whatever, and they say, "Thank you," it helps a lot. Or even a smile. It makes me want to do more for them. And it helps them, too. They really respond to kindness. Doctors will tell you that kindness helps people get well.

So I never neglected my work. But I always found reasons to be in Bruce's room. Or we'd go for walks in the hall, whatever the excuse, just to talk. If I had to walk from one room to the other, or bring something down the hall, I'd go, "Bruce, c'mon, take a walk with me." Even if it was just thirty feet, we'd manage somehow.

Then we just kind of fell into things. One day there was a sort of semikiss. We both turned red, and I slapped him. *(Laughs.)* Then the first time it really happened, he was lying in bed, and I was sitting right next to him, talking. You know the first kiss, how it is? I'm sure you remember your first one. I was like 14 all over again. I just leaned over, and he came forward, and it just kind of happened. We both turned red. I said, "I'd better go." And he said, "Yes, you'd better." Really weird! *(Laughs.)* Because we didn't want to get caught. But gradually after that, we would kiss each other good night. Always, that kiss good night.

Then his attending physician wanted to give him this experimental chemo, and he was going to have to stay in the hospital longer for it. He was walking around, he was feeling good, but he had failed the regular protocol treatment. It didn't work, and he still had leukemic cells in his bone marrow. So his attending said, "We have this other drug to give you."

At that time, the drug, Amsa, was still highly experimental.* They had given it to five people. I think four had died, and one had gone into remission, only to die later from other complications. Bruce knew all that, but it was his only hope. I kept saying, "Bruce, wait to take that drug. Get out of the hospital for a while. Just wait to take it." And he goes, "Yeah, I want to get out of here for a while." Because we both knew, deep in our hearts, that if it didn't work he was going to die. And if he waited, we'd at least have that time together before he started it.

But his doctor wanted to give it to him right away and, to get him ready for it, gave Bruce a private room. We were great, you know, glorifying everything. Even that room. *(Laughs.)* Because there, at least, we could be alone, and he could continue his painting. In the double room, he'd written in his journal and done a lot of drawing, but no painting. So now his family brought him all his paints, and he began a picture for a stained glass window in a church.

He used to get out on pass, and often went to the Catholic church on Sixty-ninth Street. He wasn't especially religious, and it wasn't so much that he didn't believe in God. He didn't know how he felt. So he used to sit

---

* This drug has since been proved effective in treating leukemic victims. Experimental drugs are given to humans only after exhaustive trials in animals for their toxic side effects, and only upon final approval by the U.S. Food and Drug Administration. They are given when there is no other known possible cure and only with the patient's full consent after all possible risks have been explained. These clinical trials have advanced cancer chemotherapy to its present high-level cure rate.

there and wonder about it, and also think about a stained glass window for that church.

Then he'd come back to his private room, which was his studio and, in a crazy way, also our little home. My roommate, Janine, was also close to Bruce, and she'd come, and we'd watch *Saturday Night Live,* get pizzas, hang out. The hell with the supervisors. No one would come into the room because I let it be known that I was going to stay. So in other words, "Fuck you, I'm staying. I don't care what you have to say. Fire me. I don't care." There was a feverish passion between us, and we were always kissing, but that was all. We never went beyond it, we never made love there. We felt we had a right to love each other, but not to do that.

Oh God, we had such plans, what we'd do and how we'd live together when he was in remission. I knew he'd become a famous artist because he was tremendous, he had so much. But deep down inside, I think we always knew he wouldn't live—except you don't know this because you never really acknowledge these feelings. I thought I had enough life for both of us. He'd say, "I don't know how much life I have in me anymore," and I'd say, "I have enough for both of us, don't worry."

All this time, he was painting. I think it's the first time that a room in Memorial became a painter's studio. It didn't seem real, and very soon it wasn't anymore. One day, I was standing in the medication room when he walked by with this sad look on his face. I asked, "What's the matter?" He said, "I'm leaving, I'm being discharged." I go, "What are you talking about?" He says, "My doctor says I can wait three months before I take the drug because I'm feeling so good."

At first, I was disappointed because I was so used to seeing him every day. He smiled and said, "But we'll still see each other." I asked him, "Will you promise to come and see me and promise I can come to Brooklyn?" I was to go to Brooklyn to meet his family, and he would come to Manhattan to me.

So he was discharged on a Friday, and we called each other three, four times a day. We knew time was precious, and there was no time for bullshit. Like, you know, "Maybe I'll call you, or you call me." There was no time for that. Every moment was important. Every moment was precious. And everything was so natural, so easy, so calm. We didn't have to pretend. With us, it was "I like you, you like me, so let's not hide it. I'm not afraid to admit it, neither are you." We knew what we wanted, and we just went with it.

On Monday, he came to see me in Manhattan. We went down to SoHo to the galleries, walked around, and went to Chinatown. We did all the things we'd always talked about, and then we came back to my apartment.

That was the first time we made love. I had always said to him in the hospital, "Do you think you'll be able to do it?" And he'd say, "Yeah, I think so." But at first it was really difficult because he didn't feel he could. He had never thought about making love to a woman again. He never thought of even being in love. He wanted to do things for me, but he said, "I don't think I can." I said, "Yes, you can, let me try for you." We gave it a good shot, and finally things worked. Then it became easier for him, and he was a marvelous lover. He made me very, very happy.

He was about a month out of the hospital when one day he said, "Come to Brooklyn." That was always the big thing. I would come to Brooklyn to meet his grandmother, whom he loved and adored. So I went and met the whole family. Later, I learned the grandmother liked me because I made Bruce happy. All these things were very important to him that day. I should have realized what it was, but I didn't.

Then he took me down to the basement where he had his studio. I once asked him to paint me a pretty picture because all his paintings had this overwhelming sadness, like Edvard Munch. You know, that feeling of something tragic, of terrible loss, of death, or whatever. So I got aggravated, and I said, "Bruce, will you paint me something pretty?" Well, he took my hand, and I'll never forget it . . . *(pauses)* and brought me before this painting which was very beautiful. People who come to my apartment, those who understand art, always stare at it and ask about Bruce Costas. It reminds me of Andrew Wyeth's *Christina's World*. There is a woman with black hair in the wheat fields of Iowa, the colors are pink, blue, and gray, all coming together in the background of the sky. It's a picture of longing and searching, of not knowing, of just wondering where everything is going. He asked, "Do you like it?" I said, "It's beautiful." Then he said, "I want you to have it."

I'll never forget that, what I saw, because it was Bruce free of cancer, of the threat of death. This was how he would be when he was in remission, when he could be his own natural self, full of joy and wondering about life *(sighs)* and how it would be when we lived together. I hugged him, and for a moment, I thought it would really work. He would get well, he was not going to die, and I could have him all my life.

I was the only one he had ever loved, and he was the first man that I ever loved so completely, so freely, so givingly, and expected nothing in return. Nothing because he didn't have that much to give. His love, sure, but as far as spending money for things, like the cost of going out, especially in a city like New York, none of that mattered. It was so unimportant. I gave, expecting nothing—just him, his person. Nothing else mattered.

After we left his family, we went for a walk and stopped in a restaurant. It was like one or two in the morning. We were just sitting there, looking at each other, and drinking hot chocolate. We used to spend silent moments together, and it was wonderful. You know you really like someone when you are comfortable with silence between you, when you know the silence isn't a sign of "I don't like him," or "I don't want to talk to you." You're just comfortable with each other, and you can be quiet, as you are often quiet with your own self.

I remember he suddenly said, "Well, Maureen, I guess this sort of wraps things up." I go, "Yeah, I know, but you're not going back into the hospital; you have another two months." He said, "I know." But he had this faraway look in his eyes, and he said, "You know, Maureen, I'm not going to make it." I said, "Don't say that. You are." He goes, "No, there is a good possibility that I'm going to die." When he said it, I knew it was true, but I wasn't going to say it back to him. I said, "No, you're not. You can't and won't. You're going to make it. I'll be there, don't worry." He replied, "I'm not, but already we've had a lifetime together." I said, "We've only started. It's not over yet, it's not a lifetime." My heart was breaking, and I wanted him to stop. "Yes, it is," he said. "We've done everything and had it all on extra time, thanks to you, to our love. I've never worked better, we've never known anything like this, we've never loved anyone this way, the way we do. We've had everything, except babies. Does that make you sad? It does me, very much, because I love you so much, Maureen." I didn't cry. I didn't want him to see me crying, because he would know that I believed him.

That was Friday, and on the following Monday he got sick and was readmitted to the hospital with a high fever. They gave him antibiotics, and he was fine. He wanted to go home, but his attending said, "No, I want to give you this drug now." I remember I cried that night. I said, "Bruce, don't take it. Wait." Because it was the first time that I really acknowledged my fears. I felt he was going to die, as he had said. But if it was going to happen, I didn't want him to die then. If he could wait for the drug, then wait. And he wanted to wait. He said, "Yeah, what difference does it make if I take it now, or take it later?" We wanted to do so many things. We wanted to go to the Hamptons, we wanted . . . *(Stops, unable to continue.)*

"Well, the doctor said he couldn't wait. He had to decide now, otherwise it'd be too late. So Bruce had to either go with his doctor—or refuse him. At that point, I began to worry about spoiling his one chance, no matter how slim. Also, if Bruce was convinced he was not going to make it, maybe he would feel different with the drug.

"Chemo always brings some hope, even to people who've lost it. Patients will yell at you, 'I hate the stuff!' Or they'll say, 'You call it chemo, I call it poison.' But they want it. They'll take it because they know it's their only hope. You hear people saying, 'I'll never take chemo because I know how horrible it is.' But they eventually take it anyway, to prolong their life. You might think, 'Oh, he's 80, what difference does a few months or years make?' Well, it makes a big difference if you're the patient. No matter how sick the patient is, offer them anything with hope attached to it, and they'll take it. I sit on the oustide, and I know it's not a sure thing, it may not work, and everyone else knows the same. But you also know you have to offer something unless there's absolutely no hope. And some hope is always there, even when it's hopeless because that's the way people are."

So I finally said, "Okay, Bruce, take it now. You'll be in remission and better off in the long run." But I didn't believe it, not really, not deep in my heart. I knew how horrible this drug was. They hadn't had any real successes with it yet, except for this one woman on the floor who went into remission, and I held onto that to make us feel better. I said, "If she went into remission, you probably will too."

I remember he got a pass to go out of the hospital, and that was the last time he ever went home to his family. He had dinner with them, then came back, and we were together. The next day he got the drug, Amsa. It completely wipes out your bone marrow, and four days later he got a fever.

The intern was coming down to the fourth floor to see him. Finally he said, "Look, this kid's so sick I want him up on the sixth floor." So that's where he went, and he was off my floor. I was working evenings, so I would come in and spend the morning with him, go home, then back to work, go to bed, come back in the mornings, and stay with him again.

Every day he got sicker and sicker. My own life hadn't ever been easy, but somehow, no matter how bad things were, they always worked out. That's how I looked at Bruce. I could never believe, in my heart, that he would die because nobody'd ever died that I cared about. Nothing like this had ever happened to me. I'd think, "I'm invincible, so it's not going to happen to him." But there were times when I was scared of being hurt so much. It's different if you lose someone because you had a fight and broke up. Death is permanent, and I wasn't ready for it.

I was spending like sixteen hours a day with Bruce, and it was getting to me. He was dying, and I was going into it with him. That was hard enough, but making it even harder was seeing pity in the eyes of the others, the staff who worked with me. I wanted to say, "Don't feel sorry, that hurts more," but I said nothing to them, and they all thought I couldn't handle it. They thought, "She's not coping." They expected me to cry more, to break down more, to do something they could relate to. But I didn't. I just held onto myself and what was left of Bruce.

The supervisor called me into her office, and it went like this: "Are you involved with Bruce Costas?" "No." "I don't believe you. Maybe you can't cope with it?" "No, I'm all right." "Well, you don't talk much." "What is there to say?" "If you ever want to talk, talk to me." "I don't want to talk to anyone, I'm okay."

It wasn't until a few days before Bruce died that I finally accepted that it was going to happen. And even then, even when he was dying, I still went on hoping for a miracle. Now I understand how it is when a patient is dying, and the family says, "Oh, he's going to make it." I know he's going to die, and they know it, too. But they still go on hoping for a miracle, and now I know how they feel.

I know what they're going through. When I see blood being hung on a patient who's practically dead, I know how much it can mean, even though it'll never save him. Because if it isn't there, and they're awake or semialert and don't see anything being done for them, they know they're expected to die. It's a horrible, frightening feeling. Bruce, when he was dying, said, "These doctors have all given up on me." Because there was nothing there, they didn't want to do anything else for him.

I got angry, too, and asked the intern, "Why aren't you giving him more blood or platelets?" He said, "It's not going to do him any good." I said, "How do you know? One pint of blood hanging in the air will make him feel less desperate, and it'll ease the family's fear that we're doing nothing." He said, "We're not treating families." I got real angry and said, "You're supposed to be *treating* a dying man, not *abandoning* him. More red cells will help him breathe better, and it'll give him greater peace of mind in dying. If he's going to die, let him sink gradually, don't drop him into it."

He was furious, but I didn't care anymore, and later the attending said I was perfectly right. At Memorial, they fight for the patient to the last breath, and everything is done to relieve the trauma of dying. That intern was an asshole. But it taught me a lot. Now I know how the families of other people feel. I know the anger, the frustration, the sorrow so well, so unbelievably well.

Gradually Bruce lost his blood count and began bleeding internally. He bled into his brain and his eyes, and one night toward the end his family brought motion pictures to show on the wall of the hospital room. The movie was going, and Bruce said, "You know, I can't really see it."

He had gone blind. They turned off the movie, and Bruce tried to help them by singing a song, "The Circle Game." Everyone in the family knew it, so we all joined hands around him and sang it together. Then he said, "I just want you all to know that I love you very much. I'm not afraid anymore. I'm ready."

That's when we all knew that it was over, and we were so happy by that time, because we were exhausted by the dying process, the ups and downs.

That evening, Tuesday, he was sleeping, and his mother was in the room. I came in, and he woke up, saying, "Where's Maureen?" His mother said, "Maureen's here." He waved his arm, to indicate he wanted everyone out of the room, except me. I said, "I know you can't see me." He said, "No, I can't," and I just kind of laughed it off. He said, "Talk to me," and I said, "Okay," and just starting laughing. I told him, "This dying is killing us all, definitely." I paused and said, "I look good." "Oh yeah?" and I say, "Yeah." He says, "How do you look, what're you wearing?" I say, "Don't get excited." Then I tell him I have on the jeans that he liked, they're real tight, and the shirt he gave me, and he just kind of smiled.

We were always going to take a boat trip together, the Circle Line around Manhattan because it was the easiest one. "You know, Bruce, I'm going to take the Circle Line, and you're not going to be with me, but you really are. You won't be there, by my side, but we'll still be together." He says, "I know, I know." And I said, "I just want you to know that I . . . love . . . you." And he told me, "I want you to know that I love you." That was the last thing he said to anyone, except for answering my question, "Do you want to go to sleep now?" He said, "Yeah," and that night he lapsed into a coma.

All day Wednesday he was in a coma, and I think about one o'clock his parents left. His two brothers, Alex and Keith, were sleeping on the floor, and I put two chairs together to sleep by the bed. I was holding his hand, and for the first time through the whole thing I began to pray. I was just praying that he would die. Enough is enough. I would say prayers and take his pulse and check to see if he was weaker. I guess I must have fallen asleep taking his pulse and praying, "God, let him die, let it be over, no more now."

Then I looked up, and his doctor was in the room. I guess the nurse had looked in and seen that Bruce wasn't breathing. I was still holding his hand, and I looked at the doctor and said, "Is this it?" He said, "Yes, Maureen, this is it. And it's all okay, you can go now."

I didn't kiss Bruce good-bye. I just looked back and thought, "Thank God . . . for him, for us, for everyone." Then, looking at him for the last time, I had the strange feeling that I had known this man long before I ever met him, and also that I would meet him again somewhere. That's how I left the room. Knowing I was not leaving him.

POSTSCRIPT: No one at Memorial Hospital approved of Maureen Roden's involvement with Bruce Costas. Her supervisors made it clear they would not tolerate another such case. But they did not fire her. It was a tribute to her, to their belief in her professional ability and her performance under extreme duress. They had all suffered through similar emotional conflicts, if not so extreme. It was one of the dangers inherent in the job of caring for people.

A year later, Maureen Roden left Memorial and is now a private-duty nurse.

THREE

LUCK

Fortune is the arbiter of one-half of our actions, but she still leaves us to direct the other half—or perhaps a little less.

Niccolò Machiavelli
The Prince

There is a tide in the affairs of men,
Which, taken at the flood, leads on to fortune;
Omitted, all the voyage of their life
Is bound in shallows and in miseries.

William Shakespeare
Julius Caesar

One of these patients is told he has a spot on his lung—but it's very small. His surgeon says, "You're a lucky man." The patient, a New York cop, replies, "Lucky? What the hell's lucky about this? I'd be lucky if I didn't have the damn thing."

Yet when the surgeon says he must leave town and can only perform the operation two weeks hence, the cop stiffens. "Wait a minute. If I've been so damn lucky, let's take this out while we're ahead of the game. Why risk losing everything while you're out of town?"

It is just this—the phenomenon of delayed recognition of what is perceived as luck, followed by a grappling for it in a stream of life-threatening events—which makes luck such an intriguing and dramatic factor in cancer survival. In this way, the stories here suggest that fortune is, indeed, the arbiter of one half of our lives—at least for these protagonists who also struggle to take what they may at flood tide.

In principle, we know what luck is or is supposed to be—a force that seems to operate for good or ill in a person's life. For the Greeks, it was personified by the goddess Tyche whom Athenians claimed as preferring to live among them. They portrayed her with a horn of plenty in one arm and in the other a double steering oar, to indicate the rapid turns and rolls of fortune.

For many who so believe, little has changed since then. Lady Luck still possesses the inconstant and unpredictable nature of the Greek goddess. She comes and goes, often too swift to be seen—appearing variously in a race of champions, in wind on a sail, in the trajectory of a bullet, in the heart of a storm, in the reach for love. It is claimed that she can outsmart the devil, outshoot Cupid, and outrun the moon. Or, simulating moonlight, she can slip into the camps of sleeping soldiers, through traps of spider webs, into command cabins of spacecraft, and onto the pathways of the lost, the lonely, and those who are ill.

To ward her off at those times when she brings only bad luck, millions of people wear amulets, charms against the evil eye, crosses, crescents, skin tattoos, bones of many sorts, and spiraled bull horns. They hang horseshoes, avoid slanting ladders and black cats, carry a rabbit's foot, touch their testicles, and place the image of protective saints in cars, trucks, airplanes, elevators—or almost anywhere that human beings are in motion and so subject to danger.

Nothing seems to diminish the belief and trust in such trinkets and symbols, in the faiths and fetishes which we find scattered around the world, from forest tribes to urban families. Those who view them as ridiculous—sad endeavors to anthropomorphize or otherwise control nature—argue that nature is neither malevolent nor benevolent, but merely *indifferent* to *Homo sapiens,* much as a tree is to an apple or a hen to an egg. This indifference, they say, is so obvious and so inimical to the concept of self-determination that a series of favorable fictions naturally arise—including Lady Luck.

So they tell us. Yet even though nature may be indifferent to us, we can hardly be so in return. For, unlike apples or animals, we are uniquely equipped to perceive our role in nature. With the gift of self-consciousness, we alone are aware of our inevitable decline and death in life's cycle. It is our essential paradox. A union of opposites, caught between the beasts and the angels, we are unable to live as one or the other. Nor are we able to renounce either—to extinguish our godlike vision and spirit, or flee from the terror of life and the fear of death. In this predicament, we naturally seek to control what we may, and luck—or its many variants—serves handily to encapsulate and buffer all that cannot be controlled.

The concept of luck becomes an ongoing and often intense affair in the lives of millions. For them, it can be a real help, especially in bringing relief from the anxiety and dread of what our minds can conceive—yet may not see or control. That seems to be the minimum that most of them hope for: that luck ward off the unforeseen, the malevolent, and so help to create a small, safe margin for living—little more.

Jack Snyder, a lung cancer survivor, looked for his luck with that in mind. "A bit of good fortune, being lucky, is always needed, if for no other reason than not to fall victim to a confluence of bad breaks. Being lucky means the cosmos stays neutral."

However one may feel about this—about luck as a real or imagined force—we witness here a series of unforeseen and often unexplainable interventions in the lives of patients who believe that these events were crucial to their survival. Among them:

A 6-year-old boy, after nearly drowning, is x-rayed for residual water in the lungs—revealing a fast-growing tumor that threatened leg paralysis within a few weeks.

A New York policeman's lung cancer is discovered in a random, city-wide screening for lung disease—five months after his regular checkup showed he was in good health.

A commercial artist, with little chance for survival, makes a last minute phone call—leading him to a surgeon who did a pioneer operation that saved his life.

A young man, stricken with leukemia in Mexico is forced by a worried friend to board a plane for the United States—arriving by chance at Memorial Hospital twenty-four hours before a crisis that would otherwise have claimed his life.

These patients fight back, as do all other victors in this book. They differ, however, in believing that luck played a crucial or positive role in the initial phase of their illness. As a result, they seek to hold onto it—as did the New York cop—for continued support in their struggle to survive.

A housewife describes how she was able to "catch a lucky moment" in a run of a "special kind of luck" that enabled her and her husband to survive three attacks of cancer. A former pro-football player, feeling his luck turning against him, breaks loose like a gorilla in the operating room, seeking to find it again at a better moment. A medical student, close to death, recites a litany of lucky moments—before talking to "the Man Upstairs." A father, feeling his son's luck borders on the miraculous, reaches beyond it in his despair—turning to God for some answer and help.

None of this seems other than quite normal—given the world's back-handed belief in luck and the particularly profound crises in which these people find themselves. Whether or not they are all cognizant of the indifference of nature or the cosmos to their fate—as some indicate—they all do one thing in common:

Taking what faith they can, from whatever incident or source, each one makes a personal and supreme act of willing the improbable. This stance, based on aggression and even anger, says, "Nothing is going to kill me. I shall *not* submit."

At this point, one turns to the growing body of evidence that emotions can influence every human ailment. Through a mind-body link—described further in the introduction to the chapter "Self"—the emotional state is believed to affect the immunologic defense system directly and so influence the course of the disease.

Here we appear to have further evidence to support this concept. In the act of willing the improbable—strengthened by a belief in their luck or a faith in related forces—these patients may well have altered conditions affecting the course of their disease and, in doing so, to have triumphed over it.

We were out at Montauk fishing, and they have a pool out there. Joey—he was only 5 then—was at the pool with my wife, but then she left him to go and look at a shark they'd pulled up on the beach. When she got back, he was floating facedown in the water.

He's 41, his parents came from Italy, and he works as a longshoreman at the Brooklyn docks, checking cargo. "I worked hard all my life. I never knew any other way. I play the guitar, and I've been a part-time musician for twenty years. I was always away weekends, so I never saw my girls grow up because I led this very active life. I never rested. That's been part of my problem, not resting—that is, up until this happened to my little boy, Joey."

We are in the kitchen of the Igneri single family home in East Flatbush, New York. With us at the table is Joe's wife, Joanne.

JOANNE: *(Interrupts)* Wait a minute. I didn't leave him alone. I left him with my friend Shelley. I was in the lounge chair by the pool, and Shelley was on the steps going into the pool, sitting there with her own baby and my little Joey. They were all there together when I heard some shouting and saw them bringing in this big shark. You could see everything from the pool area, and I watched them hanging it up. Then I told Shelley I'd be right back and went down to look at that stupid shark. It was very big, and I decided to get Joey, so he could see it. Then I see Shelley, and she's out of the water with her baby. I said, "Shelley, where's Joseph?" She said, "Didn't he come down with you?" I said, "No, he was with you and the baby."

I began to run toward the pool. Then I saw him. He looked like a little boy swimming, except he wasn't moving. Just floating there, facedown in the water. I just knew it was him, and I remember screaming, "God, no!" *(Turns to Joe.)* You don't remember hearing it, but that's what made you turn around.

JOE: *(Interrupts)* It's possible I heard her, but I don't recall it. I remember turning on instinct. Something just told me to turn around, and I saw her, like a mask on her face, petrified with panic, just frozen there and doing nothing—and I knew something terrible was happening.

I ran up the beach and leaped over a fence by the pool. Coming down, I hit a lounge chair, and it nearly broke my back, and eventually I had to go to the hospital for two weeks.

Joanne is screaming like crazy, yelling Joey's name and pointing toward the pool. Her friend Shelley was back in the water, swimming toward the edge of the pool and shoving Joey in front of her. So when I got there, I reached down and grabbed him and threw him down on the concrete and began to try to resuscitate him.

I used the back pressure method they taught us in the Navy. I was working on him maybe thirty seconds—it seemed like thirty years—when the water came out of his mouth, and he jumped up, looking at us in shock, and I said, "My God, he's back."

An ambulance appeared, but with Joey now okay, there didn't seem to be any need for it. Then I had a sort of instinctive feeling, and said, "No, he's swallowed a lot of water, maybe we'd better check it out." So we brought him to the hospital—Southampton General. They took X rays to check for possible pneumonia development because of the water in him. Then the radiologist, Dr. McLaughlin, called me in to see the pictures. "There's a mass there," he said, showing me where it was located at the top of the lung. You could see how it had even twisted a tiny rib, bending it out of place. I thought, "My God, if this thing can bend a rib, it can kill him." I was afraid to say the word, and I asked the doctor, "You said it was a mass. What do you really mean?" He said, "It looks like a tumor, but don't get alarmed. It might be benign with a child this age. You can't tell." Then he gave me the X rays and said, "Take your little boy home and get a tumor specialist. Get the best you can find." You can imagine my shock. Suddenly this . . .

JOANNE: *(Interrupts)* Looking at him, you'd never have known it. He was a perfectly normal, active child. No symptoms of anything—nothing, zero. Extremely overactive, in fact. I mean, his back was as straight as a pin.

JOE: Yeah, always on bikes, fences, climb, jump—all over the place. And now this mass, sitting there inside him, a tumor bending his bones like it was going to take his life away while nobody knew anything about it.

So we took the X rays to my wife's Uncle Tony, who's director of radiology at Brooklyn Hospital. He ran a whole new series, and he said the first man had been right. It was a tumor, but he couldn't say whether it was malignant or benign. "It just might very well be benign," he said. "You can't tell, but you have to get yourselves ready in case it isn't." That meant we needed a top cancer surgeon, one specializing in pediatric surgery, and he arranged for us to go to Dr. Exelby at Memorial.*

Well, he looked at all the X rays and began his own series of tests,

---

* Philip R. Exelby, B.M., B.Ch., attending surgeon, chief of Pediatric Surgical Service, Department of Surgery, Memorial Hospital.

including a myelogram.† And that's when we learned the tumor had invaded his spinal column. It was that big. It went from the lungs to the spinal canal, so we were going to need another surgeon, Dr. Galicich, to work on the spinal cord.‡

JOANNE: *(Interjects)* That's when Joe and I got really scared. They told us not to worry. Dr. Galicich said, "You're lucky we discovered this now. It's fairly extensive, but I think we're in time to get it out okay." And Dr. Exelby said the tumor might be benign and not to worry until he operated and saw what was there. But Joe was upset, more than I was because I could stay at the hospital, while he had to run back and forth between the docks and Memorial, taking care of the girls at home, and getting no sleep.

JOE: By this time, I'm going crazy. Two surgeons are going to work on little Joey, one on the spinal column, and if anything goes wrong, if that's damaged, he'll be paralyzed in the legs for life.

This is my only son, and I keep thinking it's lights out for me. I'd go into his room at the hospital, trying not to let him see how I really felt—you know, kidding around like it was nothing. Joanne had bought him a lot of games and toys, and they have a great recreation room there for kids where he could play. Then he'd stop and look at me, his little dark eyes watching me, not saying anything, except those eyes were saying he knew something serious was happening—and how he trusted me, how he knew his Daddy would fix it up for him and take him home. He thought all his trouble came from falling in the deep water, and he would say, "I won't go in the deep water anymore, I promise, Daddy." Each time he'd say that, it would break me up. I'd have to go out of the room.

Finally the big day came. They operated on Joey early in the morning, and I got off work to be there with Joanne.

"While it was going on, we went across the street to pray in church. I was working on one thought—that all of this was a little miracle from God, his way of saving my son. Joey had fallen in two other swimming pools, one in our backyard and one at the neighbor's. Both times he'd been pulled out after only swallowing a little water, which was no big deal. But this third time at Montauk caused him to be brought to the hospital where the tumor was discovered. It was a big tumor, so it was there, growing larger, each time

---

† Electromyography (EMG)—a neurologic test, recording electrical activity in muscles and nerves, used to ascertain whether an illness directly affects the spinal cord, muscles, or peripheral nerves.

‡ Joseph H. Galicich, M.D., attending surgeon, chief of Neurosurgical Service, Department of Surgery, Memorial Hospital.

Joey fell into a pool. I told myself that this could only mean that God was helping me, trying to save Joey.

"In the church, I looked at an image of the Virgin Mary and began to pray. Many times, when I'm concentrated in prayer, I can see her face— smiling and understanding me. But this time I couldn't see her. There was no sign from her or anything else on how it was going with Joey. That scared me, and I went back to the hospital full of fear."

JOANNE: Dr. Galicich came to us first and said the operation was a success. He was able to get the tumor out of the spine. Then Dr. Exelby came and said it was all okay with him, too. But when Joe asked him if it was cancer or not, he told us he wouldn't be able to say until he'd had a final report the next day.

JOE: The operation was something to write up in scientific journals. Dr. Galicich opened up the spine and got hold of two vital nerves to free them from the tumor. It had even grown onto a nerve root, and he got that free, too. That's how he saved Joey. In fact, he said it was just in time. If the tumor had pushed any further into the spine, Joey would have become a paraplegic, paralyzed in the legs.

Exelby went into the lung, working on the other side of Joey, taking his part of the tumor out of the chest. Then they both worked on the middle part, and in the end, they'd made a tunnel through Joey, so they could see each other from one side to the other. The tumor was that big, from front to back. Of course, they didn't tell us all this right away. We learned it later.

JOANNE: The next day came the bad news. There were some scattered cancer cells in the tumor, and Joey was going to need to take a chemotherapy cure to make sure those cells didn't start it all over again.

JOE: That's when I flipped out. It wasn't benign like they'd said it might be, like we'd hoped. God's miracle wasn't working, it was an illusion because Joey wasn't anywhere near being saved. He had cancer, and he was going to have the poison stuff shot into him until he was like other kids we'd seen coming in—no hair, no eyebrows, their bodies all thin and brittle and white, looking at you like they were haunted. *(Shakes head.)* Yeah, like being haunted. We'd had a great surgical team, they'd done the best possible, probably better than anywhere else in the world—and we were still behind a goddamn eight ball. No, I just flipped out.

I got so locked up with this that I couldn't even talk to my wife. She felt guilty in one way, and I felt it, too, but couldn't talk about it. I didn't know that parents of children with cancer tend to blame each other. They take it out on the partner, their feeling of guilt and anger. There's a very high divorce rate among parents whose kids have cancer. If they had something wrong before it happened, it'll come out in a big way with the cancer problem.

Quite frankly, we're not much different than many other couples. We've had our troubles, and now they really began to seem too much to handle, with both of us shut off from the other.

JOANNE: *(Laughs)* He'd sit up at night reading the Bible. He didn't say what he was reading. He wouldn't even talk to me, like I just didn't exist. So I began to talk to a social worker at the hospital, and he went to Father Zona.

JOE: In a crisis, you can seek help from your friends, and they can say, "Sure, I know how you feel. It's really rough." But that doesn't give you the strength you need to lean on. You need something more, to rekindle your faith in your religion. At least I felt that way.

So I went to our parish priest, Father Zona. He'd helped me before in our marriage. He was the kind of person you admired. Like your favorite baseball player or football coach, you've got your favorite minister. I said to him, "Why is all this happening? I thought it was a miracle, but it's not. If there's a God and He is good, why does this happen to an innocent child?"

Father Zona had just been mugged in broad daylight—at a traffic light in his own parish. It was the first time for him, and he was shaken by it. So at first he said, "We all ask that question. Why me? Why a little child? Why an innocent mother wronged or a crook rewarded?" He then said, "There's no answer to the question—no direct or immediate one. But after a while, even if we don't learn exactly why, we are often rewarded in another way, a way we could never have foreseen." I asked him for an example, and he said, "Well, take my being robbed, my anger at what happened to me, a priest, in my own car, in the middle of my parish. This could be telling me a lot of things, not only about people who are driven to do that, but also about myself, to help me remember my mission, to see that my sorrow and anger is nothing compared to yours for your son. And how our sorrows are nothing compared to that of a Man who died for us all—or to millions of other men and women who have suffered and died for their families, their country, or for ideals that you and I believe in."

I asked him how a child afflicted with cancer could be rewarding in any way, and he said, "I don't know, nor do you. But maybe you'll see it someday. Maybe not. Anyway, you said you believed Joey's falling in the pool was a miracle—a gift from God. Maybe He has more in the pipeline for you."

After that, we prayed together, and I felt a little better. But it didn't give me an answer to my question until about six weeks after Joey came home.

He was wearing a metal brace until his spine grew back in place, and he'd lost his hair and eyebrows in the chemo treatment. Dr. Galicich said that maybe Joey would be a bit wobbly on his feet because of the spine operation. But he was walking fine and straight, and he was riding a bike, too. So I decided to test his coordination with a bit of stickball.

We went out in the back, and I began to toss the ball at him. *(Laughs, shakes head.)* You've never seen anything like it—a 6-year-old kid connecting every time, even with that metal brace on him! He was laughing each time he beaned the ball, and I began to laugh, too. Suddenly I realized that maybe God was on our side, that Joey was really being saved, that he would get well—and this was the reward that Father Zona had talked about. I was having fun with my kid, laughing with him and getting a real thrill from it. I was closer to my son now, closer to my daughters, and to my wife.

Maybe it comes when you stop being angry with God, or maybe after you've gotten angry and figured it out a little bit, so you're no longer angry with your wife or even yourself. Anyway, it's been six years now, Joey's strong and well, and we're all okay—except I've changed. I don't know exactly what it is, but I don't feel the urge to play the guitar on weekends —that is, play for other people, like I used to. I'd rather stay home now, watch my kids grow up, and play a bit for them.

When I tell people I had lung cancer, they look at me like, "You gotta be kidding." They don't believe it because the first thing you think about, what comes to everyone's mind when you mention cancer, is death. They say, "You really had it?" I tell them, "You think I'd make up something like that? Do I look crazy?"

He's 54, with large hands and the face of a onetime boxer—dark eyes recessed under heavy brows, wide cheekbones, a broad nose, and large mouth. A New York policeman for twenty-five years, he has recently retired and now works as bartender and headwaiter in a private club.

We're in the ground-floor living room of the Ciccarelli duplex in Yonkers, New York, whose second floor is occupied by one of their three daughters. Pat's wife, Vita, brings in coffee and a homemade coconut cake.

I was in the street crime unit on Randalls Island when this circular comes floating through the department, and I just happened to see it. They wanted volunteers for a lung program to detect cancer in a cross section of the population—including policemen. You had to be over 45 and a cigarette smoker. I'd smoked for thirty years, a couple packs a day—maybe more because you don't count when you're playing cards or drinking and partying.*

It was a take it or leave it proposition. I told myself. "You don't need this. You had an X ray five months ago, and it was okay—why get into another hassle?" So I pushed it aside and forgot about it. Then I happened across it again in a free moment, and on an impulse, I signed up. That was my lucky moment because, if I'd been as busy as usual, it might never have happened. I had no ill effects from smoking—you know, the smoker's hacking cough. None of that business. No chest pains or anything. I considered myself in good health for a guy my age, and still do. Maybe I'd get winded from smoking, but I was always active, playing softball or anything else. No problems.

So because of all that, I wasn't too worried when they called me to come in for the X ray at the Lung Program Center in the Strang Clinic on 34th Street. Well, damn if it didn't show a spot on my lung about the size of a

---

* The American Cancer Society estimates that cigarette smoking is responsible for 83 percent of lung cancer cases among men and 43 percent among women—more than 75 percent over all. It is estimated that in 1984, lung cancer will exceed breast cancer as a leading cause of death from cancer among women.

nickel. So they sent me up to Memorial Hospital for more tests by a radiologist.

He messed around with me for over an hour, trying to get a piece of it out of my lung, using a long needle guided by an x-ray screen. Either because of my muscle structure back there, or maybe because I was breathing when you're supposed to hold your breath—whatever it was, he didn't get it. He couldn't get the needle into the small spot.

Finally, they called Dr. Martini, and once again I was in luck, only I didn't know how lucky I was.† Martini is the hospital's top thoracic surgeon, and by chance, he wasn't operating or tied up. So he came down right away. He's a very quiet, laid-back sort of guy—but also very smart. He looks at my X rays on a glass with a light behind them, and he says to the radiologist, "You see? The lung program's worthwhile." Then he turns to me and says, "You're a lucky man." I said, "Lucky? What the hell's lucky about this? I'd be lucky if I didn't have the damn thing." He said, "Maybe, but you're lucky to know about it now, before it's any bigger." So I thought, "Maybe he's right. You gotta know how to read your luck. Mine started when I signed up for the lung program."

I didn't know at the time, but he'd seen enough on the X ray to know what it was—except he wasn't telling me until he was certain. So he said, "I don't want you to go home. I want you to stay here so we can get a clearer picture of this."

I'd taken a couple hours off work to go to the clinic. My wife didn't even know I was at Memorial, and everything was happening too fast. So I said, "Why can't I go home and come back? What's the matter, Doc? You think I'll take a powder?" He laughed and said, "No, I'm going on vacation, and if we both go away, I'll worry about it. I don't want to worry—okay?" I said, "Okay." So they had me admitted to the hospital and put in an upstairs room.

The next day they did a lot more tests. By this time, my wife, Vita, had come—also my daughters. They tried to pretend it was nothing, that it wasn't cancer, but I could see they were really worried. It was in their eyes. The mouth can say one thing, with the eyes saying something else. That's how it was, me getting this double-talk between words and eyes. Because they loved me, they were saying it was all okay, but their eyes were full of fear that I had lung cancer—and that maybe I was going to die.

---

† Nael Martini, M.D., attending surgeon, chief of Thoracic Service, Department of Surgery, Memorial Hospital.

*Vita interrupts: "Come on, Pat. I kept telling you that your mother had
cancer and got well. She did all right. She had half her stomach cut away
when she was 25, and now she's 87 and still okay—except for that broken
hip that makes it hard for her to walk. That was all true, it wasn't any
double-talk."*

Okay, okay, but frankly that didn't help much. In fact, it made me more
pessimistic because I knew lung cancer was the biggest killer—far more
than the stomach.‡

Anyway, Dr. Martini comes in the next day and says, "We're not totally
sure what that spot is, but it doesn't belong there, and it has to come out."
I figured he knew from the tests that it was probably malignant, but he
wasn't telling me because he didn't know for sure. Then he says, "In a day
or two, I'm going on vacation for a couple weeks, so we'll take it out when
I get back."

I was a little upset at this, and I said, "Wait a minute. If I've been so
damn lucky, let's take this out while we're ahead of the game. Why risk
losing everything while you're out of town?" He laughed a little, and I
said, "I don't want to go home and stew around for two weeks with this—
cancer." I waited for him to say that I was jumping to conclusions, that
maybe I didn't have cancer. But he only nodded, and that's how I knew
what he really thought. Then he agreed to try and squeeze me into his
schedule before leaving.

After he'd gone, I felt I was right. If I was going to survive, now was my
chance. Also, I didn't want to go home and face more of it—more people,
especially those I loved, trying to be brave and full of cheer, but unable to
hide their fears that I was a goner. I was very upset, needless to say. I
didn't know what the hell to think except that maybe I was going to die—
and, if it had to happen, damn it, let's get it over with. Yeah, I was crying
and everything.

Dr. Martini finally said okay, he could do me, and the next day they put
me through some tests prior to operating. Also, they tell you what to
expect and what you have to do afterward. You'll have to force yourself to
cough up phlegm, you'll have tubes draining your chest, you'll feel pain
and discomfort in breathing—but the more you force yourself through the
paces, the sooner it'll be over.

That night before the operation, I was alone, waiting for the next morning. A priest came by, a nice guy, and we had a talk. Then I got to

---

‡ Among males, lung cancer takes the greatest toll—34 percent of all cancer deaths,
against 4 percent for stomach cancer.

thinking that people were no longer close to each other like they should be. They'd lost contact—parents with kids, with their neighbors, with other people on the job, and with God maybe. That's why the world is going to hell in a basket.

"We'd lost it, too—the police, I mean. The old foot patrol knew everyone in the neighborhood. They could help the widows, the old people, the young kids, and they also helped the detectives sometimes. But they were disbanded for squad car patrols. Now how in the hell can you know a neighborhood from a squad car? Same thing with the detective squads. They were taken out of the boroughs, where they knew every alley and crap game, and put inside one headquarters. So now you got a guy from Brooklyn, stationed in Manhattan—and what the hell does he know about the Bronx?

"The way it is now, nothing's holding together. Take street crime. We got 10- and 12-year-old kids running around with guns all over the place. They've seceded from the union, from the human race, and the courts don't know how to bring them back, or what to do with them. The correctional homes are goddamn zoos.

"Never mind the kids, the courts can't even handle the other bums. There are so many, they let them plea-bargain to get rid of them. A guy with a gun or knife takes your money, and that's armed robbery—a felony which could bring a stiff sentence. But to speed it up, they're allowed to plead guilty to petty larceny—and back they go to the streets, mugging and pushing heroin. So you're back to square one, only now they know you—and maybe you're on a hit list.

"Then there's that other bunch of cancer cells running loose in the city— the welfare people who're turning the Bronx into a goddamn jungle. I was born there, it was a nice place with A-one buildings. My mother's still there and won't move, even though they're burning the place down around her. Okay, some landlords burn for the insurance money because their property's going downhill. But mostly it's done by the Spanish-speaking families— who're living off welfare. If you're burnt out, the city pays for you to move, for new clothes and new furniture. So it's a business, from generation to generation, people who've never worked. Okay, these people have very special problems adjusting to our society, and some of them on welfare really need it—but many of them don't. You see them driving up to the welfare office at 161st Street in Cadillacs and everything. They're living a better life than I am. If their rent's four hundred dollars, they pay one hundred and the state pays the rest—and nobody's doing a damn thing about trimming off the fat.

"That's how I saw it, lying there in the hospital. It's not just the cops— everybody's riding around in some kind of a squad car, if you know what I mean. We're closed off, when we ought to be walking again, getting to know

each other better. How the hell are you gonna do it, beats me. Maybe the city has to get as sick as I was then, not knowing whether I was going to live or die, before it'll do something or accept some radical surgery. And maybe like me, if it waits too long, it'll be too late."

The next morning, Dr. Martini operated on me. I don't know how long I was down there, but it was a long time because I stayed in intensive care overnight. To make sure he got it all out, he removed one entire lobe of my left lung. The rest of the left and the right lung were okay. But the cancer had already begun to spread, and he found microscopic particles of it in some lymph glands. So he also took them out. He showed me on the X ray how he tied off the little veins with tiny silver clips.*

I said, "It's strange how I never had any pain or anything." And he said, "You're a lucky guy. In a couple more months, you would have had pain, but then it would have been too late because it would have spread." He also told me, "You're also double lucky in getting on that lung program and in being called early instead of late."

They gave me some radiation—not much, about 4,000 rads—and for a while I took a cytotoxin pill every day. After that, nothing.

It's been seven years now. I have no troubles, except when it rains or the weather's changing, and I feel some chest pains where he made the incisions. Dr. Martini kids me, says, "If you don't have that, how're you going to remember me?" He's one helluva fellow. He saved my life, but like he says, I was also lucky to be on that lung program. If I had waited for the once a year checkup, I'd probably be dead today.

I think about that sometimes. Not that I'm living on borrowed time, but more like I was given some extra time to realize how much my family means to me—how much everybody should mean to everybody else. How we ought to get closer to each other, help each other in some way, instead of going it all alone with a needle or a gun—or looking at people you're supposed to help from a squad car.

---

* Pat Ciccarelli had adenocarcinoma, which accounts for 40 percent of all lung cancers. Three other prevalent types are epidermoid or squamous cell carcinoma, with 35 percent of all cases, large cell carcinoma, 10 percent, and a small cell or oat cell carcinoma, 15 percent —this being the most deadly, generally found in heavy cigarette smokers as are most other types of lung cancer.

Luck plays such a major role in anybody's life. It's one thing you don't usually consider, but our lives are as random as hell. I get well, and the next guy dies. Can you really say why? If you consider the time of my existence and the space I occupy, the species that I belong to, the body I exist in, the exquisite circumstances that would produce a tumor on my right kidney, the warning blood that appeared, no doctor at all, then the right doctor to recommend a great surgeon who, in turn, operated on me at Memorial, then the love, the need, and so on—all of this, as far as I can see, is just a series of random events. It's anybody's luck, or whatever you want to call it.

He's 72 but looks much younger—receding gray hair, soft brown eyes, a bristling white Hapsburg mustache, and the virile look of an aging athlete. "Yep, I played football at Northwestern, then was quarterback with the Chicago Bears for a year, until I maimed both my knees. They couldn't repair that sort of thing then, so I went to work eventually as an artist, doing fashion sketches for Marshall Field's in Chicago. I did illustrations for McCall's, Ladies' Home Journal, *you name it. Then, at* Esquire, *I did their pinup girls for several years. That's when I realized how much of the world lives on fantasy. I'd get letters from guys all over the place—Korea, Africa, Jordan—asking, 'Is that girl engaged?' or 'Is that a real ring?' or 'We think you probably draw these girls in the nude, then put clothes on them—do you really?' They expected me to reply, 'Of course, I draw them nude, screw them, then turn them loose!' "* (Laughs.)

We are in the study of his home at Lakeville, Connecticut. Outside the bay window, a private pond is teeming with wild birds, drawn by nesting poles near the water. He points out starlings, blackbirds, wood ducks, a bluebird, and an angry red-tailed hawk. His wife, Mary Moore—a tall, erect woman with white hair—can be seen on the lawn, nervously watching the hawk. Al Moore says, "Today is special. It's our forty-seventh wedding anniversary."

Listen, I'm not saying I lay back and trusted luck to lick the cancer, because I didn't. I'm a member of a successful species that fights to live. Over the centuries, we have developed new and elaborate procedures, including surgery, to prolong life. It's like breathing. You can't intellectualize it—you simply do it to live. If something threatens to cut it off, you fight back with all you've got. That's what happened to me after the first paralyzing shock when I thought I was going to die.

I took a leak and passed nothing but blood. A woman's used to the sight of blood, but it's a most frightening thing for a man. I stopped when I saw what was happening, which of course didn't do any good. I went back to my office and looked out the window at the street below, thinking, "I could lift that and dive out, now's a good time." Then it was as if there was another person there, a second one, looking at me, saying, "Don't be ridiculous. What the hell are you trying to do—fink out?"

I went to the phone and called our house doctor. He fumbled around and finally sent me to Flower Fifth Avenue Hospital. This was very early in the morning, and I sat there until eleven o'clock. Nobody came to see me, a nurse or anyone. I didn't know what to do, and I was afraid to urinate because I'd see blood again.

Then I remembered an old fraternity brother from college—Dr. Guy Robbins, who I knew was at Memorial.* So I put a nickel in the phone and was lucky enough to catch him. He said, "Al, it doesn't sound good. So, I'll tell you what to do. Put your clothes back on and walk out of the hospital—then come on over to Memorial Hospital." *(Laughs.)*

So that's what I did, and Guy had it all set up with Dr. Whitmore.† He was just a young man then but considered a genius and an absolute whiz in his field, urology. They did a lot of tests and saw I had a very large tumor on the kidney.

Somewhere along the line, they decided to try a new operating technique, a new method of getting at the kidney. Instead of going in through the loin, they planned to go down through the thorax, the chest, because it would give them a clearer field to tie off the tumor and clean up everything linked to it. That's how I understood it. It meant taking out one or two ribs, so they would have a thoracic surgeon, Dr. Pool.‡ He would make the first opening, then Whitmore would take over and go after the tumor. My fraternity brother, Guy Robbins, was going to be there as an observer only, since his specialty was breast surgery. I asked Guy, "If they've never done this before, why do I have to be the guinea pig?" He said, "It'll give them greater ability to clean out the whole tumor." In short, he recommended it for guinea pigs, and me.* *(Laughs.)*

---

* Guy F. Robbins, M.D., then attending surgeon, now consultant, Breast Service, Department of Surgery, Memorial Hospital.

† Willet F. Whitmore, Jr., M.D., attending surgeon, chief of Urology Service, Department of Surgery, Memorial Hospital.

‡ John L. Pool, M.D., then attending surgeon, now consultant, Thoracic Service, Department of Surgery, Memorial Hospital.

* This was the first thoracoabdominal radical nephrectomy to be performed at Memorial Hospital—an innovative procedure in 1949—although it had been performed a year earlier

When you're facing something like this, you prepare for the worst, with all the symbols of returning to the earth. You make out a will for your wife, your children, your husband, your lover—whatever. You give instructions on what to do with your possessions, and the spare parts of your body, whether you want to be buried or cremated, and so on. By that time, you need some sort of emotional way through it.

My defense was to mentally remove myself, as though I was two people with one of them watching me, to see how I was going to react to this. It was sort of a challenge between myself, who I thought I was, and whoever I might be under such a trial. So as they prepared me for the operation, I kept psyching myself into thinking I was two people. One was about to be operated on, and then there was me *(laughs)* who was watching this to see if I turned fink and, for example, reverted to religion at the last minute. You understand what I mean? It was a chance to see what was there. If I was going to die, would I find I was a hypocrite underneath it all?

Before the operation, my Dracula nurse came, and instead of taking more blood, she put stuff into me. So with this dope working on me, I set my mind to watch myself as they rolled me down to the operating room and put me into position on the table.

Everybody was in green with masks, and while getting ready, they seemed quite jolly and full of talk as the surgeons came in, holding up their washed hands, getting the gloves pulled on—and there I was, lying there on the line. I remember the anesthetist saying, "Oh, you'll like this" —then putting a mask over my face. I could see the light above me, and hear the anesthetic being metered out, going "ding . . . ding . . . ding."

Are you aware of the London Records album with FFRR on the cover? It has the same sound for an approaching train. So I was lying there, convinced I was two people with one of me watching over everything, while this "ding . . . ding . . . ding," was like a railroad train coming closer and closer toward me. I thought, "My luck's running out—that damn train's gonna hit me any minute. Am I going to take this crap, or do something about it?"

I decided to get the hell out of there before the train hit me, so I pulled off the mask and sat up. The anesthetist tried to grab me, but I knocked him to the side and started for the door.

I don't remember a thing, but they say I came charging through like I was back with the Chicago Bears in a line of scrimmage. I was still in

---

by the Australian surgeon, Henry Mortensen. The previous procedure was to go through the flank or the chest. The new approach, opening both chest and abdominal cavity, allowed for larger exposure of the diseased area and greater ability to resect it.

pretty good shape then. They had to call in other people from the hall to bring me down. *(Laughs.)* It was a great scene, but it blew the operation, and they had to reschedule it for that afternoon.

When they finally did it, I came out the same way, on the same layer of consciousness, and started fighting again. The nurse said, "You're going to hurt yourself," and called in some others. So, they tied my arms down until I had time to emerge from the effect of the drugs and realize I was acting like a damn fool, since I could very well hurt myself.

"The tumor was larger than the kidney. They showed it to me some five weeks later at a conference of doctors that had been called to evaluate this new procedure. Whitmore showed slides, and the doctors questioned me. At this point, I guess you can call the operation a success since it happened thirty-two years ago, and I haven't had any trouble from it or any cancer since then."

They sent me home seven days after the operation. I told Whitmore it was too damn soon. With a rib gone, I had trouble breathing. He said, "Your chart says you're okay and fit to start running for a touchdown somewhere else." *(Laughs.)* I said, "Doc, you cut me halfway around my body. How can you send me away with such a big cut?" He laughed and told me, "Don't worry, you heal from side to side, not lengthwise. A long one heals as fast as a little one." *(Laughs.)* I think he also felt secure about my leaving then, because my wife is a voluntary nurse and could care for me. Also, they needed the bed. They always need the beds at Memorial. People from all over the world want to get in there.

My wife drove me to Kent, Connecticut, and I was a wreck when we got home—but I picked up fast. I had to because I was doing advertising work in New York, and they were on top of me, hollering for layout projects. After leaving *Esquire,* I'd come to New York as a fashion artist for Galey & Lord, at that time a very famous cotton manufacturer.

So I picked up where I'd left off the day I found I was bleeding—barely a month later. But now it wasn't the same. Nothing was the same anymore, though I wasn't aware of it right away, probably because I was still under the shadow of cancer. I had to check with Whitmore every month, then every six months to make sure I was free of a recurrence. Gradually, as I pulled free of it, free of losing my other kidney or of the disease grabbing me somewhere else, I began to realize that something big had happened to me.

I'd come through this thing whole, I'd been given back the gift of life— but I wasn't doing anything with it. I was on the same old treadmill, and I wanted off. Life had to have some other meaning for me, other than selling another man's merchandise. I began to think about doing something of my own, something that might endure longer than a fashion sketch.

"I remembered the first time I met Billy Rose. I was standing by his desk after being introduced, and he said, 'I started out to make six million dollars, I've made that and eighteen more. You see that Rembrandt over there? It's mine.' I didn't know what the hell he was talking about. Then he said, 'The most money I ever made was with the Aquacade. Those girls in their tank suits, you could actually see the outline of their genitals, their nipples and everything. But we always had a row reserved for the clergy, free of charge. That's the way to go. They'll accept that. Nobody'll bitch as long as there's an excuse for it.' Then I realized he was telling me a great truth. If you don't stake it out, if you don't envisage what you want, you can never get much of anything.

"Then I gave him one for his books. There had been one helluva windstorm that day and he says, 'I see you come from Connecticut. How many trees did you lose?' Again, I didn't know what the hell he meant. I was looking around and saw a row of pills on his desk, thousands of them. He was writing in shorthand, faster than I could talk, and I knew he'd been secretary to great men like Bernard Baruch before going into show business. In fact, he'd won the national shorthand championship with a broken hand, holding a pen stuck into a potato.

"Suddenly, he says, 'For chrissake how many trees did you lose? I lost a thousand in my place at Mount Kisco.' I said, 'Well, Mr. Rose, if you don't own any trees, you don't lose any.' He looked at me like I was crazy, then broke out laughing. He'd come up hungry, running fast, from the Lower East Side. I guess it was the first time he ever heard that acquiring things— thousands of trees, pills, chorus girls, sculpture, or whatever—might not be as good as having none of them."

In this period of indecision, of knowing I wanted something else, I began to think about doing sculpture. I always liked working with materials, and I began to experiment with various forms. But whatever I did always seemed to assume a shape that enclosed space. So I began to think about creating a universal frame or skeleton that could be adapted to any human use. If you look at any skeleton, you see it is adapted to the use expected of it. For example, your human skeleton can stand and walk upright, or run or sit down, and so forth. A horse is something else, and so is a snake.

Then one day I fell across it—a concept for a universal frame structure which could assume any size and cost little to build or heat. It's like a fishnet with triangular webbing, made of metal or wood, and built on a double curve like a parabola or a dome. Most building starts with the box, but mine are natural forms like your skull or an egg or a melon. You can see in the evolution of all nature's forms that the best way to contain volume and protection is either tubular or double curved. Take an egg. You can poke a hole in it, but you can't very well crush it. Many of the problems in construction deal with crushing forces—exterior and interior. So the curved form is stronger, cheaper—and uses less fuel.

I've done a number of homes, factories, and a warehouse. The idea is catching on; a Swedish firm is going to use them, and the *New York Times* wrote it up.

I'm very excited about all this. I've created a sculpture form that people can live in, work in. I feel like I'm doing something of value, which I didn't feel before. In school there was always the feeling that, in doing good work as an artist, you were somebody of intrinsic worth. I have that feeling again. I don't know how I managed to live so long without it.

Listen, we've had it three times with us. First, my husband, Phil, had a malignant tumor in his kidney thirteen years ago. We never told him what it was. I felt if he knew, it would finish him. So I told the doctors if they let him know, I'd kill them. *(Laughs.)* Then I got it in the uterus, and he got it again in the throat. Now we're free of it, thank God. We had the best doctors in the world, we love each other like crazy, we've been fighting to do what we want all our lives—but to come through this three times, and come out a winner, let me tell you, you've got to have some special kind of luck going for you.

She is seated in a wicker chair on the veranda of her seaside home at Guilford, Connecticut. She's blond, 53, and a bit overweight. Yet she has the assurance of a woman who has been good-looking all her life. Told this, she laughs, "Come on, I look like hell—what do you expect?"

It had been a hectic week—the first one in the Turitzes' newly acquired home. She had brought in new furniture from New York, dealt with the servants and the gardener, and earlier that afternoon had received a first cautious visit from her neighbors—two ladies from the traditionally WASP community of Guilford. The Turitzes are Jews. "The previous owner was Jewish," Arlynne says. "I don't see any problems there."

No problems, that is, compared to the ones that Phillip and Arlynne Turitz have overcome defeating cancer three times while climbing upward from the Seventh Avenue clothing district to this stately old manor by the sea. With a large residence in Englewood, New Jersey, already in their possession, the summer home is Arlynne's dream come true. She puts down her wine glass and throws open her arms. "I can't believe it! I keep waiting for the ax to fall any minute!"

Below us lies a small harbor with joggling boats. Beyond the jetty, a scattering of sails lean into the wind at different intervals. Seagulls soar in a blue sky, their high-pitched, lonely cries borne landward by a soft breeze off the sea.

Phil's tumor was thirteen years ago, more or less. I can't remember exact dates the way some people do. I can remember faces and what was said, and how close it was to something else, but not the exact day and year.

Overnight, he had a pain, and so into the hospital and the next thing, the doctors say, "He's got a tumor in his kidney. It's not a cyst, it's a tumor. We have to take out the kidney." I knew Phil would fall apart if he knew he had cancer. So I decided to not tell him, at least until after the operation, and I told the doctor not to reveal it.

Well, it was a clear-cell adenocarcinoma, luckily encapsulated in the kidney. They took the whole thing out, and there was no need for follow-up treatment. So I told Phil he had a nephrectomy, a kidney removal, and nothing more. I told everyone else, "I'll kill the first person who tells him anything." *(Laughs.)* Finally, he got it into his head that he lost his kidney from drinking too much coffee, though I don't know what he really thought. God knows, I never told him that he had cancer or that it was malignant.

He got better, and I thought that was the end of it—except it wasn't. You see, he'd been a cutter in the garment business all his life, and he hated it. So he had chucked it all to become a salesman—anything but a cutter. To do it, we had moved from Connecticut back to New York, heavily in debt. My God, what a scene! When he got sick, he was just finding his way as a coat salesman—a really lousy job for him.

When he went back to work, after losing his kidney, our local doctor said, "Listen, Mrs. Turitz, do not have a baby. For five years, do not buy a bigger house. And for God's sake don't let your husband go into business, because for five years, you will never know. This is a very sticky thing."

I believed him. Dr. Vogel, Arthur Vogel, was a good man, a wonderful man, everybody in Englewood loved him. Anyway, two weeks later Phil comes home one night and says, "Listen, I'm going into business." I say, "I don't believe it!" He says, "Don't you have any confidence in me?" How could I tell him Dr. Vogel had said not to go into business? He still didn't know he was recovering from cancer. So I said, "That's very nice, I'm very pleased. But, honey, we'll have to borrow money for this, and you're still all taped up from surgery. Maybe we'd better wait until some other time."

Of course that didn't stop him. He said, "We have to borrow five thousand dollars. That's all we need to get the business going." We had a house, but we didn't have five thousand dollars cash. Raymond Naptali, the man he'd taken in as partner, already had his share of the money, so we began to gather up our share. Some people cosigned notes, some lent us five hundred dollars or less. I tell you, we scrounged to our last nickel—still owing the doctors, still owing the hospital. By now, it was impossible to tell him about the cancer. He wanted this, and I thought, "To hell with it. Let him do it. It's his life." That's where we were lucky again. If I hadn't lied to him, I would have told him what Vogel said—and we might never have caught the lucky moment when it all began to happen for us.

At the time, I was working at Columbia Presbyterian Medical Center as Dr. Dana Atchley's secretary. He was one of the most famous internists in the world, so I asked him, "Our doctor says Phil shouldn't go into business or take any risks for five years." Dr. Atchley said, "There's no courage in that. You let him do what he wants."

So we did, and at first it was very rough. Each partner—there was a third one by then—was drawing only a hundred dollars a week. We weren't doing so well. We could hardly pay the rent. Then, all of a sudden, by the end of the first year, they were doing fine, and now, twelve years later, my husband and his partners have rolled themselves into a forty-million dollar business. It's called Peabody House. . . .

"So Phil built his business without ever knowing he had cancer—or that he wasn't supposed to risk what he was doing. Then, after a year and a half, the boys decided to take out insurance, in case one died. You have to do that if you're in business. So they all applied, and Phil got an application form. It asked: 'Did you ever have surgery?' Phil wrote: Yes. 'What was wrong with you?' Phil wrote: Nephrectomy, because I told him it was that. 'Did you ever have cancer?' No. 'Are you in good shape?' Yes, 100 percent.

"Well, of course he was put in a nationwide dropout pool immediately. When the other two guys got their insurance, they learned Phil had been rejected because he had had cancer. They didn't know what to do about that. Should they tell him or not? Finally, they decided to say nothing.

"Then one day, Phil is poking through the bookkeeping system and sees his partners have insurance, but he doesn't. So he says, 'Hey, what's this?' They said, 'Well, Phil, we didn't know how to tell you, or who to talk to. We didn't want to ask Arlynne, but they said you had cancer.' 'Me?' he shouts. 'You're crazy!' Then he phones me from the office. 'Arlynne! Did I have cancer?' He was screaming. I said, 'Well, yes, you did.' " (Laughs.) *" 'Why didn't you tell me?' he asks, and I said, 'What good would it have done? It would have sickened you.' So he found out a year and a half later and never had a minute's discomfort over it."*

Then I got it, about four years later. I began to feel a loss of energy and thought I was having a change of life. I always have a very high energy level and feel terrific, but now I was logy. So I went to the local doctor in Englewood. I wasn't too worried. The bleeding and all that is not important in the natural phenomena of a woman's menstrual cycle. But I felt something was off.

The doctor said, "Listen, you need a D&C. Go right to the hospital this minute." So I went to the little Englewood hospital, and the next morning it was done. In the late afternoon, flowers came, friends came, and everything was swell.

Around about ten o'clock that night, Dr. Saphier, the local doctor, came into my room and said, "Listen, I hear you are very strong—you have cancer." "Acchh!" I said. "Am I going to die?" I remember that moment. He said, "No, you're not going to die, we're going to take care of it. You need a hysterectomy right away." I said, "Is that so?"—without knowing what I was saying.

After he left, I was all alone, and I didn't call anyone. I looked out the window and saw my brand-new Mercedes in the parking lot. I can't believe this! There was maybe a hundred miles on her—the first time in my life I have a Mercedes. Anyway, the next morning an oncologist told Phil, "She has a very rare thing called a hydatidiform mole." This little guy in Englewood! One in eight thousand women get it, and this remote doctor spots it right away! How's that for luck? Then he said, "There's a fellow by the name of John Lewis* over at Sloan-Kettering who's a specialist in this. He's done more research on it than anybody. If he'll have you, I think you should go there."

So they called John Lewis, and he said, "Sure, bring her down." That was Friday, and Sunday morning they had a bed for me, and I went over there. It was in the old wing of Memorial Hospital, an ugly place with a bare light bulb in the ceiling and eight in a room.† So dismal, and nobody talks about how you feel. They say, "Well, where have you got it?" That's some way to have a dialogue with people!

I perked everybody up and told them that we're all going to be fine and also I couldn't wait to meet this John Lewis. But he didn't come until the day before surgery, and before I knew it, the surgery was over.

I had chemotherapy before surgery and also afterward. Toward the end of the week, I was lying in bed, thinking, "My hair doesn't look pretty today, I need a touch-up." I have wonderful hair. I do nothing to it, and it just grows. Not that it looks so great, but it gives me no grief. So I was feeling better and began to brush my hair. Acchh! With one brush, a whole section lifted off. What is this? I thought if I pull it, everything will come off. So I didn't do anything. The nurse said, "You're going to lose your hair." I said, "You're telling me?" It was coming out at the roots!

I didn't take it too seriously, even though it was shocking because the next morning all the hair was gone—gone! Then my husband, who's not a shopper and seldom buys me anything, you know what he did? So touching. Bought me a wig. Went to a shop with my daughter and bought one of

---

* John L. Lewis, Jr., M.D., chief attending surgeon, Gynecological Service, Memorial Hospital. "Sloan-Kettering" is a common euphemism for Memorial Hospital, which is part of the Memorial Sloan-Kettering Cancer Center.

† The new Memorial wing, with a 565-bed facility, has modern rooms, each with one or two beds.

those thirty-five-dollar numbers off the hook. I was so touched, and it was so needed. I put the wig on my head and didn't look back.

After I went home, I got some kind of terrible infection and had to go back to the hospital. I wasn't depressed about it. I had a lot of living to do, and I got rid of it. But the treatment went on and on. A year later, I'm still doing chemotherapy. Three times I went bald, first in the hospital, then twice later. I was nine times in the hospital during four years.

At first, I came every two weeks to see Dr. Lewis, and he used to interview me. "How do you feel?" "Marvelous!" But one time I remember telling him that I'm Jewish, and I feel like the women collaborators during the war, that I was being punished from the past. He said, "Foolish girl, that means the treatment is working." You know, he's a man who always knew the right thing to say, and I hung onto his words. Whenever I felt that I needed something, it's incredible how I heard it from him. He said, "You're going to be okay," and I believed him. I wanted to, I guess.

We'd planned to go to a New Year's Eve dinner, at one hundred dollars a ticket. I'd just had chemotherapy, was feeling fine, but I was afraid to spend the money. We were going with another couple, so it was four hundred dollars. I called Dr. Lewis and said, "Am I going to be alive and well? It's a hundred dollars apiece." He laughed and told me, "Go right ahead and get it."

One day he saw my diamond ring and immediately asked me, "Where'd you get that diamond ring?" I said, "I showed it to you last year." He was relieved and said, "When my patients start buying big things, I get nervous. It's as if they think they're going to die, and it's all over. How do you feel?" "Terrific!" I said. "But why didn't you notice this lovely ring last year?"

Another time, he asked me, "Anything bothering you?" I said, "Yes, my daughter's fading away before my very eyes. They think she has anorexia."‡ He said, "I know you by now, and I know you're not crazy. An anorexic girl usually has a disturbed family, and I don't see you as a disturbed family. Let's look at her before we put a label on her." So he had me see the top hematologist at Sloan-Kettering. He did a workup on her, and it helped to turn her around. After that, Dr. Lewis became part of the family. He even went to my daughter's wedding. He was so happy for us, for what we'd been through.

I decided to take my wig off for that occasion. My hair was just growing

---

‡ Anorexia nervosa: a nervous condition confined mainly to young women who refuse to eat, sleep very little, yet remain very active. Emaciation may become severe and even result in death.

in and felt funny, like I was bare, but everyone said it looked beautiful. When hair comes in new, it's very curly and lovely and fresh. It hasn't been beat up by the sun and bleach. People began to stop me on the street and say, "Who does your hair?" It happened so often, I had a standard reply: "Sloan-Kettering!"

When cancer struck again, this time in Phil's throat, Arlynne was not immediately aware of it. "My brother was dying in California, and it upset me so that I failed to see what was happening to my husband. My brother had had emphysema for a hundred years, but suddenly in December they rushed him to the hospital.

I flew out to see him, and this time his lungs are shot. He's all through. *(Sighs.)* I don't know why, but when you're terminal, they do everything to keep you alive. He's worth about two million, and they're doing all kinds of dramatics on him. He has a tube down him, and he's hooked up to a respirator with three round-the-clock nurses going on and on, adjusting and pulling, tightening and fixing, and he can't speak anymore—he's just hanging there in a kind of never-ending nightmare.

I'm desperately unhappy, because my brother and I were always so close. I know he isn't going to live, and *(begins to sob)* he has these two lovely children, young and married and pregnant—his son's wife in her seventh month, his daughter in her eighth. This is terrible. It's on me so much, I can think of little else.

When I get back home, I hear people teasing me. "You're such a doctor, you seem to know so much about medicine, why don't you see what's wrong with Phil's voice?" He'd been hoarse for over a month. So we went to see a doctor I knew at Columbia, Dr. Savetsky, and he said, "There's nothing wrong with him. It'll probably go away. But come back in six weeks if it doesn't." Well, six weeks came and went. I went out to see my poor brother who was still in the hospital, still on the respirator, and came back to find Phil had no voice.

I told Dr. Lewis, and he said, "You'd better get him seen by our man here, Dr. Strong."* What a marvelous guy! He looks Phil over and says, "I don't see anything either, but you come into the hospital overnight, and we'll take a good look at what's down there." So we get him into the hospital, and there I was waiting in that lounge I know so well, when Dr. Strong comes down and says, "I've found a polyp." I was so relieved

---

* Elliot W. Strong, M.D., chief attending surgeon, Head and Neck Service, Memorial Hospital.

because, when he didn't say any more, I thought everything was fine, it was all over. I later learned that he felt certain it was malignant, but did not want to say so until he got the final biopsy reports. We went home, and forty-eight hours later, Dr. Strong called me and said, "I've found enough evidence that we're going to have to put your husband through a course of radiation." I can't believe it. Poor Phil, it was the first time I ever saw him cry.

Still, he faced it like the man he is. He got thirty-six treatments and went to work every day. By now, I'm going back and forth to my brother in California while Dr. Strong is saying, "Your husband's going to be okay. It's localized and hasn't gone anyplace." Dr. Lewis again was right in there, detailing and interpreting for me, saying Phil was going to be okay. So I minimized it, maybe too much, but I was thinking of my brother who was going to die.

Poor Phil, he has claustrophobia, and for his treatment, they put a mask over his head and screwed him down to a table. That was the worst bit. But also when he'd go to the hospital to face this, he'd find people waiting. With radiation, it's not possible to have fixed, orderly appointments. So he'd sit there, sometimes for an hour or more. Finally, he got restless and —you know Phil, how attractive he is—he gave the nurses a number to call him when they were ready for him.

It was a bar on First Avenue where he'd have a drink, watch television, and talk to people, lab assistants or whoever. I caught him there and started shouting. He said, "You're really beautiful," and I thought, what the hell, each of us goes at this his own way. He certainly didn't load it on me. He'd come home, have a drink and dinner, and say nothing about it. I looked at him, sitting there alone in that bar, and I thought I could never love anyone in the world as much as this man.

After it was over, he had no voice left. But he went to a golf camp with his buddies, using a writing pad instead of his voice. On the seventh day of this golf thing, his voice came back like a miracle. He called me on the phone and said, "Hi,"—and I began to cry, I was so happy.

The next day, I learned my brother had died, and I thought how you can never know about happiness. How sometimes it can be just in having something that can be cured.

I was in Mexico, studying medicine at the University of Monterrey, when it first appeared. If it hadn't been for my closest friend, I would have died there—or on the way back to the U.S. It's just one stroke of luck among many, that explains why I'm alive today.

He's 30 and a resident urologist at Albert Einstein School of Medicine in New York—a handsome youth with delicate hands and features, fair skin, gray-blue eyes, curly brown hair, and a neat, light-brown mustache. He speaks carefully, eyes occasionally closing in an effort to recall every detail in the first trauma of the event nearly eight years ago.

We are in the living room of the Storch apartment at Hartsdale, New York, with a hilltop view of White Plains in the evening. His wife, Barbara, brings in wine and cheese with a soft drink for her husband, then sits in a sofa chair to join us.

It was in March of '76, during my second year in medicine, when I first noticed some enlarged lymph nodes in my neck. I thought it was nothing to get alarmed about. I felt well. I was studying a lot, working at the hospital, and very active. I was running every day, and on weekends I would play basketball four hours at a clip, nonstop.

The next weekend, I began to fatigue earlier but still didn't think it was abnormal—just an off day. However, two weeks later the swollen lymph nodes hadn't gone away—in fact, they'd gotten a bit larger.

So I went to one of the professors at the hospital. He said, "Don't worry about it. If they haven't changed in a couple of weeks, we'll do a biopsy or something." He wasn't too concerned, so I wasn't.

I waited, and more nodes appeared—now under my chin. Also, I began to feel a little fatigued just doing daily affairs. And I noticed, on inspiration, a slight pain in the left upper abdomen, in the area of the spleen. I looked in my book and figured I had mono—mononucleosis. I was fatigued, I had lymph nodes and an enlarged spleen—classical mono. It was not a bad diagnosis . . . *(smiles)* except it was wrong.

Unfortunately, one of the top professors, who was also highly respected in Mexico, agreed with me. After a full physical, he said, "You know, you're probably right. It's most likely mono." However, when he received my white blood count the next day, it was 80,000 above normal—too high for mono—and it had many immature forms. That alarmed him, and he called me to come in right away for a bone marrow aspiration.

During the next two days, while waiting for the results of that test, I began to get sick. I was running a fever, getting weaker, and the pain in

my side increased, with the left upper abdomen distending from the enlarged spleen. Also, pinpoint hemorrhages appeared on my ankles—pete-
chiae—indicating a rapidly dropping platelet count, so my blood was not
clotting as it should.

When the lab results came back, the professor called me in again. He
was very upset, but he didn't want to tell me exactly what it was. He
merely said, "I want you in the hospital." The attitude down there is not
as straightforward as it is up here. So I asked him point-blank: "How'd the
bone marrow turn out?" He said, "It was abnormal." I said, "You mean it
was malignant?" He sort of hedged: "I think so, it could possibly be."

At that point, I could figure it out for myself. I was only a fledgling
medical student, but I knew I probably had leukemia, and I had to be
hospitalized right away, as the professor said.

I went into the hospital stunned, like a zombie, figuring this was it. I
would probably die—not right away, but somewhere down the line. You
know, you see movies and read books about people with leukemia who live
for months or years. So I didn't know. I had no clinical experience with it,
and my medical knowledge was quite narrow at the time.

My plan was to return home, without alarming my family or telling
them what was wrong until I got there. After that, I'd go somewhere for
treatment, and take whatever time I had left. I didn't want them to watch
me die. So, I'd sort of disappear somewhere. Rather immature attitude, I
suppose, but that was the way I saw it at the time.

So I called my folks and said, "I'm in the hospital because I have an
enlarged spleen, and they don't know why." I asked them to find a place in
another hospital when I returned. There was no rush—they could expect
me in about a week or so.

As I said, I didn't want to alarm them. But I also didn't know how
rapidly the disease could advance, or how fast I was deteriorating in the
hospital. Fortunately, my close friend, John Garofalo—who was also a
med student there—recognized the extreme gravity and urgency of my
situation much better than I did. Unknown to me, he called my folks right
after I did and told them I was full of bullshit. He said, "Don't believe a
word Sam tells you. He's seriously ill and probably has acute leukemia.
Get him a bed in the finest cancer hospital you can find, and take him
there straight from the airplane, which is going to be the first one I can get
him on." *(Pauses, overcome.)* I owe my life to that man. If he hadn't moved
me out then, I would have never survived. It was a race against time, and
every hour counted.

*"The next morning, he checks me out of the hospital, and we start for the
airport. It's about thirty miles outside the city, the plane is leaving in an*

hour, and we take a French Connection ride through downtown Monterrey like you'd never believe. (Laughs.) John had a little Mustang, and, I swear to God, he was going ninety to a hundred miles an hour down the street, on the sidewalks, up one-way streets, through red lights. Monterrey has about a million people, and you see some crazy drivers—but nobody'd ever seen anything like this, ever. John's wife is huddled under the back seat, absolutely frightened to death. And I'm so mixed up and frightened about myself, I think, 'What the hell, this is a lot better than going the slow way with cancer.'

"I flew into New York, and they took me straight from the plane to Memorial. My mother's cousin is a neurosurgeon who knows the head of hematology at Memorial, Bayard Clarkson.* He told him: 'Listen, my cousin is flying in from Mexico with leukemia, he needs immediate treatment, can you get him a bed?' That's not easy to do at Memorial, to get a bed immediately, but Clarkson was able to arrange it—one more piece of luck in the run of things."

Twelve hours later, I went absolutely critical. I couldn't move. The spleen was now so large it was distending my abdomen like a football. And, my God, the pain. I've had operations and injuries, but nothing equal to that. The splenic capsule is very sensitive. Acutely stretched to those limits, it made any movement, even breathing, an excruciating experience. Lying in bed, I could barely move enough air back and forth to maintain a level of consciousness. One more day in Mexico, with all the complications resulting from the delay, and I would have been a goner.

Even at Memorial, it was touch and go. Starting on Sunday, it became progressively more critical, and that evening they expected to lose me at any moment from a ruptured spleen and internal hemorrhaging. One way to prevent this, of course, is to operate and remove the spleen. But my white cell count was over 300,000—an unheard of number—and my platelet count was virtually zero, meaning they risked uncontrollable bleeding if they operated. So they were caught between the devil and the deep blue sea. Leave it in, and I would rupture and bleed to death. Take it out, and I'd bleed to death.

I was to be in the care of one of the senior hematologists at the time, Monroe Dowling. But I'd come in on the weekend, and he hadn't even seen me. Also, at the time of admittance, I didn't look terribly ill. So nobody expected this to happen—that is, for me to become so rapidly

---

* Bayard D. Clarkson, M.D., chief attending physician, Hematology-Lymphoma Service, Department of Medicine, Memorial Hospital.

critical. Now it was a full-blown crisis, and they began to phone all over the place for Dr. Dowling to decide which way to go.

"At the most critical moment, my parents walked into the room, and of all things, I threw them out. I thought I was probably going to die, and I didn't want them to remember me like that. So I asked them to leave. It was one of the toughest things I ever had to do. Physically, just to speak was difficult—but, even worse, it broke my heart to ask them to go. I can still see them there. Every pain I felt was reflected in their faces. (Pauses.) I couldn't stand to see that, to have them suffer so in looking at me.

"As they turned to leave, my father grabbed my hand. I wanted to offer him something, and I said, without believing it: 'I'm gonna make it'—sort of hissing it out between my teeth. He squeezed my hand so hard he could have popped my fingers off, and said, 'You're damn right you're gonna make it.' I could see he didn't believe it either, but he wanted me to think he did. We were both trying to help the other, and both of us were full of shit. It was really one desperate situation.

"Late that night they decided to get ready to take out the spleen anyway, in case it became the only chance. So they rolled me downstairs for a preoperative X ray. On the elevator going down, a priest got on—not for me, he was going somewhere else. (Laughs dryly.) It's funny. I couldn't speak. I could hardly breathe, but in my mind I was saying, 'You got the wrong guy, buddy. I'm not ready yet.' It's strange where you find humor in times like that.

"But when they left me for a few minutes in the corridor, waiting for the X ray, I realized suddenly that I could die right there, in an empty corridor, without anybody being around. I'd just pop off, and they'd find me there.

"That was one of the times, during the thick of things, that I had a few conversations with the Man Upstairs. Very carefully so. I figured if I was going to meet Him real soon, I'd better introduce myself first. Did I speak to him in Hebrew? No, English. We don't have a religious home. My folks are active in the Temple, but mostly on a cultural, social basis.

"I just lay there, trying to get a focus on what might happen, not saying anything out loud, just thinking how much I'd wanted to be a doctor, how that was my one dream—to live and help other people to live, not to die like this in an empty corridor for no reason at all. I started to feel somewhat bitter and angry about this, and then they came and took me away."

In the middle of all of these crises, there was a doctor on call, a hematology fellow. I'll never forget him—Dr. Drapkin, a little fellow who reminded me of Toulouse-Lautrec—very serious with soft, sad eyes. In all the years I spent there, I never saw the guy smile once. But he's the second person I owe my life to—unless you also count my relative and Dr. Clarkson for getting me into Memorial on that critical weekend.

Drapkin took the bull by the horns. Since he was unable to find my attending physician, it became an emergency where any qualified physician can act. So he said, "We can't wait any longer, we have to do something for this kid. Even if the chances are nil, it's better to do something than nothing." By then, I was telling myself that I'd been lucky up to this point, every step of the way—it could not leave me now.

So he drilled my bone marrow a couple of times, made an initial diagnosis, and began to treat me with vincristine and allopurinol—my first chemotherapy. By the time they found Dr. Dowling—and this is not to say anything against him, for he eventually did everything for me—I was already responding to the therapy, thank God.

The next day, the spleen began to recede, as did the risk of spontaneous rupture. So I had passed my first, immediate crisis. But I still had no insurance that I was going to live. In fact, I began to realize I had very little chance. I had a very severe type of leukemia—acute lymphoblastic leukemia of the T cell type—which carries the worst prognosis of all adult leukemias. At that time, only one in ten made it.† That left me with a lot of unanswered questions, and very little to hang onto.

"Then one evening something tremendous happened. I think it was in the evening. This was a period when things were not very clear to me. There was a lot of emotional stress.

"A young man came into my room. He had blond, curly hair like mine, and he was sort of smiling. I don't know who he was. I think he was a resident of some sort, but he wasn't assigned to my case. Whatever it was, he walked in and saw me lying in bed. Then he came over and grabbed my hand, and said, 'Don't give up. You have a curable disease.' (Pauses, shakes head.) *Nobody had said that to me. They were all working on me, taking care of this and that—but nobody told me that I had a chance or that there was something I might be able to hope for.*

---

† At Memorial, however, the L-2 and the L-10 protocols were to raise the survival rate dramatically to one in two. Leukemia means "white blood" but it is not, as commonly called, a blood cancer. It is a cancer of the tissues in which blood is formed—mainly bone marrow, as well as lymph nodes and spleen. In the United States, it currently strikes 24,000 persons annually, claiming 16,700 lives. Though generally considered a childhood disease, it actually invests more adults each year (21,500) than children (2,500). Acute lymphocytic leukemia accounts for 1,800 cases annually among children, while the two most common forms in adults are acute granulocytic (6,800 cases annually) and chronic lymphocytic (7,600 cases).

"This guy comes, and in five seconds he grabs my hand and gives me the most precious thing I needed—hope. Just a little ray of hope to hang onto. 'Don't give up, you can be cured. . . .' (Pauses again, overwhelmed.) A few seconds later, he walks out, and I never saw him again.

"This gave me the drive to get through that first tough period. It came from a figure of authority, a doctor—and I believed him. It's hard for doctors to know what patients need because most doctors haven't been patients. There's a tremendous difference in the point of view from one side of the bed to the other. It's a rare doctor who can understand a patient, and it's a rare patient who truly understands the doctor."

I also had a lot of help from someone else during the early phase of my consolidation treatments when I was going through hell, with nausea and vomiting. I could hardly stand up, and I felt like I was going to die—mainly from toxicities and side effects of the drugs. I began to think, "My God, is it worth it?"—becoming more and more desperate, without saying anything. But Dr. Dowling, who was very perceptive, saw it.

One day he came into the clinic with a young fellow about my age, saying, "This is So-and-So. He's had your same leukemia, he's had several relapses, but now he's okay." I could hardly believe it. The guy looked like a million bucks, like nothing had ever happened to him.

So we talked, and he told me how he got through it, how rough it was at the beginning, but how you just have to hold on and hang in there. And now, he'd been off therapy for over a year and was feeling great.

That was a big thing for me. It gave me a goal to shoot for, and it helped me through that particularly rough period. Subsequently, I was able to do that for someone else, and it was very moving to pass along something that had been given to me, like a torch or a staff in a relay race.

"You learn in other ways, too, though not so pleasant. I'm talking about getting it from those who don't make it. Like I had a roommate once, a young fellow who had melanoma. My age or maybe a year or two older. His name was Michael, and when I first met him, he looked pretty good. His disease was widely disseminated, however, and they were trying to save him with immunotherapy of a radical nature.

"We became pretty close in the short time we spent together. Michael knew his outlook was bleak. He knew this was his last chance, and if it didn't work this time, he probably wouldn't live out the summer. Yet he always had a smile for everyone. He never had a cross word, even though he was always in significant pain.

"They have patient meetings at the hospital to help patients cope with the illness—or, rather, the disease as an illness, if you consider the disease as a

clinical entity, and the illness as its impact on the patient's entire social life as well as his family's. For these people, it was a big help to be there, because they had others like themselves to talk to. Afterwards they'd say, 'Gee, I feel better.' They saw they weren't alone or the only person—that this disease was all part of life, and their path in life had taken an unexpected turn.

"At these meetings, however, some people would stand up and cry out, 'I can't take anymore!' You'd try and tell them, 'Have a little hope, have a little more drive.' But they would reply, 'It's easy for you to talk. You're going to live, you have a chance!' It was real heavy.

"Michael never did that. In the end, he knew he was going to die, but he never laid it on anybody. He would sort of smile at you, like you both shared a secret that explained everything. Then, one day, he died. . . . (Pauses.) *sort of quietly slipping away. He taught me a lot. . . .* (Frowns.) *. . . except it's not easy to explain. Courage, yes. Not buckling under, yes. But there was much more.* (Smiles.) *. . . I have a picture his girlfriend sent me afterward. I was never as close to another patient again. It was too frightening."*

They put me on the L-10 protocol, which is a complex chemotherapy treatment, using drugs that are quite toxic. In the induction phase, they give the maximum dosage your body can take, so that they kill as much of the leukemia as possible within the limits of your body's tolerance.‡

After five weeks of this, the leukemia has been blasted into temporary remission, and you are then ready for the next two phases, aimed at total

---

‡ The L-10 and L-10M, developed at Memorial by Bayard Clarkson and his colleagues, was a refinement of the earlier, successful L-2 protocol (course of treatment). Multidrug chemotherapies, they all depend essentially upon the proper orchestration of three factors: (1) the specific *drugs,* (2) the *time* at which they are administered (since the leukemic cell is variously vulnerable to different drugs during intervals of its growth cycle), and (3) the *method* of injection (intravenous, oral, or intrathecal). This last path, into the spinal or brain fluid, is necessary in order to bypass the body's blood-brain barrier, which otherwise blocks any foreign element. These protocols were further refined into the more recent L-17 and L-17M.

The treatment is three-phased. *Induction:* The patient receives vincristine, prednisone, and adriamycin in maximally tolerated doses for a period of five weeks. *Consolidation:* Patient receives alternate cycles of further drugs for approximately six months, with inpatient intervals. *Eradication:* Drugs given on outpatient basis for twenty-two to twenty-eight months. Total treatment time: two and a half to three and a half years.

In a Memorial survey over a thirteen-year period (1969–82), the long-term survival rates of 135 previously untreated adults with acute lymphoblastic leukemia were as follows: L-2 (twenty-two patients) 27 percent, and L-10/10M (sixty-nine patients) 50 percent. It is hoped that the more recent L-17/17M (forty-four patients) will further extend these hitherto unmatched survival rates.

eradication of all cells, which will take another two or three years. The first phase is the hardest, the most destructive to the leukemia and your own body. Your bone marrow is so severely diminished that you end up looking like a concentration camp survivor. I'm sure you've seen patients in this premorbid condition—so emaciated and weak they can't even pick themselves up off the bed. That was my condition. I came in looking relatively fit, but that's how I ended up—being carried around wherever I had to go, even to the bathroom.

I'll tell you something. In that short period of time, I lost all feeling of self-worth and self-confidence. I was just a bag of bones, a burden on everyone—stripped of any feeling of self-esteem. Physical energy is easier to replace than emotional psychic energy, and it took a long time to regenerate mine, even after my physical condition began to improve.

I went home for a week before starting the second phase of the protocol, and it was really rough. My family had to come up to my room because I couldn't get out of bed. A couple of days later, they carried me down to the den, and I tried to make a good show of it. But I was desperate. Where before I'd been independent, now I was back in my parents' house—totally helpless. I felt ashamed and worthless. I knew I shouldn't feel that way, but I couldn't help it.

At the same time, I had to do something else that further diminished me —withdraw my application to half a dozen medical schools. I was too weak to take the National Board exams.* So it was only right to withdraw and leave my place for someone else. Next year, I could reapply. In the letters, I explained it was for personal reasons, without mentioning cancer. But I knew I was marked now—inside and out. It could not be hidden. It was going to follow me. No matter how good I was, the cancer was going to be two strikes against me wherever I went in pursuit of becoming a doctor. It's hard to explain the terror of this unless you've had it, unless it's been put on you.

---

* Seeking uniform medical competence in the United States, the National Board of Medical Examiners requires all students to undergo three-stage examinations. The first comes after the second year in medical school, the second after the fourth year, the third upon completion of a requisite internship in a hospital. After passing all exams, anyone with a recognized medical degree is eligible for license in most of the United States. The Co-Trans program uses the first-stage exam to evaluate transfer of a foreign student to an American medical school, and the competition is fierce. Foreign students study months, night and day—far harder than American students, who need only passing marks. Result: 90 percent of the highest scores come from students trained abroad—like Sam Storch.

"When you're down, when you've nothing to offer and need people, that's when you find out who your real friends are. Some people, who I thought were very close, just disappeared, and it hurt. But there were others who surprised me.

"Also, my mother. That was something else. I spent a hundred days in the hospital, on and off, that first year. She was there every single day—from the moment visiting hours began until they kicked her out at night. My mother is the type of person with two hundred pairs of shoes in the closet, but she didn't buy a single pair of shoes that year. She gave up her life— every aspect of her life. She'd sit there in the corner. If I wanted to talk, she'd talk. If I didn't, she'd sit there and knit. If I wanted to play cards, she'd play cards. How can you ever explain something like that?"

BARBARA: *(Dryly)* I didn't even know Sam was here. I thought he was still in Mexico, practicing his Spanish on the local talent.

SAM: *(Smiling)* You see? She always suspects the worst. Anyway, when I'd put on some weight and didn't look like such a horror, I started to get in touch with people. *(Glances at Barbara.)* So I took a deep breath and called her, figuring, "Here it goes again . . . maybe."

BARBARA: It was in June, on his birthday. I said, "You sound awfully close, where are you?" He said, "I'm in New York, at my folks'." I said, "Aren't you supposed to be in Mexico?" He said, "Yes, but I got sick and I'm home."

SAM: *(Quickly)* Her first reaction was also typical of my cheeky wife. "What'd you get, some strange venereal disease?" I replied, "Oh no . . . if it were only true." *(Pause.)* If you want to know where all this began, it was at Great Neck North Senior High. She was a junior, I was a senior.

BARBARA: I obediently wore his class ring, and we took some ski trip weekends that were something else.

SAM: *(Interrupting)* We thought we were the best thing after cream cheese. We had all the answers. Then I went to college at Rochester, and she went to George Washington in D.C. I became a hippie, and that was it, because Barbara's just too straight and narrow to be believed. So we became just friends—social friends. Then, when I was in school in Mexico, my father told me she'd called, asking for me, and it aroused all my base instincts.

BARBARA: To be expected, I suppose. I'd been dating this guy who was a real turd, and I started to remember Sam—how he was always nice to me, even in college. So, after I called his father, I got a letter and the first three words were *"¿Qué pasa, chula?"*—meaning, "What's up, cutie?" Obviously, he wasn't spending all his time in medical books. Then he came up for a vacation, and we spent a marvelous weekend together. But after that, he never wrote from Mexico—four letters maybe.

SAM: *(Interjects)* That's four times more than never, as you put it, and a lot for me. Anyway, for some weird reason, you just couldn't hack it.

BARBARA: *(Coolly)* I realized I wasn't the only *chula* around, so I told you to forget it. The next thing I know, you're calling me to say you have leukemia. Jesus!

SAM: I realize it was quite a bomb to lay on anyone. That's why I waited so long.

BARBARA: We talked a long time, and I said, "Sam, this is a pretty heavy trip. I'll come to see you, but not right away, not until I can get it all together. Otherwise, it'll only depress both of us." For about a week, I guess, I was destroyed. I went to St. Stephen Martyr in Washington, and lit a candle for him. In a moment of weakness, I'd gone back to the same cruddy boyfriend, but now I kicked him out of my life. I didn't analyze it then, but I guess I was still in love with Sam.

A month later, Barbara came to New York. It was the July Fourth weekend of 1976—the bicentennial. A friend of Sam's, with a Riverside Drive penthouse, threw a party, and everyone watched the Tall Ships sail the Hudson. After that, they became quite close again. Since Sam was regularly in and out of Memorial on the consolidation phase of his chemotherapy, Barbara usually came up from Washington, where she worked as a lobbyist for a telephone trade association. Four months later, on a Thanksgiving weekend, they became engaged.

SAM: My folks were not surprised, since we'd been going together on and off since high school. But they couldn't understand why any girl would get engaged to a guy who might be dead in a year. And anybody could see that was possible. I was a skinhead for most of my two and a half years in chemotherapy. Intermittently, the hair would grow back to very short levels. Then, after the next treatment, it would fall out again. I felt like a dog that shed in seasons. People looked at me like a Hare Krishna freak, like asking, "Where'd you leave your finger cymbals?" I developed a rather morbid sense of humor about it. I'd say, "Under a rock in Central Park, come and see us on Sunday!" *(Laughs.)*

The truth is, I still had the cancer, and nobody could say whether I would live or die. I was walking around, dating Barbara, but the first phase had only knocked out the disease. There were still leukemia cells lurking in parts of my body—in the bone marrow, especially—dormant but ready to spring up again if there was any letup in the chemo treatments. At the time, I was in the third phase of my therapy, the eradication phase—a long-drawn-out process of eliminating the last leukemia cells, wherever they might be.

That meant taking pills orally every day and coming in every two weeks, or every month, for injections. The most painful were the spinal taps, to inject the methotrexate into my spine in order for it to reach the brain. Otherwise, it would be blocked by the blood-brain barrier.† A normal spinal tap takes about a minute, but after a while, I became so scarred it was a major hassle to get through. They were hitting nerves, and it was like electric shocks to my legs. That's when it starts to become dangerous, especially if a patient is low on platelets. You can hemorrhage into the spinal fluid and risk severe nerve damage.

So they decided to give me direct injection into the brain. To do this, they put in an Ommaya reservoir—one of three surgeries I had during my leukemia. They drilled a hole through the skull, and put a catheter or tube into one of the brain's cisterns, or chambers, which is part of the circulatory system. Then they connected this to a self-sealing plastic bag that was implanted directly under the scalp where the small section of skull had been removed. After that, any time they needed to inject methotrexate into the cerebrospinal fluid, they stuck a needle through the scalp into the bag. It was one of the greatest things they ever did for me. I hated those spinal taps. You never knew what was going to happen.

All of this was going on when Barbara and I got engaged and—

BARBARA: *(Interrupting)* Your parents thought I was crazy.

SAM: Everybody thought you were crazy. I thought you were crazy.

BARBARA: *(Pensively)* I knew Sam could die, as much as anybody else. But I didn't really know what that was, I hadn't experienced it—or been near it. Everybody in my family was living to nearly a hundred. So I'd never seen anybody die, and I really didn't know what I was getting into.

SAM: If you had, you probably wouldn't have done it.

BARBARA: I don't know. I have no idea. Probably yes, because I wanted you so much. *(Smiles brightly.)* I loved you.

They had been engaged six months when Sam finally began preparing to take the National Board exams to obtain credit for his two years of medical studies in Mexico. He passed with high marks—but the joy was short-lived. His letters to American schools, reapplying for third-year entry, were not

---

† A physiological and physical barrier to the entry of certain molecules into the brain which might be toxic to it, thereby insulating it against most chemotherapeutic drugs when injected into the bloodstream. Thus the direct injection into the spine or into the brain.

answered. His deepest fears were being confirmed. The cancer not only threatened his life; it was a real danger to his career as a physician.

SAM: Before I became sick, several schools had called me for interviews. But now, with cancer on my record, I was being dropped everywhere. I had more going for me now—two years of medical studies, and I'd passed the board exams with good marks. But from their point of view, that didn't matter.

They were going to invest a lot of time and money in my education. They wanted to see it pay off with a guy who'd live to become a successful physician of some type. But here I was, facing two more years of chemotherapy before anybody could say whether I was going to live or die—if then. Who'd want to risk it?

I began to fear my career was destroyed. Okay, I'm stubborn, and I didn't give up. I told myself I would make it somehow. But inside of me, there was a lot of buried rage. Once, visiting my folks, we were watching *60 Minutes* on television and—wouldn't you know it?—there was a report on American medical students overseas having great difficulty in transferring back to the U.S. Med schools in this country are overcrowded and a lot more expensive, so foreign schools are the only chance for a lot of students.

I watched it a few minutes, thinking, "This is me, I'm getting the same raw deal." So I got up, and I went into the bedroom where I started to open the trundle bed. The roller got stuck, it wouldn't open—and that was the last straw. I went absolutely berserk and tore the damn thing apart. It was blind rage, and the bed was a wreck. I remember looking over my shoulder, and there's Barbara and my father staring at me like I've gone absolutely insane.

Obviously, it was a major crisis. I wanted nothing more in life than to practice medicine. It was my dream. Yet here I was, having it robbed from me by something out of my control.

BARBARA: You tore up that bed *after* we were married.

SAM: *(Shrugs)* Yes, it probably was.

BARBARA: Sam said he didn't want to get married until he was out of medical school. We'd been engaged seven months already. So I said, "Send me a postcard when it happens."

SAM: I didn't want to lose her the third time. So we were married by the town judge in Great Neck. It was very nice. Very private with just the family. I even had a little bit of hair for the occasion.

BARBARA: But he'd taken adriamycin a couple of days before, and on our wedding night his hair started falling out. *(Laughs.)* The first week of my married life, I vacuumed Sam's hair out of the furniture.

SAM: As I said, I was like an old dog. So then we decided to move to Washington, where Barbara had an excellent job. My therapy down there could be controlled from Memorial by Zal Arlin who'd taken over my case —a great guy who became a good friend.‡

"Washington was a good idea. With my basic training, I was able to get a job as a cardiovascular technician at Georgetown Hospital, doing catheterizations, cardiac monitoring, and pacemakers. That was perfect because I could work and get my therapy at the same place.

"It was a low-paying job, but one of the greatest things that ever happened to me. For the first time since I got sick, I was productive again. I was earning a living, helping others. For a long time, even when I was dating Barbara, when we got married and afterward, I had no self-confidence. I was afraid to be seen, and it wasn't because I had no hair.

"Something was gone from me. I was afraid to talk to people, I was like a man who'd been stripped bare. Outwardly, I sort of compensated, but inside there were great insecurities. That's why getting this job and re-joining the world in a worthwhile way helped me feel like myself again.

"The job also turned out to be a major step in my career. I became rather well-known to Georgetown physicians—in particular, a cardiac and thoracic surgeon, whom I frequently assisted in my work and who happened to be on the Georgetown admission committee.

"So when I once again reapplied for admissions to other medical schools, I included Georgetown, since they knew me. They knew I had leukemia, but they could see I was beating it. I was able to function. I held a job at the hospital, and the only time I missed was when I had to have chest surgery, which was my own stupidity."

A number of my fellow technicians were out on vacation, and I was doing fifty-sixty hours a week, as well as taking therapy, and I began to cough and run a fever but didn't pay any attention to it. Barbara was bugging me, "Go see your doctor." I'd say, "It's nothing at all," even though the coughing increased until it was almost constant. I just refused to pay it any mind.

I worked very hard, and on one shift, I went eighteen hours straight— an emergency, with no one else to cover. When I got home, I collapsed on the couch.

---

‡ Zalmen A. Arlin, M.D., formerly with Memorial Hospital's Hematology-Lymphoma Service, now professor of medicine, chief of Neoplastic Diseases, N.Y. Medical College, Valhalla, N.Y.

BARBARA: *(Interrupts)* He's lying on the couch, and I said, "Sam, you look lousy. I'm taking your temperature." He said, "I don't have any fever." I said, "Nonsense," and stuck the thermometer in his mouth—and it's one hundred and five! I pulled the phone across the room and told him, "Call the hospital." He should've known better.

SAM: Both lungs were completely inflamed. They had to do a thoracotomy, that is, open them up to get a tissue sample, because they feared it might be a possibly fatal infection for someone like myself—an immunosuppressed patient taking toxic drugs. Thank God, it wasn't and we eventually got it under control.

But Barbara's wrong. I did know better—only I denied it. It was a stupid denial. I'd done it twice before—this denial of illness—when I was in New York and got the shingles, and also when I reached the point where they had to remove my spleen. I knew better but refused to look at it and at what was happening to me. I had a great deal of denial.

When you're a cancer patient, you suddenly become different from anybody else. You want only to be normal, just like everybody else. You start to hate yourself because it's you. There's something in you, in your body, that's making you different. It's a very complex emotional struggle.

I had a great deal of this hatred and denial. As a result, I refused to look at my illness—any illness that came along. So I would overcompensate. I would work day and night, I'd push myself more than any normal individual.

"Then came the big day, the greatest day of my life. I'm sitting in the coronary care unit, watching the monitors—the blip on the screens—to make sure nobody has life-threatening arrhythmias. Then somebody says, 'Sam, there's a call for you.' On the phone, I hear, 'Hello, Mr. Storch? This is Dean Stangeart, dean of admissions at Georgetown.' I thought, 'What's wrong now? What's missing on my application?' Finally I hear, 'We have been authorized to offer you a spot in the third-year class this fall.' I said, 'I'll take it,' and hung up the phone calmly, like slow motion. Then I asked somebody to relieve me. I figured if I screamed right there, in the coronary care unit, I'd have three heart attacks on my hands.

"I had finally gotten back into school. I realized now that if I could just keep going—if I stayed in remission without a relapse—nothing would stop me. It was a tremendous feeling. I walked out of there floating on air."

To succeed in medical school, I gave up my job. We managed okay on what Barbara made, with my father paying the rent. But I couldn't give up chemotherapy. So I scheduled the heavily toxic drugs—the ones that caused nausea and vomiting—for Friday so I could recover over the weekend.

Toward the end of that year, in November of '78, I began to have difficulty tolerating the medication, particularly problems with liver toxicity. Each time they gave me the therapy, my enzyme count indicated liver damage, and they began to fear I would develop irreversible liver damage —a uniformly fatal condition. They tried holding off and starting again. They tried substituting similar medication. But they couldn't get around it, and this was now a real crisis.

The protocol stipulated three and a half years of chemotherapy in order to eradicate all the leukemic cells that might still be in my body. Patients who did not go that length of time did not do as well as others. They had relapses, they died. I still had one more year, but there was nothing to do about it. Dr. Arlin felt that all other alternatives were not yet sufficiently proven and too risky. So he finally decided to bag the whole thing and hope for the best.

"For years I had yearned for this—the last day of chemotherapy. I'd said, 'What a beautiful day it will be!' But when it happened, I was scared down to my very soul. I had suddenly lost my crutch. As much as I hated taking the drugs, as much as I couldn't wait for it to be over, it was a sort of insurance policy. It kept me well.

"Suddenly, I felt I was left bare. I was walking on thin ice, wondering, 'When will it break? When will I fall in?'

"It took a long time to get over that. No, I must be honest. I guess I'll never really get over it, even though I've now gone six years without a relapse, and I'm considered clinically cured. Despite this, I'm constantly aware that there's no guarantee it won't come back in some way. It's a very frightening prospect, and I try not to think about it. But it's with me, always in the back of my mind.

"On the other hand, it brings you immense understanding of others. I am closer to patients because of it, and maybe I'm also a better doctor. I am bound in a special way to them, as if I was part of every patient. Especially when I see some with malignancy who aren't doing well, I think, 'There I am—but for the grace of God.'"

I don't want to sound pretentious, or like I did in my old hippie days, but this has profoundly changed my priorities. It's brought me closer to the cosmos—to my small part in the general scheme of nature. It's made me more appreciative of the real worth of simple basic things. Like walking out today and taking a simple breath of fresh air without feeling pain. I once dreamed, I once prayed to be able to do just that, and now it's an utter joy.

I think it's really difficult to understand these things—this joy of living again, of being able to live without cancer—unless you've gone through it yourself. But I certainly wouldn't recommend that anyone undergo such an experience, such emotional and physical demands, to attain this understanding.

Maybe my story, or others like mine, will help in this way, will indicate what is possible—not only to those facing illness, but all those who are like I was before this happened to me.

POSTSCRIPT: Seven years, four months, and sixteen days after Sam Storch feared he would die alone in a corridor of Memorial Hospital—after telling "the Man Upstairs" that he was holding onto a dream to live in order to care for other people—he returned to Memorial. No longer a patient, Dr. Samuel J. Storch came as resident urologist in the Urology Service, Department of Surgery at Memorial.

We are in the head nurse's glass-enclosed station on the sixteenth floor of
Memorial Hospital, following our initial encounter. See page 131.

Some people survive cancer, and others don't. If they all get the same
treatment, what makes the difference? I believe a lot has to do with how
and when they get here. Just think about it—about that particular moment when they are picked out of the crowd and brought to this special
hospital, to get the right person at the right time to do the right thing. It's
an incredible series of coincidences, especially when you're dealing with
biology. That's one factor, all of these events coming together. In a way,
you can call it luck—just being plain lucky.

The second is the spirit of the person. I've seen many people with the
right fighting spirit, but for different reasons. Some have it because they're
so angry at something that happened to them that they are determined to
survive to rectify the wrong.

I don't want to one-case you to death, but I had a fellow here with his
bladder burned away by a radiation therapist in another hospital—a hole
burned into his body by inappropriate therapy. His wife, in the middle of
the crisis, took everything out of his apartment—everything, clothes, television, paintings—everything except his clothes, and then she left him.
Took his son, too. Just walked out. Here's a guy on the brink of death. He
got so mad that he swore he was going to survive to get even with her.
And he's alive today. The hole is closed up, and he's starting a normal life
again.*

So he made it with a fighting spirit. But also he was lucky to finally get a
doctor to cure him, Horace Whitely, after all the bad luck with other
doctors who just about killed him. So luck is always there, playing a part
in it.

He was in Vietnam for thirteen months, drafted into the 1st Air Cavalry.
"Did you see Apocalypse Now? *It was like our unit. I read Conrad's* Heart
of Darkness *before going to see the movie. It was based on that book.*
Underneath the helicopter, it says, Death from Above. *I was looking*
through my top drawer the other day and saw that written on scarfs they
gave us.

"I was shot three times in the back, arm, wrist—superficial wounds, but I
was pretty messed up in the head when I came home . . . didn't know

---

* Melvin Schlossberg, p. 220.

what I wanted to do with myself. I came back to a cultural and social structure, you know, where your friends tell you to collect unemployment for sixty-five weeks. So you get drunk all the time. You know, the typical teen-age approach to living. But the odd thing was that I was about 100 years old. I was so much older than everybody around me, because I'd just come from another heart of darkness. It took me a long time to get over that. I was hurt. It was typical.

"I come from a civil service family. My father's a cop, my brother's a cop. I could've gone into the police department, but I'd been too injured to pass their medical exam, which was a blessing. Don't get me wrong—I don't have anything against cops. It's just that I'm glad I stumbled into this.

"I met my future wife a week or two after I came home from Vietnam. I was working in a restaurant, getting into a lot of trouble. Then I was out of work. Catherine was a nursing student at St. Clare's Hospital, in Hell's Kitchen. She got me a job there as an orderly. Then I went to Roosevelt Hospital School for Nursing, graduated, came here for training, and just stayed on."

When I started here, I took a book and wrote down the names of patients I'd like to remember. I have three hundred and eighty-five, in five and a half years. It's funny how I can go down the list now and recall where they come from, what happened to them, why I remember them. For some reason, some kind of relationship developed between the patient and me, or the family and me.

That kind of helps to keep it all in perspective. My father-in-law is an old-time sort of country doctor, a G.P. He once told me, "You have to remember, when you're dealing with somebody who's critically ill, that it's the most important, the most serious thing that's ever happened to them. This is the apex of their life. They've never been in a position where several doctors will walk in, just to talk to them about their own life."

We have to remember that here, because we see it all the time, the same story, the same diseases—another colon cancer, another stomach cancer, another liver tumor. For us, it's just one more cancer case, but for them, it's the most important thing in their life.

I try to keep that in mind when I talk to patients. It's important to spend time with them. A lot of nurses say, "Why do nurses make beds? It's unprofessional. Get an aide to do it." They don't realize it gives you contact with people, it brings you together. They're sick. You've stripped them of their clothes, and they're sitting in a chair. Now you can talk to them. You say, "What'd you do for a living?" A retired man will say, "I don't do a damn thing, I'm retired." So you say, "But you must've done something before you retired." Then you get the whole story and how he wound up in this place. It's invariably like that.

There was a guy in here recently, his name was Bowe or something like that. He was a writer, spoke several languages and had translated Dante's *Inferno.* I was in his room, making his bed, and started to talk to him. After a ten-minute conversation, he said he'd told me more about himself than he had told anybody in his entire life. He wanted to know how I did that. I said, "I didn't do it. I'm in a perfect position for it to happen. You are trapped in an environment, waiting for someone to come in and say the magic word, so you can finally get all those things off your chest that've been bothering you."

There's an altruistic side to all people that they don't talk about. I think it's part of our nature to try to be that way. It's almost impossible to be totally altruistic, but I think we have that in us. The names on my list help me to remember that. They also remind me that I'm just part of the process here, that there were hundreds of people before me, and that hundreds more will soon pass me. And to remind me in dealing with people, who need you right then and there, that they have particular feelings, that they are in pain or angry or mad at their wives, or a whole bunch of things that make them this way. You have to deal with their particular situation.

For example, a lot of the names on my list were terminally ill. They were approaching the end of their life, but it wasn't always a lifetime. You can speak in terms of five- or ten-year cures. But if you have an 18-year-old boy with osteogenic sarcoma, and you tell him he's gonna live five years, that will make him 23. That's not a lifetime when you're 18 years old. When you're 73, another five years may be a lifetime.

You never know how some people will react. Take this fellow, Henry de Cicco, an author and an antitechnocrat, teaching at the New School for Social Research. He was against technology at its worst. You know, what we've done to our society with automation and TV. Then he comes to Memorial Hospital near the end of his life. He was a philosopher and a mathematician, and he kept talking this antitechnology thing, yet the only way we would treat him was with a pump, one of the most technological things we do. He was opposed to technology, but it kept him alive. His wife was very interesting. She struggled with the dichotomy that Henry created. She didn't want him to die, but she also knew this violated his thinking, this acceptance of what he denied. Fascinating. Finally, they reached the point where this man, who was an atheist and didn't believe in God his whole life, converted to Catholicism a day or two before he died. From his deathbed, he gave me a lecture on the mystical body of Jesus

Christ, drawing it up probably from something he had read twenty years before that moment. It touched me in a way that I've never been touched before.

I'm not very religious, though I once was when I was young. I got married in a church because my wife's family wanted it. It had nothing to do with me. But I've always been interested in how people respond to stress in terms of religion.

In Vietnam as a soldier, I saw people under great stress, and I watched how they responded to God and religion before the fear of death. When I came here, I expected it to be the same, especially with the young rejecting and the older ones accepting. But it wasn't always so.

We had Cornelius Ryan here, the guy who wrote *The Longest Day*. I took care of him the day he died. A priest came into his room and tried to get him to confess. They seldom do it like that, but this one did. Ryan was a lapsed Catholic and an agnostic, and he refused everything. Wanting none of it, he refused the priest on his deathbed. Unbelievable. The courage he had to hold onto his beliefs under such pressure.

Then you see the opposite thing happen with Henry de Cicco, who was just country cool about the whole thing. He moved me more because he was willing to change his view and take an even broader leap of faith. Most of us never change our view. We get bogged down in intellectualism and processes to where we can't change. But he changed. That takes another, special kind of courage, to change as he did. And that moved me.

FOUR

NEED

Unless we prefer to be made fools of by our illusions, we shall, by carefully analyzing every fascination, extract from it a portion of our own personality, like a quintessence, and slowly come to recognize that we meet ourselves time and again in a thousand disguises on the path of life.

Carl Jung
The Psychology of the Transference

"Close! Stand close to me, Starbuck. Let me look into a human eye. It is better than to gaze into sea or sky, better than to gaze upon God."

Herman Melville
Moby Dick

As with love, the role of need—that is, having need and being needed—is visible throughout this book. At first glance, it appears to be the most protean, all-engulfing of the five survival factors.

We find, for example, that need often supersedes love as a bonding factor between people or as a force for individual transfiguration. We also discover that it can outreach the role of self in embracing the totality of these people under duress. It would appear, however, that this is because need is actually an extension of both love and self—that is, a transference of these two states of the human condition into day-to-day living.

As used here, total human need means more than being needed by someone or having needs that must be met. It also includes the need to release something of value from ourselves, to create or give in some way that will satisfy an innate sense of continuity or meaning of life.

In this way, it also has the power of connecting dualities or opposites. Need, for example, can encompass Eros—the ontological drive to develop oneself, to create something unique—while also enveloping Agape—the opposing human drive to group oneself with others or through others in a shared experiencing of the cosmic process of nature or life. As a result, it links these two opposite expressions of love—a holy spirit within love's trinity.

Finally, as we see in these stories, the web of need creates personal and social contracts which force upon us a recognition of necessity. This, in turn, provides a semblance of freedom as we act or live with increased resolve and courage before the terrorizing totality of life.

In this section, we witness need in various ways. Nelle Harris has "healing moments" when faced with the need to save her husband and family. Julius Binetti, an insurance salesman, holds onto a thin thread of life— convinced his wife could not survive his loss. John Corbalis, a telephone operator and aspirant actor, must learn to speak again—or lose his job as well as the dreams which sustain him. Melvin Schlossberg swears nothing can kill him until he gains custody of his son and gets even with his wife who walked out on him.

How this occurs elsewhere, among other patients, is described by the first witness in this section. Sister Rosemary Moynihan draws upon many years' experience as a social worker in exploring the role of need—not only as a factor in holding onto life, but also in allowing for the release of an essential goodness which she sees as existing in all human beings, regardless of their faith or quality of life.

As a witness of the multiple forms of need, she shows how they manage to enrich many lives and even help people to live and die in ways which sometimes assume heroic dimensions. As a religious sister in a cancer ward, working with human beings under extreme duress—doctors and hospital staff as well as patients—her testimonial is also a rather moving credo on the worth and potential greatness of human life.

Some people survive cancer with a good quality of life, and often claim it is even better than before their illness. Then there are those that barely make it. They hang on, grasping life with their fingernails. In both types, but especially the more desperate ones, you find patients claiming they cannot die because they are needed by someone, or they need to live to a certain date for any number of reasons.

We are seated in the coffee shop at Memorial Hospital. After discussing the role of love in survival (page 118), Sister Rosemary relates her experiences with another powerful force in fighting the disease.

In my interviews, I'll hear a patient say, "I need to live to March." Then they'll invest that date with an arbitrary meaning that has great importance for them, such as "March will make it one year since I was diagnosed. If I can make it to one year, then I can probably make it to two." After that, the patient has a date to live for, a future victory day.

The need is usually linked to the family. One woman refused to die, saying she wanted to see her grandchild born. Well, she managed it. She lived until the child was born, then she advanced her needs to a later date. "I want to see him at home. I want to hold him. I want him to have some kind of affection for me, even though he'll never know me."

There is a basic human drive to stay alive. But as you get to know these people, you see it isn't only a grasping at life, against the pull of death. It also comes from a tremendous potential in people. Now and then, you get an insight into it. It's what they wanted to do but have been unable to do. It's the longing for relationships to be good, the longing to do something worthwhile, to make their mark doing something for a better society, to help the lives of those around them. And it's a desire to be remembered in the lives of their children, which will reverberate down through the generations. Some patients say, "If I go through this Christmas, maybe they'll remember that." What they are really saying is, "If I can articulate my faith, my love, my values through them, then maybe they will remember me."

Some of them talk about the need to finish painting the house—or something else, like building a boat or maybe redecorating their home. But many talk about their family or their spouses—how they want to be remembered by them. Even if they fought through an entire marriage, they don't want the other one to be left alone or otherwise be helpless. They're able to identify the very vulnerable parts of their healthy spouse. They'll say, "She—or he—has difficulty with finances, never filled out a checkbook. How will she manage?" In one way, this means, "I shouldn't die, I should stay around to help her do this." When they're able to work through this anxiety over separation, they often feel better if there is a plan to take care of their survivors. They don't want someone to take their place, naturally, as much as to have some appropriate support left for their survivors—in a way, an extended form of themselves after death.

Even in the most conflict-ridden relationships, they try to reach out to the other person. At such time, emotions can be mixed. There can be sadness over having to die and some anger at the other's health. But there's always that thread of real concern, of real integrity coming from the human potential for goodness. I'm not being naive. It's *there*.

There was this woman, Eileen, with breast cancer that had metastasized to her lungs. She had six children at home, and her husband was recently out of work. He had been an executive and was suddenly dropped. She was agitated and having recurrent nightmares, which is why they referred her to me.

She was on chemotherapy and had lost her hair. In her nightmare, she dreamed she would go home from the hospital and put a sign on her door, saying, "Please look beyond my bald head and talk to me." Her neighbors and friends would come to the door and read the sign, then turn and walk away. They would leave her alone. That was her constant dream and nightmare.

In the initial contact, we helped her understand a little bit of what it meant. In talking about this, she was also able to talk about her dying. The talks vacillated between concern over her shortness of breath, the chemotherapy, her wanting to live, and her greatest fear that she was going to die and leave her work as a parent unfinished. You always deal with life as well as dying.

So we looked at the fact that she was still alive and not helpless—and what was she really most concerned about? She said it was leaving her husband alone, with six children in need. They were young—five boys and a girl—and each one had their own problems. What was she going to do since her job wasn't finished?

She was in the hospital two months, and we met daily to talk about her mothering role. How could she still be a mother when she didn't feel well and had only a limited life ahead? She decided she could talk to her children and tell each one the sorts of things she wanted them to carry through life. We spent weeks going over each one. Tommy, for example, had large ears and thought he was ugly. He thought the girls wouldn't ever like him. What could she do to help Tommy think better of himself? Someone else was having trouble in school, and what could she do to help him understand that? Someone else was shy, and another one was going to get married.

Not only did she go through her tasks with each one, but she also figured out how to approach them. Tommy, for example, wouldn't ever sit still long enough to listen. Eileen wondered, "How can I ever get him to talk to me?" Then she came up with a special strategy for Tommy. "He'll sit for hours if I scratch his back. So when he comes into my bedroom, I'll scratch his back. Then I can say some of the things I want to say to him."

We went though this over and over again. Gradually, Eileen became less anxious, and her husband became more relaxed and was less worried because she was more comfortable with herself. Then she went home, and I would get little messages by mail, such as, "Well, I talked to Tommy, and he listened." And she would go through each one. So she did something that would nurture them, enable them to grow, and also something they could remember her by. She taught them to cook, each one, knowing they would be better off because they would be able to eat well. And here, once again, she wouldn't ever be forgotten, no other woman would completely take her place—at least in the kitchen.

We were playing backgammon, and my wife noticed my skin looked discolored. I said, "It's nothing, just suntan." She said, "No, it looks yellow." So I told her, "Nonsense, everything's all right."

Next thing you know, I'm waking up at night with indigestion and an acid stomach, and I can't understand what's what. Then people in my office start asking, "Have you lost weight?" Of course, I don't hop on the scales, so I don't know—like some dumb ostrich with its head in the sand.

Then I'm out laying stones in the patio, and my wife says, "Your eyeballs are yellow." I said, "Oh c'mon." At that, she gets real upset and says, "No, you have to call a doctor and find out why you're turning yellow." This is on a Saturday, and I tell her, "We're not gonna get hold of any doctor today." "Never mind," she says. "Just get on the phone and tell them you have hepatitis."

That's what happened, and right away, I got to see our family doctor who took one look at me and suspected the worst. "Yes," he said. "You'd better get into the hospital as soon as you can."

He was born in Trieste fifty-seven years ago with the fair complexion of a northern Italian, the rugged face of an Alpine, soft hazel eyes, and dark hair turning gray. He's an insurance salesman and is wearing a blue cashmere sweater, blue-gray tie, and gray slacks. He jokes and laughs easily, yet when the laughter subsides, there are glimpses of the private man—the defenseless face he would see in the morning mirror, the eyes appearing to be especially vulnerable.

We are drinking a beer in the patio garden of the Binetti suburban home at Pompton Lakes, New Jersey. His wife, Edmée—a slender, taut woman with blond hair and delicate features—sits with us in a deck chair. Julius, who is diabetic now as a result of his illness, says, "I have to be careful with beer. But from the way I began to crave it after my operation, I figure it must have some kind of digestive enzyme that's good for me." Edmée shakes her head: "He'll talk himself into anything he wants, especially if it's forbidden fruit."

So I went up to the local hospital where my daughter Claudette is a nurse —Chilton Memorial, near Pompton Plains. They conducted all kinds of tests—X rays and everything else. Somebody said they couldn't see the pancreas, and I made a joke of it: "Hey, just a minute, I came in here with one, so it must be there." Little did I know that a tumor was hiding it on the X ray.

After about a week, the doctor came in and talked first with my wife and daughters. Then he came into my room and told me the big news. The word he mentioned was "cancer" and then "pancreas." In my experience with insurance, I'd never heard of anybody licking cancer of the pancreas. So this was it, the end of the road, and I really broke down.

When that happens, boy, you see a big hole, and you're in it, and somebody's throwing dirt in your face. From then on, it's like you're living in a dream world. You say, "It can't be me. I heard it wrong, it's not right." You just can't believe it, so you try and put it out of your mind.

That's when Dr. Koenig, who used to be chief of surgery at Chilton, suggested I go to Dr. Fortner at Memorial where they have more sophisticated equipment and know more about it.*

So I went to New York and saw Fortner. He took my X rays and looked at one and said, "Aha!" I asked him, "Is that a good *aha!* or a bad *aha!?*" He sort of laughed and said, "Don't worry about it." Then he went into the corner with his partner in crime, his associate. They talked a bit, then he said, "Okay, bring him in"—like I was already in a stretcher. I said, "Don't bother, I can still walk. But how am I going out?" He laughed and said, "I think it's a good prognosis."

Later I learned they can never really know if the cancer has spread to the lymph glands and the rest of the body—not until they open you up. God bless Fortner. He never told me it could be hopeless. He was always positive. Believe me, that helped a lot—the feeling he gave me that we were going to lick this thing.

"I got help in another way, too. When they put me on the sixteenth floor, I was still asking, 'Why me?' There was an orderly there named Ben, and he said, 'Look at me. I'm black—why me?' I thought, 'Hey, wait a minute. He's got something there.' After that, my attitude changed. I still resented it; I wished to hell it'd never happened, but I began to admit that I had it and that I had to lick the damn thing in one way or another.

"I had a double room and a lot of bunkies. It started with Ganz, the first guy, the difficult one. Talk about prima donnas! He's staring at the ceiling and says, 'Don't talk to me, I'm busy.' Some help he was. Then they moved in this guy Jerry, who had his girlfriend visit him one day and his wife the next day. I said, 'What's gonna happen when they both meet?' He said, 'Listen, what you're seeing now is the same situation I had before I came in here, only more speeded up.' (Laughs.) Then he said, 'I couldn't turn them off before I got into this mess, so how the hell can I do it now? The only

---

* Joseph G. Fortner, M.D., attending surgeon, Gastric and Mixed Tumor Service, Department of Surgery, Memorial Hospital.

thing is to try and regulate them and hope to God they don't collide.'
(Laughs.) *Then I thought, 'Hey, when you're laid out like we are, you need
all the loving you can get. So you don't turn it off, no matter where it comes
from.' "*

Before you know it, they did the first operation, which was to put a T tube
into me to drain off the bile. I had so much backed up, I was a surgical
risk, and they had to get rid of it before going further. So I came out of
this first one with the T tube draining into a hanging bag.

I went home for a couple of weeks, taking special pills and eating a
special diet. At this point, you can't stand the smell of coffee, of milk, of
meat—of anything. Everything is against you. But after two weeks, I was
in better shape, I wasn't so yellow, and I went back to the hospital for the
big operation.

This time I know more, so it's harder. I know I have a growth in the
head of the pancreas . . . *(hesitates)* a cancer. It's blocking the bile duct,
and Fortner's going for broke. Either he gets it all out—or else, if it's
spread, that'll be the end of it for me. *(Pauses, nods.)* So I'm a lot more
tense than I was the first time—you follow?

EDMÉE: *(Interjects)* Only tense? He went into real shock. I walked in,
and he's shaking in his boots.

JULIUS: *(Frowns)* I don't remember that. . . . What boots? I was in
my pajamas! *(Laughs.)*

EDMÉE: *(Unheeding)* Joan, my friend, became so upset that she left the
room. Me, I'm so frightened in hospitals to begin with, I don't know what
to do. Then one of Fortner's doctors came in and explained, as Fortner
had, what was going to be done. *(Nods toward husband.)* But since he was
so upset and worried, this doctor tried to get past it by being funny.
"You'll do fine," he said, "but the next day you'll feel like a truck hit you."
Julius is all ears now, and no longer thinking about the operation. "Oh?"
he says, "what'll we do about that?" The doctor says, "We'll get the license number." *(Laughter.)*

JULIUS: No, you're scared because you're going to have it done the next
morning, and you don't know what they will find—I mean, whether or not
it's spread to the whole body. I even had a new will drawn up, and all that
jazz. You think, "Somebody else may survive, but I might not make it."
Then the fighter inside you says, "No, this won't happen." So you go back
and forth between "Yes, it's going to happen" and "No, it won't." It's a
very hard way to be.

EDMÉE: I kept saying he was a marvelous man, he was going to come
out on top like he always did, even when everything was against him. I
shouldn't say this, but I will. *(Pauses.)* His family was not very nice to

him. They left him in Italy when they came over, and he's very proud of what he did with his life after that.

JULIUS: *(Uneasily)* Yes, well my father left me to go to the U.S. when I had only six months, and my mother followed him when I was three. So I was left with her sister, my aunt.

EDMÉE: *(Angrily)* And whoever else wanted to take care of him—foster homes, you name it! I think that was his difficulty when he became ill. His feeling of "What's going to happen to me?" was a reverting back to when he was a little one and used to say, "Who's going to take care of me?"

JULIUS: I remember being a child and crying. It wasn't about my mother or father being gone, but about my aunt. I kept asking, "What's going to happen to me when she dies?"—not realizing, of course, that I would be older then and able to take care of myself. Finally, my father got the papers together to bring me over here—because, you know, there was a quota on how many people could come. Otherwise, you sat there and waited—or you came, and jumped the old boat.

EDMÉE: *(Quickly)* Like his parents did. They jumped the boat.

JULIUS: I came over on the *Roma,* an old liner sunk during the war. I remember getting up early and missing breakfast just to see the Statue of Liberty. When you see that for the first time, standing up in the sky, holding that big lamp for all of us coming over the water—boy!—you don't know what to think. *(Shakes head.)* I get the shivers just thinking about it now, would you believe it?

I was so small—I was only ten—they were keeping me until someone came to get me. There was this big table, and the purser or some officer was there with me, and there were lots of people around us. To help find my father, I had an old photo of him standing next to a racing bicycle. But he recognized me first. I heard him shouting my name, "Giulio!"—that's Julius in Italian—and then he's picking me up and kissing me, and he's crying, and I'm very happy to have a father again. *(Shakes head sadly.)*

"My father had a panel truck, and we drove to Baltimore where they had an apartment over a grocery store where he worked. Have you ever been to Baltimore? All the houses and steps look alike. If you're a little kid, or maybe drunk, you can get really lost there. After a week, I had to start school, and on the first day my father took me in the truck to show me how many streets to go down, and how to count the trolley tracks.

"The next day I started out, and of course I got mixed up and wound up in downtown Baltimore. Talk about scared! I had to go back all the way until I finally found the school. Then this teacher is yelling at me that I'm late. I know I'm late, but how do you answer her if you can't talk the language, to say that you missed the street? There were three Chinese kids

in the same condition like me, and we used to play together and, during lunch hour, we'd visit Chinese laundries.

"My mother paid this woman who ran an Americanization class to teach me English—spelling and writing. That was a big thing. In those days, you were proud to learn English—not like it is today in a few places. You were also proud to be a U.S. citizen, and when I graduated from high school, I planned to take out citizenship papers. But I got to working for a construction company, and before you know it, we're in World War II, and the draft board grabs me: 'Okay, buster, you're in the army now.' I told them 'Hey, wait a minute, I'm not even a citizen!' They laughed and said, 'Don't worry, we'll fix that.' Then they took a whole mess of us down to Louisiana, put us in a room, made us raise our right hands—and that's it! (Laughs.) We became American citizens right then and there."

For the big operation the next morning, they give you a shot so you're a little fuzzy. Then they take you down to the coldest damn place in the hospital—the staging area next to the operating room. They got you laying there, with nothing on but your sheet. Cold as hell. Next thing, the anesthesiologist—she'd already been up to my room—comes out saying, "Hi! Here we are again." She starts explaining what she'll be doing. But by now your mouth's like cotton, you're real groggy, and you can't focus too well.

Next, you're being wheeled into the operating room, and there's the big overhead light you always see on TV, and you say, "Oh, I'm under it now." On the wall, there's a big clock, and you're thinking, "That's funny, they said, this'd start at eight, and it's eight, right on the button. Boy, they sure don't mess around in this place!"

Dr. Fortner comes in, and even with his mask, you know he's smiling. He leans over and says, "Here I am, we're all ready." Then he touches my arm and says something I'll never forget. . . . *(Pauses.)* "Don't worry, you'll do fine!" God bless him. Those few words meant everything to me. I began to let go, to drift off, and I'm telling myself, "This guy's going to get it all out, he's going to fix me up, I'm going to walk out of here and go home—back to Edmée and the girls who need me and are waiting there. . . . *(Chokes up.)* That's funny, it still gets me, just talking about it.

Next you know, I'm coming to in the recovery room, and a nurse is yelling, "Wake up, Mr. Binetti! Everything's all right!" I wonder what the hell she means—*all right?* I've got a tube down my throat, so I can't talk. I can't see, either, because everything's fuzzy. I know the nurse is there, but all I can make out is her curly hair. Then, gradually, I can see this huge room with beds all over the place. It reminds you of the movie *Coma*, with bodies hanging in the air. After that, I pass out again.

The next time I wake up, I'm in a smaller room with white curtains around my bed, and I wonder, "Hey, what is this—a morgue?" There's a tube in my nose and one coming out of my stomach. I've got one arm strapped down with needles in it, and wires fixed to my chest and legs. You can hear *beep-beep* sounds from a lot of TV heart monitors, all going at the same time like a bunch of cooped-up canaries, and I think, "Holy smoke, I go from the *Coma* room with the hanging bodies, to a heart failure terminal. God help us."

My heart starts going like mad, skipping beats, and I panic and start banging the bed rail with my ring, yelling for help.

The nurse comes running and tries to quiet me: "You're in the intensive care unit, it's the same as the recovery room, only more so." I ask, "What for—did my ticker stop?" She says, "No, your heart's fine, you're doing all right." It sounds like a runaround, and I tell her, "Everybody says I'm all right, but, if that's so, why the hell am I here and not in my room?" I can feel the panic rising. "Didn't Fortner get it all out?" "You have to ask him that," she says. "He was just here, and he's coming back."

I can see past my curtains to another bed where there's some guy moaning and groaning like he is going to kick the bucket any minute, and I ask: "Why's he making so damn much noise—is he dying?" She says, "No, there's nothing wrong with him, he just thinks there is."

So I'm lying there, listening to this guy moaning and thinking, "What the hell's going on here? That poor bastard really feels bad, and that's probably how I'm gonna be in no time." Suddenly the curtain is pulled back, and it's Fortner, wearing his green operating room clothes. He doesn't look worried at all. In fact, he seems pleased and asks me: "How're you feeling?" I tell him not so good: "Your assistant said I'd feel like a truck had hit me. The damn thing must've backed up and run over me three or four times." He laughs a little, and says, "I've got good news. The cancer had not spread, and I think we got it all out. You're a lucky man." I didn't feel lucky in that place and asked, "Why am I here—heart trouble?" He looked offended and said, "Hell no, you're right where you belong."

It seems they had told me to expect this, but I didn't listen to them— that I would need intensive care after the operation. To begin with, I was now a diabetic. Without a pancreas, I couldn't produce insulin to control the sugar balance in my blood. So I needed special care until my body got back in balance. Also, besides the pancreas, Fortner had taken out my gallbladder, spleen, duodenum, half the stomach, part of the intestines— you name it. I asked, "Gee how come we took so much stuff out?" He said, "Would you like to come back two years from now?" "Oh, no, thanks," I said. "In fact, if you want anything else, now that you're at it, just help yourself." *(Laughs.)*†

EDMÉE: *(Interrupts)* They told me to stay home, and they'd let me know. I kept praying and hoping, and then Dr. Fortner called to tell me they'd caught it in time, so it hadn't spread to any vital organs.

JULIUS: It was too much for her. She collapsed.

EDMÉE: *(Quickly)* Only because of what was happening to Julius. I was nauseous. I couldn't eat, I couldn't get out of bed.

JULIUS: She doesn't take too well to hospitals. She has deep—what do you call it? *(Looks at wife.)*

EDMÉE: Anxiety.

JULIUS: Yes, anxiety. She doesn't like to see anyone suffer. If she does, you never know what'll happen. When our daughter Claudette had her teeth extracted—four impacted wisdom teeth—my God! It was like a comedy of errors. We come in, and there's the sick daughter who's passed out and doesn't know which end is up. My wife takes one look, and she passes out—*ka-lump!*—down she goes between two beds. Then, of course, my younger daughter begins to roll back her eyes and moan, "Daddy, I don't feel so good"—like she's going to the floor, too. So I start swearing, "Hey, wait a minute, what is this—a circus? Is everybody gonna pass out? What am I gonna do with all the bodies?" *(Laughs.)*

That's why she never made it to the intensive care unit. We knew what'd happen—you follow me? I look more dead than alive with all the tubes coming out of me, and my heart's bumping up and down across the TV screen. Just imagine—she walks in, takes one look at me and—*ka-lump!*—down she goes to the floor again. They would have had both of us in intensive care, and I would have had to worry about her as well as myself. You understand? That's why we all told her not to come until they moved me back to my regular room.

My daughters came every day—especially Claudette, who's a nurse—and every day the girls told Edmée, "Dad's doing fine." But she didn't believe them. In some mysterious way, she knew I was having a rough time. . . .

---

† The tumor was extensive. Located in the head of the pancreas, it surrounded both the common bile duct and the main pancreatic duct, extending into the tissue immediately surrounding the pancreas. Dr. Fortner performed a regional total pancreatectomy, removing gallbladder, bile ducts up to the right and left hepatic duction near the liver, all the pancreas, the duodenum, lower half of the stomach, the spleen, and the pancreatic segment of the portal vein. Fortunately, the lymph nodes were negative, indicating no metastasis beyond the area. To safeguard, however, there was also a regional lymph node dissection.

EDMÉE: *(Interrupts)* Mysterious? You didn't phone me, so what else could I think?

JULIUS: Oh yeah, the phone. There weren't any next to the beds—only one phone that the nurses used. So it happens that I get real sick, because the fluid isn't draining from where they'd re-joined my stomach. It's backing up, and Fortner doesn't want it to go into the lungs. So they take me back to the operating room for another go at it.

This time, when I get back to intensive care, I'm like the guy I saw the first day. I've got a fever, I don't know where I am, and I dream that Edmée is also in the hospital. She's calling for me, "Help! Julius! Help me!" At that point, I wake up yelling, "Where's my wife? I want my wife!"

Two nurses come running and tell me no wives are allowed in at three o'clock in the morning. *(Laughs.)* I guess I had a fever because I explained that my wife was already there, somewhere in the hospital, calling for me. They try and tell me I'm imagining it, but I don't believe a damn word they're saying, and I try to get up with all the tubes pulling on me. *(Laughs.)* They jump on me, trying to hold me down, and I start yelling for Fortner to save me, when the night doctor comes running in, saying, "You're waking up the whole hospital! What the hell's going on?" I tell him, and he says my wife isn't there, but I don't believe him either and start yelling again for Fortner until one nurse says, "If we call your wife and get her on the phone, will you quiet down and stop waking up all the patients?"

They call Edmée, and I insist they let me talk to her. So they pull me up, with all the tubes and wires, until I can reach the phone line. My poor wife, I guess I scared the bejesus out of her.

EDMÉE: I expected the worst at that hour—who wouldn't? I thought he was dying and wanted to see me before he died. Then I hear him say, "Tell me that you're there," and I got even more mixed up. Where else would I be? I'm sitting up in bed, holding the phone—where does he think I am? I can hear other voices, like he's struggling to keep holding onto the phone, and I decide he's really delirious, very ill, and trying to say his last words to me. So I begin to cry and ask him to tell me that he's not dying.

JULIUS: *(Interrupting)* I went crazy and began to yell at her, "For chrissake, will you shut up and listen to me? I'm not dying, dammit!" This offends her, of course, and suddenly I hear nothing—just silence. I think maybe she's gone down to the floor again and I start yelling, "Edmée! Speak to me! Are you all right?"

EDMÉE: *(Coolly)* I said I was fine, except he woke me up at three in the morning.

JULIUS: After I hung up, I started to tell the doctor and nurses that she was okay—but I sort of broke down and couldn't go on. Maybe it was the fever or something—but, you know, I was happy that she was safe at home and not in the hospital like me. *(Pause.)* It sounds funny, I guess, but we'd come such a long way together, and she needed me so much now.

They had met at Le Petit Pavillon, a beach club in Marseilles across the street from where he was billeted as a noncommissioned officer, a T-4 with the army engineers. "The club was off-limits to G.I.s because the army said the water was polluted. But they didn't say anything about the girls being polluted so we'd sneak over during our lunch hour. One day I spot Edmée in one of those skimpy French bikinis, and I think, 'Holy smoke, that's some mademoiselle if I ever saw one.' "

She knew he was an American, even though he spoke French like an Italian: "His swimming trunks were very funny. They came down to his knees." *After meeting several times at the beach, she agreed to a regular date, and later he joked about the evening:* "I hardly recognized her with her clothes on!" *She softened his name to "Julie," and he called her "co-cotte"—his little chicken. One night, walking home from a dance, he kissed her many times and said,* "Listen, when I get out of the army, I'll have to look for a job, and it might be rough for a while—could you take something like that?" *She held him close and said,* "I think so, Julie, if you're with me." *After that, there was little more to be said.*

Her father was a master saddle maker and owned a livery and leather goods store. Horses were disappearing in the war, however, many of them being eaten, and business was very bad. "So my father became a policeman to help support us. My mother was ill with tuberculosis, and there were three children to care for. It was very sad. When he heard Julie wanted to marry me and take me to America, it broke his heart. Poor Papa. After he finally agreed, the army sent around some Red Cross ladies to find out if our family had been German collaborators—and my father threw them out. I thought he would have a heart attack. The next day the army chaplain phoned, asking me, 'What is this—a wedding or an anti-American riot?' " (Laughs.)

Back from the war with his French bride, Julius eventually got a job managing a steel products warehouse in Elizabeth, New Jersey. They lived in a furnished room, and he enrolled at Rutgers University for evening studies under the G.I. Bill of Rights: "I was pushing thirty, and the kids in my class used to say, 'What're you doing here? You're as old as Jack Benny!' (Laughs.) *For eight years, I worked by day, went to school at night, and studied on the weekends. I'll tell you, that's doing it the hard way—and Edmée stuck by me. We couldn't afford a good time, no matter what. I had my nose in a book, and she had to take care of the kids to make sure they kept quiet and didn't run around, so Daddy could be a college graduate and get a better job."*

On graduation day, Edmée sat with hundreds of proud parents in the university stadium, to witness Julius Binetti—the abandoned boy immigrant and World War II veteran—receive his Bachelor of Science degree in business administration, Rutgers University Class of '56. A dream had come true, and a few months later, it became a further reality when he was accepted as a trainee by the State Farm Insurance Company—eventually to become one of their top salesmen.

After I got out of intensive care and was back in my room, I began to pick up fast, and pretty soon I was feeling a lot more like my old self. I made a couple of calls to my office, then they started calling me, and before you know it, I'm calling customers from my hospital room. It was better than lying around in bed, doing nothing. So why not? I figured it'd get the juices going, the adrenalin pumping, and maybe even get me out of there sooner.

Another thing—our company has a convention every year for those of us who've sold half a million dollars worth of insurance. I'd always made it and wasn't about to be left out this year just because I'd been sick. I wasn't sick any longer, at least with cancer, and the sooner they knew it, the better. So, by the time they let me go home in October, I was off and running with a lot of personal calls to make. That's where it counts. On the phone, people will say, "Yes, yes," but you haven't got them sold until the name's on the policy and the money's there—you follow me?

That meant a lot of hustling, and during November and December, I sold a quarter of a million dollars worth of insurance. It put me well over my quota, and my manager could hardly believe it. He said, "I'd written you off as being unable to do anything. That was some comeback, nobody expected it. You must've had some great doctor—or was it the nurses?" *(Laughs.)*

I like that, setting goals for myself and making them. I also like giving people straight advice on insurance: get with a good company that has a reputation, and get an agent you can trust, one who's been in the business for a while and can give you good advice.

"Once I got home, my biggest problem was learning how to eat right and live as a diabetic. As I said, if you lose your pancreas, your body has no insulin to regulate the blood sugar level. So you have to do it yourself and do it right—or get into trouble and maybe end up in the hospital. Too much sugar in the blood, and you zoom up to a crazy high. Too little, and you get

disoriented and have the shakes. In five minutes, you can go from a dizzy high down to what I call a babbling idiot.

"So you become a sort of high wire trapeze artist in the food department, and you also learn to doctor yourself with insulin shots every morning and evening. My wife, God bless her, gives them to me in the leg—or else, I do it myself, in the stomach. It doesn't much matter where you do it, as long as it's in the muscle and not a vein.

"You regulate your insulin intake by measuring your blood sugar level with an instrument—the Ames Glucometer. You can do it in a couple of minutes—prick your finger for a drop of blood, put it in the test, and back comes the reading. If it's low, you know you must eat something to raise it. If it's high, you wait until what you've eaten wears off. Or you work it off by raking leaves or something. I can work off a high by just being in the office, by answering the phone, by being excited in what I do. As for the lows, you have to be prepared for any unexpected expenditure of energy, like staying late at a dance, bowling a few extra games, or being late for a meal because you have to eat at regular hours. You keep candy in your pocket, or crackers in the car for traffic jams, because you never know what might happen to catch you off base."

It's not as bad as it sounds, this living with diabetes. You get used to it. The tests and medication take a couple of minutes twice a day, that's all, and the diet is healthy for anybody. You don't get fat, and if you obey the rules, you feel fine most of the time.

So you learn to live with it. Only you don't live like you once did because something like this changes you, and you're different in a lot of ways. For one thing, you enjoy life more. You experience it one day at a time, like it might be your last one—if you follow me. You sit in the backyard, you watch the birds fly, the flowers grow, and you appreciate just being alive. You get a kick out of simple things you once took for granted—like waking up in the morning, looking out the window, and breathing fresh air. Something ordinary, like that. Or walking down the street and looking at people and feeling like you've known them all your life—even though you've never seen them before. *(Laughs.)* It's hard to explain and maybe it sounds a little crazy.

Something else, too. You find yourself wondering about the others who didn't make it. Right now, I'm thinking about the fellow who was in my room with me and died the day after Christmas. Or Mrs. Barrett, that nice old lady who lived down the street—she didn't make it, either. And my daughter's godfather, our best friend, Bob Frank, who lived next door—he went out, too, with stomach cancer.

Why all of them and not me? The girls at my office say God didn't want me because I needed more time to clean up my act. *(Smiles.)* Maybe. But I think a lot of it has to do with yourself. If you fight back, saying, "Dammit, I'm not going! They won't get me!"—I think it counts a lot. Especially if you have something to fight for, someone who needs you. Edmée needed me that way. She needed me so much that she became ill when I did, and when I dreamed she was in the hospital, calling for me, I went out of my mind. I guess it was then that I realized how much we needed each other, and that I was fighting to live for both of us.

She is 38, the mother of four boys—a large-boned black woman. Her great-grandmother was Cherokee, and some of this seems visible in her broad face, in the reddish hue of her brown skin, and in her unwavering, dark eyes that appear to be staring out of an old photo album.

She was never wont to complain much about herself. Two days before entering Memorial Hospital for a forequarter amputation of left arm and shoulder, she played softball with her women's team.

They didn't see anything because I wore long sleeves and a big blouse. Later they said, "Why didn't you tell us you was having trouble? You were just going after the ball, and swingin' and battin' like a fool—weren't you in pain?" I said, "Well, I really didn't think about it because if you enjoy it, if you want something, you just go ahead and forget about what's bothering you." That's how Jack feels when he plays his wheelchair basketball games.

Jack Harris, her husband, sits nearby in a wheelchair—paralyzed from the waist down, after being shot by a neighbor in an argument over a dog. Jack has the long, immobile face of Larry Holmes, the boxer. As a result of pulling himself in a wheelchair, his arms are enormous. Mark, one of four sons—tall and lean as his father was before being cut down—says: "Pop lost his legs, but he's got two new ones growin' outa his shoulders!" Everyone laughs, and Jack smiles.

We are in the small front room of the Harris home, one of many two-story, wooden frame dwellings along 120th Road in St. Albans, Queens—a predominantly black neighborhood. The Harris home is painted bright red and has a ramp at the front door to allow Jack to scoot down onto the walk and into his car.

Nelle is seated on the sofa. She wears a flower print blouse. The left sleeve hangs limp, without an arm. Beside her, on the sofa, is her battery-powered artificial shoulder and arm. During an earlier visit, the arm was elsewhere, being repaired after having a "nervous breakdown." It went out of control near the Empire State Building, grabbed Nelle's dress, and wouldn't let go. Now it lies strangely inert next to her thigh, and as she touches it, one notices it has the same color as her living hand.

Since it came back last week, it's been behavin' fine. There's no trouble with it round here. It's just in the city, with the radio waves—all those signals crisscrossing in the air. If I don't remember to turn the switch off, it feels all those signals and gets confused. *(She indicates a switch button inside the wrist, plus six chrome electrodes in a curve beneath the shoulder cap. When pressed variously by residual shoulder stump and back muscles, they cause the hand to open, close, and turn.)*

I try to keep the switch off. But going through a turnstile in the subway, a slight push can turn it on. So if I'm not careful, it'll grab onto something. . . . You wanted to see how it works, so I'll put it on. *(Picks up arm and goes into bedroom, then returns. The blouse is fuller now, the sleeve possesses an arm, and silver bracelets dangle above a flesh-colored glove masking artificial fingers.)*

Unless I wear men's clothes, the sleeves are never long enough. So I use bracelets on that hand. *(Demonstrates how the hand is able to open, close and turn. There is no mechanism, however, for raising the arm.)*

I have to do that with my other arm. *(Lifts the limb upward.)* But most people, especially from a distance, don't notice. I was crossing the street, and this little lady comes up and says, "Darling, will you help me across the street?" So I said, "Sure, I'll help you." She grabbed *this* hand. *(Laughs.)* I guess she thought it was real 'cause from a distance it does look sort of real. They did a good job in matching the glove, don't you think? This is a new one. They wear out very fast. If you cut them, it spreads like a run in a stocking. At first, I wasn't used to wearing it to work, and before you knew it, I had it covered with ink. Or if anybody hits the glove with a cigarette, it'll go right up. So I keep a spare one handy.

Some women lose a breast and feel they are no longer a whole woman for their men. You've lost nearly one quarter of your upper body. Do you feel less a woman?

(She pauses, face immobile. In his wheelchair, Jack's tree trunk arms twitch, and the chair moves an inch. Suddenly Nelle bursts into deep, easy laughter, and Jack smiles.) You know, a psychologist at the Institute* is always asking me that. Well, it never seemed to bother me. As long as I was able to get back home and be with my family and children and stuff. *(Pauses.)* I've always been a tomboy, you know *(laughs),* so it never did really bother me, 'cause I wasn't up into women's fashions, even though I like to dress up nice when we go out.

Some people ask me where I get the strength to carry on. Well, you just go on, and you find it. You never know what kind of strength you have in

---

* Rusk Institute, which helped rehabilitate Mrs. Nelle Harris, provided the artificial limb, and offered training courses that led to her current work as a telephone consultant with Blue Cross/Blue Shield.

you until you're faced with this situation. You find it when you need it, like the time Jack was shot.

Her husband was shot shortly before Christmas, when Nelle returned home from the hospital, with stomach drains from adhesions following a gallbladder operation. "I was due to stay in the hospital, but it was near Christmas, and my children needed me. I'd been away so much that, whenever I got home, I couldn't move without Jamie, my youngest one, wrappin' himself around my leg like maybe a cat or a little dog. So they taught me how to clean the stomach drains and let me come home for a short spell."

When we drove up before the house, there was this neighbor there with his dog. It was a vicious dog, never on a leash. When the dog saw my sister Betty—she was eight months pregnant—he chased her, and she ran and jumped up on top of the car. So Jack said, "Listen, man, you know her sister's pregnant. Why can't you keep that dog on a leash?" They argued out there for a few minutes, just an exchange of words. Then Jack came in and started straightening up the house for me, saying, "It's about time you go to bed because you had a hard day." After that, he went back outside with my brother-in-law, Tommy, to play Santa Claus. They'd bought two electric motorbikes for Mark and Brian and had hid them in the trunk of the car, to slip in when the kids weren't looking.

While they were doing that, I was in the back changing my stomach drains. The fluid had to come out, you know, and you had to keep sterile gauze on it all the time—when I heard Tommy shout: "Look out, Jack! He's got a gun!" Then I heard a shot, sounding like it was in the front room of the house.

I dropped the gauze and came flyin' through the house to out front, where I saw Jack on the ground behind our car, and Tommy behind his car. I began to scream at that crazy man. I said I was going to kill him myself, and he ran away.

I told myself then, "Nelle, you got to heal real fast 'cause Jack's gonna need you real bad." Well, it happened. The hospital wanted to put me back in again, but I never went back. The wound closed up, and I never had any more trouble there. It was sort of like a healing moment. Then I had that other one, another moment like that, just before they took away my arm. That's when I heard a voice speaking to me.

She is not certain where the voice came from. She just heard it. "I don't know if it was God talking to me or who was speaking. But I was in bed and a little frightened after they told me they were going to take off my arm. Dr.

Knapper† had come into my room, and he was sitting on my bed, talking to me. He explained how, before coming to Memorial, they had operated on me twice to remove tumors from my arm, then given me thirty-six cobalt treatments that burnt the area black—but it didn't halt it. Another knot had come back. So they had sent me to Dr. Knapper as a last resort. He had done a biopsy on the arm and found it was malignant all around.

"Sitting on my bed, he explained there was nothing to do but take off my arm. I'd already given consent to go further, to take off as much as needed to get me well. But that night he didn't say anything about taking off the shoulder, too, because I suspect he wasn't sure of it, and he didn't want to upset me more than necessary. But that was already enough. My arm was going to be taken away, and I was frightened. Where was this going to stop? It'd begun as a simple pimple between my elbow and my shoulder."‡

After he left, I lay there alone. I was taped all the way up to the neck after the biopsy operation and couldn't even move my arm. I wanted to just feel it a little bit longer before they took it away. But more than that, I was worried about my family, how I was going to take care of them now with only one arm. Jack had no legs, and he needed me. The boys, they needed me, too. No matter what happened, I was going to have to keep on working and making do with just one arm. I was also frightened about the pain when they took my arm away.

Then I heard those words coming to me. I've never been able to figure out exactly whether it was a voice of somebody there, or if it was just, you know, a hearing that came into me, or whatever. I was lying there, and the television was on, but I wasn't exactly looking at it. There was a sort of disappearing, a fading, and I heard the voice saying, "No need to worry, Nelle, everything's going to be okay." I got a tingling feeling all over, all the fear went away, and I went to sleep and slept very good without any problems. From that moment on, I was never afraid.

But when I woke up after the operation, Dr. Knapper says I was screamin' and goin' on, sayin' . . . *(Laughs.)* It's so silly, every time I think of it. I said, "You told me you was gonna take off my arm but you left my hand. . . ." 'Cause you know how people get the phantom pain, except I'd never heard anybody talk about it. I was prepared for everything else, but not for that. I kept saying, "Why on earth did you remove

---

† William H. Knapper, M.D., attending surgeon, Gastric and Mixed Tumor Service, Memorial Hospital.

‡ Nelle Harris had progressively recurrent fibrosarcoma—cancer of the soft tissue of her left arm. See p. 101.

my whole arm, except my hand and sew my hand to my stomach?"— 'Cause it felt like that.

Dr. Knapper came into the recovery room, and he talked to me, and it helped. Then, after I got through that night, I was okay because they have a very good program at the hospital, what they call pain control. If you join it, they have a special nurse who'll come around and talk to you, and if you really need anything for pain, she'll give it to you. That helped my whole fear of pain and eased my mind.

That place is absolutely fantastic. I'm not just saying that because you're writing a book about it. Not only the doctors and nurses, but all the others. One day a woman in a light blue gown* came in and asked me, "Is there anything you need? Anything we can help you with?" She took some plain cotton, stuck it into nylon stockings, and made me a shoulder cap. 'Cause without that—my shoulder now comes straight down, you see— my blouse isn't going to stay on. She also made other little things—a slip to help me hold my food on my tray and a nail cutter—little things that she figured would help me when I came home.

Nine days after they took the arm off, Dr. Knapper said I was doing well, and he let me come home. But then I got very restless, or more like impatient. Everybody waitin' on me hand and foot got on my nerves. It was very hot, and I put my bed on the sun porch to look out. But lookin' out wasn't the same as bein' out, you know, so after three days I finally got on my clothes and asked my sister to drive me to the store.

I just had to get away. Jack knows how I am, but he kept on saying, "Now why on earth you going to the store?" Actually, all my stitches wasn't out because they'd removed only every other one. And when I got out at the store, I wasn't really strong, but it felt good anyway to get outside. After that, I just started taking care of the necessary things around the house. Just go ahead and do it, you know. . . .

Now she's able to help others like herself. "*An occupational therapist at Rusk had me speak to one of her patients who was going to Memorial to have a lower arm amputation. She had a small baby and such fears. So I tried to convey to her that she was lucky in a way because they was only going to take a little bit above her elbow. If you have that much arm, you can cradle, you know. . . .*

"*You think you'll never survive, but you do—except for that phantom pain. It stays right after you, especially on days like today where it's cloudy.*

---

* One of 450 part- or full-time volunteers at Memorial Hospital, many of them former patients.

They told me as soon as I got the prosthesis, the phantom would disappear. I must be a rare case, 'cause it hasn't. I don't know why I never feel the arm where I used to have all the pain. I never feel that part of it. It's just the hand—mainly my fingers and my wrist. Gary, where are you going like that?" Another son, Gary, 14, is walking through the living room in short pants and an undershirt. He makes a fast retreat. Jack leans back in his wheelchair and laughs.

When the children asked to see your amputation, what did you do?

I don't think it was a matter of them wanting to see it. I just never did hide it, you know. Like in the summertime when it was too hot for robes and long sleeves, it never did embarrass me. I'd be out there, sittin' on the stoop without my shoulder cap—I never really did hide it. So if they asked questions about it, I explained. I told them about the disease. I explained it straight. There was a time when you didn't mention the word "cancer." You would just sort of whisper it. But now, it's better to say it straight, except when the children are too young to understand.

You feel as though you've beaten the cancer?

The doctors said it was localized and didn't get into the bloodstream. So I think maybe I'm free of it now. The psychologist at Rusk keeps asking what's changed for me. Well, most people would think it'd be better to have never removed the arm, but it really opened up opportunities for me.

It's hard to say you got to lose an arm before you get a lucky break, but it seems that's the way it happened for me. It was the right time at the right place or whatever, but now I got a job I like, helping subscribers to Blue Cross and Blue Shield. I'd had jobs before, but nothing I really enjoyed—just doin' work, you know. It's given me a lot more confidence, so there's a lot more to life than before.

In a nurses' lounge at Memorial, the talk turns to patients who refuse to die and, for one reason or another, manage to survive. A veteran nurse says, "You get a lot of them saying love is the big thing that pulled them through. But I knew one guy who was saved by hate. He came in here with a hole in his stomach, his intestines falling out—a really bad case of overradiation. He said, 'I'm not about to die. I'm going to live and get even with my wife. Nothing can kill me until I take care of that bitch!' And you know what? He did just that." Laughter.

The Premise:

Serious illness can strain any relationship. With cancer especially, it strikes suddenly and is intensified through a progressive series of increasingly violent and awesome stages.

Initially, there is the sudden shock of discovering the disease lurking in one's own body—a creeping, hidden enemy within, disobeying all biological laws within the body of its birth, turncoat cells now using the tactics of terrorists to kill and maim, increasing in numbers to eventually destroy the society that sustains them.

This first psychological trauma is followed by still another shock: the violation of personal privacy and proper image by the transfer of self into the hands of others in a medical protocol—a transfer that conveys more than the mere body. The mind, with hopes and dreams to live again, also goes with it. Further, this transfer is endless, for the uncertain outcome— the possibility of life or death at the end of the treatment—remains constantly in the hands of others. In the long, attenuated struggle for life, the patient lives in a limbo of endless nights and slow dawns, looking backward over a lifetime while enduring such indignities as the loss of hair, the withering of flesh, the nausea and vomit of chemotherapy. For some, there is also postsurgical disfigurement and physical impairment.

This can play havoc with marriages, love affairs, and close relationships. We see it happen in this book—couples sinking under the weight of sudden illness, crying out in anguish and pain, turning away in fear and shame. Yet most of them—as though drawing strength from some deep wellspring of life—emerge with their love or friendship strengthened and enriched by the ordeal.

Melvin and Stella Schlossberg fell apart.* The love, or what they believe to have been a love, did not hold them together. Where other wives

---

* Identities of patient and wife have been altered.

faltered and fell—yet rose up again—Stella did not rise. Where other husbands managed to hold onto their love, Melvin's slipped through his grasp.

After that, Melvin fought on alone, drawing on revenge and hate for the strength to survive—only to discover that he could never entirely let go of love.

Melvin's Story:

It came all of a sudden. I was in my office working when I went into the bathroom and urinated blood. I thought maybe I'd lifted something, and when I went back to the bathroom later in the day, it eased up. The color was turning more natural, and when I came home in the evening, it was normal. This was in May—eight years ago.

We are sitting in the living room of his flat at Borough Park in Brooklyn. He is 47, but he looks much younger, with the features of an American Indian. Mel laughs at this and says, "It must come from my Sephardic ancestors." Beneath his yellow T-shirt and blue jeans, one discerns an athletic body—a former physical wreck now rebuilt by weight lifting and gym workouts.

The next day, the same thing again. Solid blood, then it eased off in the afternoon. I told my wife, and she said, "Go to a doctor." I said, "I'll give it one more day. I think it's a strain or something."

Third day, it was again solid blood. My wife said, "Go into a doctor." So I went to one we knew, and he sent me to see a urologist in Brooklyn—Dr. Nathan Saltzman.† He took some X rays and said, "There's something there, you'll have to be hospitalized." They did a biopsy with a cytoscope, cutting out a specimen, and I waited. After a week, he said, "It's malignant, up against the wall of the bladder. We have to operate."

I told myself that at least it wasn't my heart again. I'd had heart trouble and gotten over it by slowing down and taking better care of myself. So now I was going to get over this, too. They operated, and everything was fine. Then Saltzman said, "Now you need radiation—about thirty treatments." I went every day, Monday through Friday, for six weeks. It made me very sick—so sick I had to stop for two days, with vomiting and violent stomach pains.

It almost killed me . . . *(pauses)* and it did kill my marriage. Before this, Stella and I were really in love. At least, we thought so. I remember her saying we'd never been closer in our seven years of marriage. But the

---

† Name altered.

radiation blew it. The day I started is the day I got turned off. She turned me right out of her life that day. It was too much for her. If it wasn't for that, we might still be married.

She flipped out because, when she was a little girl, her mother had cancer. She took her mother to the hospital, she saw her get blood transfusions, she saw her get chemotherapy, and—after fourteen years of this—she saw her die there.

Later, she said, "You never listened to anything I told you about my mother. We had a lack of communication." Well, there was a lack of everything else from her. As soon as the cancer started, I became another person for her—a stranger. I don't think we had sex more than three times after the radiation began, if that.

When the treatments stopped in August of '76, I had so much pain I went to the VA hospital for a checkup. They examined me and sent me back to Dr. Saltzman. He gave me Empirin and codeine and sent me away. The pain increased, and he gave me more of the same, only stronger. Finally I couldn't stand it, and in tears I went back to the VA asking for help. They sent me to their psychiatrist. This surprised me, but I knew that a lot of veterans—I was in the Korean War—came back psyched out. Or else they pretend to be that way, for some extra pay. So they get a lot of kooks. Anyway, the psychiatrist said I was normal. "If he says he's in pain, I believe he's in pain." So they sent me back to Saltzman again.

This time, he cut me open in the middle of my stomach and found extensive radiation damage. I asked, "So what do we do?" He said, "I want one more test on you—a spinal tap." "No, you don't," I said, "I've had enough. I want out." I called my wife and told her, "Pick me up tomorrow, I'm getting out fast." "All right," she said, and then she added something I'll never forget: "If you're still sick, don't expect me to take care of you."

Well, I was sick—too sick to realize she meant it. The cut Saltzman had made in my stomach would not stay closed. Because of the radiation damage, it kept opening up after I got home. I was so desperate I let Saltzman put me back in the hospital. I'm not saying he was responsible for the radiation damage, or that he was not trying to do his best. But I figured he had made this hole in my stomach, and it was his job to close it up somehow.

This time, he decided to do another cytoscope and gave me some sort of a laxative to clean me out. It blew me up, and my bowels popped out through the hole. Saltzman then said, "Now we're going to have to remove your bladder, and also give you a colostomy." Crazy? I was going to

have two bags—one for my urine and one for my bowels. I freaked out. I never expected anything like that, and in a panic I called for help.

My mother wanted to send me to Lenox Hill, but my wife said, "No, let's go to Memorial." I had a cousin who had been there as a patient of Dr. Whitely,‡ and my wife got me to see him. So I have to say that, in a way, she saved my life because Dr. Whitely operated on me just in time. But I lost my bladder, and I had a tremendous hole down there. He closed it where possible, but there was still an open space from the radiation damage. He hoped it would heal over but was not sure because, he said, he had never seen such horrendous radiation reaction on a human being.

The day after the operation, my wife comes in. "How are you?" "Fine." "I'm not fine," she says. "I put the dog to sleep." It was my dog, Buck—a gorgeous German shepherd, only 4 years old. I asked, "Why'd you do that?" She said, "It's too hard to take care of him, and I couldn't give him away, so I put him to sleep."

She said she was going out to Sag Harbor to stay with her parents—that's her father and her stepmother—and was taking our son, Daniel. This is Thursday, the day after I lost my bladder, and she would come to me Sunday. Sunday I was depressed, and I called her. I'd lost my bladder, and it seemed like everything else was gone, too. She came in and made a big stink. "I had to drive all the way from Sag Harbor to come and see you. Your son threw up in the car coming through the tunnel. He's downstairs in the car waiting, I can't stay too long."

After a month, when I was ready to come home, my wife warned me to make sure I had someone to take care of me because she couldn't cope. So they brought in a hospital bed, and a nurse came every day to clean my stomach hole. When she left in the morning, I was on my own, and it was murder. I could barely walk, and Stella had taken a job to get away from all of it. She left at seven thirty. So I had to make sure our son was properly dressed for school, make lunch for myself, and make dinner for us both. After that, Stella would come home. One day I asked her, "You leave early and come home late—why?" "Because I can't stand to be near you. It's too much."

Sometimes at night I had to ask her for help. While sleeping, you're hooked up with a tube, an ilio conduit, that runs into a jar on the floor. A few times it broke loose in my sleep, and I'd wake up with the bed soaking wet. So I had to go in for a shower at three o'clock. Stella wouldn't get up until I screamed at her to please change my sheets. She'd tear off the wet

---

‡ Horace W. Whitely, Jr., M.D., associate attending surgeon, Department of Surgery, Memorial Hospital.

ones, throw them in the corner, and throw on two others without tucking them in or making the bed, screaming back at me "You should be in a nursing home, who can stand this?"

I kept bleeding and losing weight until I was under a hundred pounds, and they put me back in the hospital to build me up. After another month, when I was to come home, Stella insisted I go into a nursing home. Dr. Whitely said, "Absolutely not, you will go home." This time, they arranged to have a woman in the house, taking care of the cooking, cleaning, and doing everything while my wife was working. Stella would not have to do anything.

The day before I was to go home, she came into the hospital room, gave me fifty dollars, the house keys, and said, "I'm leaving. I've sent Danny to my parents at Sag Harbor, and I took a little furniture." That was it—and she left.

I came home the next day, bent over, hardly able to walk and I find she's taken all the furniture, the antiques, the pictures, the stereo—anything of value. She left the couch you're sitting on, that crummy lamp over there, a busted TV in the bedroom with the bed and a lamp. That was it, plus a pile of dirt in the corner. She had never cleaned the house, just pushed it all there, never did a day's wash, emptied our checking account, except for two thousand dollars, and paid only a minimum on every bill— even though she was working and my full salary was still coming in. When the cleanup woman came from the agency, she took one look at the place and almost left immediately, saying she'd never seen such a pigpen.

I could barely walk, but the next day I staggered into the bank, changed the accounts to prevent her from stripping me of my last dime—and staggered home, swearing I was going to live. I had to live to get even with that bitch. Until I did, nothing was going to kill me—nothing.

He returned to Memorial three more times—in March, April, and October of 1977—until the bowel opening was finally closed by a muscle transplant and skin graft. During that time, he initiated divorce action for abandonment and adultery against Stella, who was now living with another man. She countersued, claiming Melvin had abandoned her, and—citing his many hospital trips and ongoing surgery—obtained temporary custody of their son. As a result, Daniel now stays with his mother all week, seeing his father only on weekends. Melvin is deeply concerned about what this is doing to his son.

I pay for everything, and she does nothing. She gets Social Security help for the boy—three hundred ninety a month. She also makes two-fifty a week working for a union. If Daniel wants a shirt or shoes, she says, "Tell your father to buy it."

It's a bad scene for my son. She screams at him about everything. And always the marijuana. He says the first thing in the morning she has to light up marijuana. He hears her moaning and groaning at night, making love to her boyfriend. Their friends come in, and he sees them stoned out of their minds. Twice, she has sent him out to live with her parents at Sag Harbor for months at a time.

The boy is suffering from this. He wrote me a letter saying he had a dream. In it, his mother comes to him and tells him that I am dying, and at the end of it, he puts a gun to himself and wants to die, too. That's why I want him with me. A boy needs a mother, but if his own mother doesn't behave like one, then he's better off with his father.

Melvin believes he and his son could live well together, as did the father and son in the film Kramer vs. Kramer. *He does not foresee another marriage for the time being.*

I'm impotent right now. The radiation killed me there, too. I'm trying to get an erection, because I still feel like I want to, but it doesn't come up. They say there's a surgical remedy for this, but I can't psych myself up for another operation right now. So I live with it. I meet a nice girl, we go to dinner, we talk, she knows the situation. If she wants to come back, fine. If not, no bad feelings.

He wears a bag to replace the bladder, but it is not a major impediment. It does not show when he is dressed, nor restrict him from swimming or any noncontact sports. Nor would it limit lovemaking. The problem for the moment is his impotence.

I know a real nice girl in this building. She asks me to come over and listen to some of her old records, like Sarah Vaughan and the others. We sit on the couch, and she literally attacks me. Pulls down my pants, wants to see my body. We tried sex, we tried everything. I just couldn't get it up. We kept seeing each other for a while, but then it wasn't there for me, so we let it ease up. That's where it stands with women right now. But I'm not desperate. I can get along, live without it—especially if I get my son.

We leave the apartment. Outside, on the sidewalk, a late sun filters through trees, creating a soft glow. Near the entrance, a young girl in a white dress says, "Hi, Melvin!" "What's new?" he asks. "Going dancing," she replies. "That's great," he says, just as three young boys come running toward him,

*yelling, "Melvie! Melvie!" They ram into him, playfully holding him
around the waist. "You got the tickets for the game Saturday, Mel?"
"Yeah." "And we're gonna have a pizza first?" "Yeah." "Yippee!" they yell,
and Melvin watches them run away through the twilight. "At least I have
that kind of loving," he says.*

<u>Stella's Story:</u>

My husband has said a lot of things about me, about what happened to us.
I want to say this. If you put down everything he says, if you write it down
in black and white, it will not always be true because there are shadings,
underlying reasons for our behavior and the situation that followed. It
isn't as plain as it seems.

Also, my husband is the type of person who has trouble expressing his
real emotions. I tend to be very aware of mine. He is not. He is not
realistic that way. He sees everything through his own special vision. So
he's never totally honest with himself.

*Stella Schlossberg is telling her version of the story during the divorce pro-
ceedings that followed. She is 41, a small well-formed woman with delicate,
sensual features. Under questioning, these transform into a tight bitter
mask, and she stiffens as though facing a physical threat. In one nervous,
birdlike gesture, she sweeps back her dark hair. Her darting, gray-brown
eyes reflect variously nostalgia, sorrow, a sense of betrayal—and, perhaps
above all else, the loneliness of one who discovers the person that she has
been living with, the human being she once loved, is now a distant stranger.*

Yes, I did leave him on the day he was to return from the hospital. But you
have to know the actions preceding that, the extenuating circumstances. A
wife would not up and leave her husband the day he's expected back from
the hospital, if there wasn't some profound reason for it.

I agonized over his illness more than he did, or more than he does
today. He has done things that have hurt me incredibly, yet if I had the
thought to hurt him, I couldn't do it, thinking of what he went through.
Really, I have such sorrow about that. He says I left because I couldn't
face the physical problem of his stomach being open, his bowels coming
out. It's not true. He also has me saying I couldn't cope with cancer or
Memorial Hospital because my mother died there of lymphoma. Well, that
has nothing to do with it. I had years of adjusting myself to that place, and
I can handle it.

The day I was born, they told my mother she had cancer—Hodgkin's
lymph node. The books at that time gave her seven years to live. At

Memorial they save people now with that, and even then they doubled her life. It was fourteen years of my life, too. I remember going through the agony with her.

Yes, it was horrifying for me to learn that Melvin had a tumor. And I insisted he go to the best place for it—Memorial. If it wasn't for that, he'd probably be dead today. I think that shows how much I cared for him, for his life.

But there were also the horrifying years before that, when he had heart attacks, one after the other. My husband is the type of person who does not seek help. So he went through a heart attack in the house where I had him on the floor, breathing life into him, mouth-to-mouth, because he was breathing so shallow. Then, when he was in the hospital for this, I went to see him every day. After that, I went through years of his taking nitroglycerin for angina—right? Even when he was healthy, it was like he was always in between attacks. So that was always a problem. We were aware of it, but it didn't come between us.

The next thing that happened to him was just awful. He threw a bag of sawdust down the incinerator on the sixth floor, and it burst into flames. So he had third-degree burns. He didn't have hands. I mean, they were so bandaged that I became his hands. I cried for a week when it happened. He didn't cry, but I cried because of how he was hurt by it. That's how it was with us.

Then he found out he had a tumor. I hope you realize I'm not the kind of woman that would leave somebody like that for no good reason. He says I turned away from him when he began radiation because I felt he was another person, and so I couldn't go the cancer route with him. That's not true. It was not me that changed—it was him, my husband. The truth is this. Once my husband became a cancer patient, he was horrified of himself. That's when it started, that's when he began to change in his relations with me—not me with him.

Some people who are sick will welcome help from others with open arms. That's normal. Some other people feel disgust for themselves, like my husband did. So they start to push you away.

That's what he began doing to me. I couldn't believe it—my own husband. He even wished cancer on me. He did it several times, saying, "You'll get cancer, too. I know you'll get it from me. How will you like that?" Here I am cleaning up urine, making his meals, actually killing myself—and he's wishing that I get cancer. I was thinking, "What's happening to this man?" It's not supposed to be contagious, they tell you it isn't—but he's wishing it on me!

Yes, he would scream at me in the night to clean up his urine and change his sheets. Yes, I hated that. I hated the ugliness of it, I hated what the illness was doing to him—but I never hated him. You must understand, I did not hate my husband. I was trying to hold on, trying to help, but he was making it harder and harder.

I told myself that I should be patient. He was taking medicines; he had a broken body. So it wasn't his fault. But then he started to get mean. He slapped me twice, brutal slaps. He says now that he doesn't remember it. But how can I forget my husband striking me? That's when I became frightened. This man was beginning to like it, to enjoy hurting me. He started saying that I wanted him to die. He knew what I was up to. So he was going to cut me out of his insurance.

I did what I could, I clung on and on, telling myself he was angry only because of his illness. He did not mean to hurt me, to destroy us. But it became worse and worse until I couldn't take no more. If I stayed any longer, I would die.

So what happened is that I did not leave him. I was driven away. After all the caring, the crying, the loving—to have nothing in return, it was too much. I did not abandon him. I was driven away.

I didn't take all the furniture. I took those things that I had bought and loved, that were mine. I didn't empty our joint account. I left two thousand dollars in it, and Melvin had eighty thousand in another account with his aunt. As for the dog, I couldn't control it. It would pull me down the avenue, and get loose and run away. I tried to find someone to take it. The superintendent of the building said he would be glad to take the dog. He would teach it to behave, he said, with the club. The thought of having Buck clubbed into submission was too much. So I had him put to sleep rather than allow him to suffer.

It doesn't matter anymore. None of it, what happened to us, it doesn't matter now. What matters for me is my son Daniel. I'm his mother, and he needs me. I know he loves me and needs me because he has been living with me.

I have lost my husband, my marriage is over—gone. But I do not want to lose my boy. I am his mother, and he needs me, to have a proper home, to be with his mother who cares for him.

Stella Schlossberg's charges that she was abused by her husband and thus forced to leave were questioned by her husband's lawyer. She was asked: "You say your husband brutally struck you twice and hurt you. How is it possible since he was in bed, hardly able to stand up, and weighed less than ninety pounds?"

Witnesses were then called with the aim of showing that Stella Schlossberg did not provide a proper home for her son, Daniel. First to testify was a young man who admitted to living in the same apartment with the mother and son—but as a boarder only. Following this, Stella's father took the stand to state he had seen this same youth in bed with his daughter. He stated also that the couple smoked marijuana and created a home scene that was unfit for a growing child. Stella's stepmother followed this with further testimony against her daughter.

Judge Rigler wasted no time in giving his opinion. "I'm going to give you the decision now," he said. "I'm going to find in behalf of the plaintiff on the grounds of adultery and abandonment. I'm not granting any alimony to the defendant. . . . The custody [of the child] will be with the plaintiff. Should the defendant change her life-style and get married—and I cannot force anybody to get married—I think the living situation would be altered on behalf of the child—whom I interviewed, by the way, and he does not have any real objection to anything I'm doing. In the event [the mother] changes her situation, she should regain custody of the child to live with her, with the continuation of the liberal visitation that the plaintiff has had in the past. Do I make myself clear?"

POSTSCRIPT: One year later, Stella Schlossberg was still unmarried and still without custody of her son. Except on rare occasions, Danny no longer sees his mother, who lives only ten minutes away. Mel often tells Danny to phone or visit his mother, but the boy replies, "Why doesn't she call me?" Stella is convinced that Melvin has turned her son away from her. "Someday, my boy will know the truth and come home to me again. No, I won't call him. It's his duty to call his mother."

It's six thirty in the morning, and I'm on my way to work when the red light stops me before I can cross the drawbridge over the Passaic River north of Jersey City. The bridge has to lift up to let some boat go by.

So I'm stitting there in my car, and it's the dream car of my life—a white Lincoln Continental with maroon seats. The radio is on KTU playing disco music, and since I'm first in line, I can see the river as the bridge rises.

Suddenly, right out of the blue, this huge truck smashes into my rear. I go up in the air and turn over, almost upside down, against the cement road divider. Everything collapses. Glass is flying all over, I'm in the middle of it, and the roof comes down—wham!—onto my head. It's a total shambles, and I'm in shock.

Then I begin to hear car and truck doors slamming, people shouting and running, and voices coming toward me. The first one I hear is a man, saying, "Don't touch him—he's dead." I must've looked that way, because I was hanging down behind the wheel. I began to move and signal that I wasn't dead. Then I heard someone else yell, "Let's get outa here, the car's gonna blow up!" Next, there's some guy's face on the passenger side, shouting, "Turn off the ignition!" The door on my side was blocked by the road divider, so he said, "Climb up here and open the window!"

Three men pulled me out, one of them the truck driver who'd hit me. He was very apologetic. "I thought I'd killed you," he said. "My brakes failed, I had to hit you or go into the river." We exchanged numbers, and he said, "I want to come and see how you are." To this day, I've never heard from this person. He's a bastard, but I suppose I can't be angry because, in hitting me and sending me to a doctor, he probably saved my life.

He's 27, with blond hair and the high forehead, full lips, and strong jaw of a puffy Marlon Brando. The blue eyes—at once intimate, then suddenly withdrawn—are also Brando's. "I wanted to be an actor. I studied it in school and in New York with Jerome Waldman. Theater is my passion." He works, however, as a telephone operator for the New Jersey Transit Authority, giving out bus and train information.

We are at a table in the Riviera Café, a popular Village hangout in Manhattan. John has arrived with his fiancée, Linda Kipper, 27. Of Irish-Lithuanian parents, she has broad Baltic cheekbones, green eyes, light blond hair, and a soft, rippling laugh. John explains: "We met at work two years ago. She's Operator Number Nineteen, and I'm Number Twenty."

A waitress comes, and John orders three spritzers—white wine with soda.

He speaks slowly, a gravelly timbre to his voice, and without much volume.
The waitress nods, "Okay . . . say, you caught a lousy cold, didn't you?"
John replies, "Just terrible. I can't get rid of it." John and Linda laugh at
this. It's a real gas.

So I got out of the car okay, but it was totaled, and I had to wait on the
bridge for a truck to come and scoop it up. It was so sad to watch it—that
beautiful car being hauled away like junk. It felt like a funeral.

The police came finally, and because I didn't seem injured, they took me
to a drive-in so I could call a friend to come and get me. Then I called
Linda and told her.

LINDA: I was already at work, wondering where John was. I don't
know how, but I knew he was in serious trouble.

JOHN: We get to River Edge Hospital, and a Dr. Griggs examined me.
He said I had suffered a whiplash in my neck and lower back from being
hit. "You're lucky," he said. "Except I don't like the way you're breathing.
I want a soft-tissue X ray of your neck."

I had that done, and he called me back the next morning, saying, "John,
I want you into the hospital immediately. There's a large growth blocking
three quarters of your windpipe." I said, "I don't believe it. I don't have
any trouble breathing." He said, "You'd better believe it and get it looked
at—like right now." I said, "I can't go today. I have tickets for
Dreamgirls." He said, "You can dream about the girls from the hospital."
(Chuckles.)

LINDA: John called to tell me he had to go into the hospital, but I
should go to *Dreamgirls* anyway. We'd waited so long for tickets, he didn't
want me to miss it. I told him, "Are you crazy? My show is on stage with
you."

JOHN: *(Smiling)* Stealing my act, as usual. She can't help it.

LINDA: *(Laughing)* All right, but you *did* have trouble breathing. You'd
had a cough for months, and that Jersey City doctor had been giving you
pills for asthma—without ever seeing the throat problem that Dr. Griggs
spotted right away. Would you believe it? That's the kind of doctor to
avoid if you want to stay alive.

JOHN: *(Interrupts)* Okay, so we go to the Pascack Valley Hospital,
where Dr. Kantor did a bronchoscope with a throat mirror. When he
pulled it out, I remember asking, "Is it serious?" He said, "Very serious,"
and sent me to the hospital's throat surgeon, Dr. Rosen, who also examined me, then scared the daylights out of Linda and myself. "You
should be operated on immediately," he said. "Otherwise, you risk being
choked by the tumor."

It was frightening, and I asked him what that meant. He said, "We'll do a tracheotomy—that is, an opening in your throat for you to breathe if it suddenly becomes difficult. At the same time, we'll take a biopsy to determine whether or not the tumor is malignant."

I'm listening to him talking like he's planning a motor drive to the country, and I don't believe it. This man's talking about destroying my life. I said, "Just a minute. I'm a telephone operator, and I'm studying acting. If you put a hole in my throat, what'll I do?" He began to talk about Elizabeth Taylor. "She had a tracheotomy, and it hasn't stopped her from talking or doing anything else. She's got a little scar, hardly visible. That's all you'll have. We'll make the opening, then plug it up, and you can go on as a telephone operator, on the stage, or sing in night clubs. That's the first stage—okay?" I asked, "Then you do the biopsy—what if it's cancer?" He said, "It might not be. Throat cancer is rare in young people your age. Besides, the growth is separate from your larnyx, so when we remove it eventually, there's a good chance it won't affect your voice—okay?" I could see he was a decent guy, trying to help me, and so I said, "Okay"—but I was shaking.

So I check into the hospital, and they're going to operate the next morning. I've never been in a hospital before, I'm nervous as a cat, and my folks are there, trying to help me. But they're real worried, too. So I end up trying to calm them down. Some comedy. Finally, all visitors have to leave, and they go—but not Linda. She hides out, to stay behind with me. I told her to go, but she wouldn't do it. *(Shakes head.)*

LINDA: We met this fabulous nurse, Monica*—who told me privately, "If the tumor is malignant, get his ass to New York." That's when I decided to spend the night with John. So I hid on the floor behind his bed, watching TV until he went to sleep. Then I took a pillow and covered myself up with my jacket and coat, so nobody would see me.

After a bit, he woke up and called my name, and I got up for a little bit to be close to him. It was risky, but we didn't care. Then he said, "You'd better go home." But I didn't want to leave him, so I lay down again on the floor, and he put his arm over the edge of the bed, touching me, until we both fell asleep.

Next thing, I hear a cleaning lady in the room, and I quickly cover my head. She's saying, "Oh, it's so messy back there, let me clean it up for you." John goes, "No, don't bother. I like it the way it is." *(Laughs.)* I thought I'd explode! Then Monica comes in and sees me, and she says "You'd better leave, or else it'll cause real trouble. The night shift is coming on. So just walk out like you belong here, and they won't ask any

---

* Name altered.

questions." I kissed John good night and told him, "I'll leave you with Monica." He said, "Nobody can take your place—ever." I wanted to cry, but I didn't let him see it.

They never expected this—to become so involved with each other. John recalls: "She was just another operator at the Transit Authority. We sit in cubicles, about thirty of us, taking two hundred calls a day. That's one every two minutes. You look at maps, time tables, the price of tickets—you don't see much else. Besides, I was focused elsewhere—toward New York and the stage." Linda recalls: "I was going to Rutgers, then an insurance school to get my license. Then one day he came in to pick up his check, and we had a coffee together—remember?" John nods: "It seemed so simple at first. We both knew what we wanted." Linda: "It was about relationships. He was not involved with anyone, neither was I. He was into his theater, I was into insurance business with my father. I said to John, 'You know, I enjoy my life, I enjoy my family and friends—and going out on casual dates. That's enough for me. I don't feel I'm lacking much without a love relationship in my life.' What I was really saying was I felt there was no one out there who could understand me. I was too abstract for anyone to understand." (Laughs.) *"Then I found out he was just as abstract as I was!" John: "I knew she wasn't seeking involvement. I wasn't, either. But after that fateful cup of coffee, I began to look at her and think about her when I went home —or to the Village where I feel most at home. When I saw a play I liked, I thought, 'Linda would like that because she knows where I'm coming from.' Finally, I said, 'I've got to try to get a date with this girl.' So we went to New York, to Chelsea's Place, and then to the Ice Palace for dancing." Linda: "I felt so silly. I hadn't been dancing in years, and I was afraid I wouldn't know how to anymore. But it was still in my blood, and all of a sudden, I remembered how."* (Laughs.) *John: "They were playing an old disco favorite, 'Hooked on Classics,' when I thought, 'This is where I sink or swim. Either she slaps me in the face—or love blossoms."* (Smiles.) *"Fortunately, I didn't get slapped!" Linda: "We were on the dance floor, and he kissed me. I was in shock. But we went on dancing all night." John: "Yes, then we opened up."*

I go through the operation and wake up and see the traditional family group with long faces—my mother, my father, and Linda, only she's smiling bravely for my benefit. I ask them, "So what is it? What'd he find out?" But nobody knows. They're waiting for the doctor to come. I can feel the trach, the opening in my throat, underneath the wrappings around my neck. I can talk okay. So maybe it's all okay.

Then Dr. Rosen came and said, "We have to have a family consultation." Right away, I know this is bad news—and it is. "The tumor is malignant," he said. "It's a rare kind, normally found in the salivary glands, but this is in the windpipe." I couldn't believe it. For me, cancer meant only one thing—curtains. I said, "What can I do?" He said he'd send a specimen to a specialist in California, to confirm the diagnosis—and to know best how to proceed.

LINDA: As soon as Dr. Rosen left, I told John, "We're getting out of here. You're going to Memorial Hospital. They saved my life, and they'll save yours." I'd had cervical cancer when I was twenty-one, and it was removed entirely, with no problems, by Dr. Clark—a marvelous man, very courteous and one of the best gynecology surgeons.† John's parents agreed, and I called Dr. Clark who said, "Bring him in."

JOHN: I'm stunned. I'm like some bum fighter in the eighth round. Just tap me, and I'll collapse. I've got a cancer growing in my windpipe. Before, I didn't feel it, but now I can feel it—or think I can.

They said it might mushroom up and choke me. Then I'll have to pull out the metal plug in my throat and breathe through my neck. I kept wondering where it would happen. While I'm out to dinner with Linda—or in bed, maybe? Or while I'm at work, answering the phones, and suddenly speechless? A nightmare.

I remembered seeing a neck breather on a train once.‡ A woman had all these bags and two little kids. The man pressed an electronic device against his throat and said, "May I help you carry a bag?" It came out like a squawk box, like the dead speaking, and the child was so scared it grabbed its mother's leg.

This is driving me crazy until I make a simple decision. I didn't tell my parents because they would've gone completely berserk—especially my mother who's very protective of myself. But I told Linda, before we all drove into New York to Memorial Hospital. I'll never forget it.

We were walking on the campus of St. Peter's College across from my house. A squirrel kept running back and forth across the walk like it wanted us to turn back. I said, "Linda, you must be ready for this. If they have to take away my voice to get rid of the cancer—forget it. I'm not going through with it."

She just nodded, like she expected it, like she knew where I was coming from. She said, "Then what?" And I said, "I'll just go some place, away

---

† Donald G. C. Clark, M.D., attending surgeon, Gynecology Service, Department of Surgery, Memorial Hospital.

‡ Following a laryngectomy (surgical removal of the larynx or voice box, performed for cancer of the larynx), the patient breathes through a stoma, or opening, in the neck.

from everybody, and wait for it to happen." She squeezed my hand, and I saw tears coming down and her lips trembling, but she isn't telling me I'm wrong. She's walking with me, and she knows I can't live as a squawk box.

LINDA: *(Softly)* Yes, but I did say, "We don't know, John. We still don't know what's going to happen."

JOHN: Right. But you didn't try and tell me I had no right to my thoughts—to my feelings. That's why I felt you were so close to me.

At Memorial, Dr. Shah took over my case.* This is not to speak badly of Dr. Rosen, who did his best for me. We just wanted to be in a major cancer center with all its support systems and without having to send a specimen to California to find out what to do next.

I liked Dr. Shah right off. He's an East Indian—very thin, very cool—like Ben Kingsley playing Gandhi against the South Africans and the British—except, for him, the foreigners, the invaders in the homeland, are cancer cells. *(Laughs.)* I told him right off how I felt. "If you have to take my voice, forget it." He nodded, like he understood, and said, "Let's see what the tests tell us." So I go through all the tests—the X rays, CAT scan, and all the rest.

On a Tuesday morning, one of Shah's assistants comes into my room, saying, "You're scheduled for surgery tomorrow." I said, "What kind of surgery?" He said, "Dr. Shah will tell you all about it." At that point, I know there's some doubt about what's going to happen. But I also know I'm not going to get any fast balls from Dr. Shah. He's meticulously honest, and later in the day, he proved it.

He comes in with three other doctors, and he starts talking in that light but very precise way that Indians have—like they don't want to force it on you, but they aren't going to change, either. So he explained it to myself. He says, "John, you know the tumor is about this much away from your voice box." He indicates about an inch, then says, "I'm going to be honest with you. I can't come to a final decision until I open you up and actually see what we can do. But I would like your consent to a possible laryngectomy, and I would also like your permission to videotape this operation because it's a very rare tumor." I said, "Fine, but I make a living as a telephone operator and I'm studying to be an actor. Both of these make life possible for me. If you take away my voice, I won't know how to live or even who I am anymore. I would prefer to leave it, just as it is, and live out what time I have left." He shook his head. "John, it can never be

---

* Jatin P. Shah, M.D., associate attending surgeon, Head & Neck Service, Department of Surgery, Memorial Hospital.

as it was, once I begin to cut into it. If I start, I'll have to go to the end—whatever it is. But, like I said, I believe you have a chance, and I'm going to do everything I can to save your voice."

It was checkmate. Either I signed the papers, or he wouldn't be able to operate on me and try to save my voice—and my life. It was a gamble, yes, but the odds were in my favor. At least, I figured they were from what he had said. So I signed the consent forms.

But after Dr. Shah left, I began to feel my chances weren't so good. I had a gut feeling. . . .

LINDA: *(Interrupts)* He began to say, "I feel it coming. I'm going to lose my voice." I also felt that he would lose it. But I never let on. I kept saying, "John, you'll come out of this talking too much—as usual."

JOHN: *(Smiles)* There was this fabulous nurse, Beth, a cute little blond number, who also tried to keep my spirits up. She'd say, "John, it's like New Year's Eve. You've got the champagne, you're having one hell of a time, but you're also making resolutions about how life's going to be better tomorrow—right?" I'd say, "Right, Beth, keep talking." Linda loved her, too. In fact, she looked a lot like her, and Linda said, "I didn't worry about you with that other nurse, Monica, but this is something else." *(Linda laughs.)* They were all kidding me that way, to make me feel better.

Then something fabulous happened. Ginny Grandinetti, my boss at the Transit Authority, showed up, this same evening before surgery, with some great Chinese food. She said, "John, no matter what happens . . ." *(Breaks up.)* Every time I think about that gal saying this to me, I choke up. She said, "No matter what happens, John, you have a job to come back to"—meaning, if I was voiceless, she would get me another job with the company.

"That night, I couldn't sleep. I kept waking up and this black nurse's aide kept coming into my room to see if I was all right. Nothing helped. I'd go on tossing and turning, and at three A.M., she put her hand on my brow. It was very warm and soothing. Her name was Anabelle, and she came from To-bago, near Trinidad, and she said, 'John, do you believe in God?' I said, 'Yes, Anabelle, but He doesn't make it easy.' She laughed, very gently, and began to sing me a spiritual. She sang it again later, and I've never forgotten one part:

> " 'Only believe,
> Only believe,
> All things are possible:
> Only believe.

No, never fear:
Whatever your luck,
He enters our room,
The doors being shut.
He never forsakes,
He never is gone,
So count on his presence,
In darkness and dawn.'

"Her voice was soft, with that Trinidad lilt of the calypso singers. When she returned to the chorus, starting with 'Only Believe,' her voice seemed to come from inside the soul, and it went soaring up and up until it was like it was hanging there, like a prayer hanging in the sky for God to pick up whenever He came along." (Laughs softly.) *"I fell asleep with her singing, and her hand on me—God bless that woman for those few hours of peace."*

The morning of surgery, Linda called, my mother called, and all my friends called—giving support. Finally, Beth came in and said, "Okay, John, they're ready for you down in surgery." She began to prepare the injection, to calm me down for the trip, saying, "Don't worry. You're going to do fine." That was some gal. Right down to the line, doing all she could for me. When they came to roll me away, she squeezed my hand to say good-bye. It was like a sister there, giving you her love.

They took me down, got me on the table, and there is Dr. Shah with a camera crew—all of them wearing green sterile suits. I said to Shah, "I'm going to be famous and in pictures—at last!" He said, "One part of you, John, will surely be a super attraction." We were sort of laughing at this, when I faded away.

Next thing you know, I'm coming to, swimming up out of the fog, and I hear this doctor yelling, "John! We couldn't save your voice!" That's all I needed to hear, and this coldness crept right over me.

"I wake up in the recovery room. There's a nurse moving back and forth over me, everything is bright yellow, and I feel all these tubes—in my arms, in my nose, in my chest. Someone says my name, then repeats it as though expecting an answer. Jesus, don't they know I can't ever speak again? Never! I roll over and go to sleep, hoping it's forever.

"I wake up again in the recovery room. At first, I think I'm underwater, struggling for air. Next, I open my eyes and still have the feeling that I'm choking to death, because there's something in my throat, and I can't swallow. Then I realize that I'm breathing okay, and this choking sensation is caused by a tube that goes through my nose, down into my throat.

"The room is now deadly still, like a morgue. Maybe it's the middle of the night. I suddenly cough and feel it tearing through the opening in my throat—just that, no sensation in the mouth. It's very weird.

"I put my hand over my mouth and breathe out. Still nothing happens. Then I take a deep breath and put my hand over my throat. This time I can feel warm air coming out through the covering over the neck opening. I touch it—a sort of gauze bib tied around my neck. Then I try something else. I clamp my hand over my mouth, like I'm trying to suffocate myself. I hold it there and go on breathing through my neck with no trouble.

"I get a chill and begin to shake. I stare at the ceiling and tell myself, 'That's it. You're one of them now. A neck breather, like that poor bastard on the train. Jesus, what happened to all the prayers? What happened to Anabelle singing 'Only Believe?' Only believe in what? In this? In being stretched out mute, like living in a grave?

"Hanging on the edge of my bed is one of those magic slates that little kids have. You write on it with anything, then pull up the plastic cover, and it cancels out. This one has a yellow border with Mickey Mouse characters on it. I think, 'That's perfect. Where before I could speak, I could play King Richard or Dracula, now I have other companions—Mickey Mouse and his dim-witted friends. I've been saved from cancer, to live in Idiotland.' "

Finally they come and wheel me back to my room. Linda is there with my parents. They know what's happened, they've been there for hours, and you can see it in their faces. Linda comes to kiss me, and I turn aside, so she kisses my cheek.

I guess I was worried about the first kiss on my lips, now that they had no air, no voice. I thought, "Christ, what's going to happen later on?" I didn't want to think about it, about my neck breathing on her, and I tried to turn off these thoughts.

My mother looks terrible. This is killing her—seeing her son with cancer. She grabs my hand and begins to cry. My father tries to carry on as usual and asks, "How're you feeling?" I want to put on a brave front for them, so I write on the Mickey Mouse slate, *Fine, I'm O.K.* My dad takes it from me and writes, *I'm glad!* I grab it back from him and write, *DAD I'M NOT DEAF!* The poor guy goes, "Oh yeah, I guess I got mixed up"— and everybody laughs.

Then they sort of stand there, not knowing what to say or do, and I thought, "Jesus, they can speak, they have voices—yet they have nothing to say."

LINDA: *(Interjects)* We had a lot to say, but we were stunned by what had been done to you.

JOHN: The sight of me would've turned anybody off.

LINDA: *(Quickly)* No, not me. But I was frightened of what this might do to us, like your turning away from a kiss—as if I was a stranger.

JOHN: Not you—me. I was a stranger to myself.

"After they leave, I no longer have to pretend, and I begin to sink into a deep depression—just going down and down toward suicidal despair.

"Beth comes bouncing in, and I grab the Mickey Mouse slate and let go with BETH THEY TOOK MY VOICE! *She said, 'John, if you cry, I'm going to cry, too—and I'm not supposed to. I'm supposed to be brave.' I could see tears in her eyes, or maybe they were just in mine. I reached out my hand, and she took it and smiled. I thought of Judy Garland singing in a spotlight, her heart breaking, singing about a lost love, about surviving all alone in the world.*

"She said, 'John, I've seen this happen to a lot of people. It's always a terrible shock. If you're angry, you should be angry. If you feel lousy, you should feel lousy. But you're a very good-looking guy, and you'll climb out of it. You'll learn to talk again—esophageal speech, or however. Didn't Dr. Shah tell you about it?' He had, of course, but I hadn't wanted to listen or think about it. Beth said, 'You'll talk again, and you'll do a lot of things.' I wrote out, Like what? *She said, 'You'll see, some of it starts right now.'*

"Then she began to show me how to use two suction tubes by the bed. One was for the mouth, since I couldn't swallow too well because of the tube in my throat, which was to get food past the point where Dr. Shah had stitched me up. Beth said, 'When the stitches heal, we'll take it out, and you'll be able to swallow okay.' The other suction tube was more flexible, to clean out the stoma—the opening in my throat. She had me cough and try it, and it wasn't too difficult.

"When we'd finished, she said, 'John, would you now do something for me?' We were close to Christmas and they were playing 'Jingle Bells' on the television. I nodded and she said, 'It's perfect for you. Sing me the chorus of "Silent Night" ' " (Laughs.) *"It broke us up. We began to laugh so much I nearly choked. That Beth was fabulous. The best."*

Linda came every day, she wanted to stay close and help me, but pretty soon we were having trouble. Doing what I had to do without a voice, I was sharing intimate things with new people—like Beth helping me take care of myself. This excluded Linda, and she became jealous. . . .

LINDA: *(Quickly)* Just a minute. I was never jealous of Beth. I thought she was perfect for your needs—a perfect nurse.

JOHN: *(Shakes head)* And the social worker, Karen Londa, also a very pretty girl. . . .

LINDA: *(Interrupts)* Hey! Not her—just your meetings with her.

JOHN: Okay, the meetings, which consisted of all the laryngectomees on the floor, plus other head/neck patients with their families. We'd talk about how to adjust to our busted lives, and Karen would give us advice.

LINDA: Other parents, wives came, but you wouldn't let any of us come. Okay, it was probably best for your mother who was under such stress, but not for me. We were intimate, we said we loved each other, but you were closing me out of your life at a time of crisis. Finally I said, "John, I don't understand this. Write me a letter and tell me what's inside you." *(Pauses.)* It was a beautiful letter.

JOHN: I told her that this was my tragedy, and I had to learn how to cope with it. I said I don't want to be selfish, but everyone has done all they can for me. It's on my shoulders now. You can come to the social worker classes, but first I have to try it alone. If I react well—fine. If not, I don't want my girlfriend and my family around at a critical moment which is part of my space.

LINDA: I accepted that, but I only understood what it meant later on, when we were about to split up.

JOHN: The trinity of life.

LINDA: Yes, in life you have three things—time, love, and space. We thought we had no problem with love, that it was easy, but we found out that it can't exist without taking care of our separate needs for space and time.

JOHN: Exactly! That means space to do what you need or feel like doing. For me in the hospital, it meant being alone to get my act together and try to communicate with other people. But it can also mean going for a walk, or hopping on the Staten Island ferry without having to answer picayune questions or punch a clock.

LINDA: Time means just the opposite. It means you return from your space trip to be with others. Where he was uptight about his space, I was jealous about time. It runs out, and you can't get it back. You know something? It's like going down a long corridor that is only so long—the length of your youth or your life or whatever—and you can never turn back. I didn't want to get to the end of it all and find that John had just hopped onto the Staten Island ferry. *(Laughs.)*

JOHN: You've got to have trust or it doesn't work. Trust when the other one is off into his or her space, and trust that you'll find each other at the end of the corridor of time.

LINDA: The saddest part of his letter, the most moving, was when he told me I could leave him.

JOHN: I said to her, I love you. My sickness can't change my love for you. But it certainly can change yours for me. I said I'm trying to believe you'll still want me as a man, but I also worry about you. Our world collapsed overnight. My dreams, the future goals I set for us, have dissolved.

I said I realize I have no rights to keep you down with me. You don't deserve it. If you meet another young man who can give you a future you want, I cannot possibly feel angry towards you. We've had some very beautiful moments, and I'll always have those memories. . . .

LINDA: *(Interrupts)* That's where I cried. It must have hurt you to write that. Why did you do it?

JOHN: *(Waves hand)* I had to.

LINDA: *(Insists)* But why? You saw in my face I was suffering. You knew that I loved you, and you loved me. So why tell me I can go off with someone else?

JOHN: I don't know why. Maybe I wanted to hear you say that you'd never leave me. I think I was calling out from my prison of silence.

"A couple of days after the operation, another woman enters my life. She comes into my room, saying, 'Hi! I'm Elaine Harris.' She's a slender gal, with dark hair and eyes sort of like daisies—except that, with this one, you just know it's not all daisies and clover. She says, 'I'm a speech therapist. I teach people like you to speak again.' I wrote out, How? *and she said, 'Various ways, but the main one is called alaryngeal or esophageal speech.'*

"For the first time, I listened to this possibility of speaking again by regurgitating air and using the esophagus to replace the larynx—the voice box. She gave me some pamphlets from her briefcase about the technique and the people who had mastered it. Then she said, 'I'll send you a couple of people who will show you what it's like—what can be done.'

"After that, three people came—three laryngectomees. The first was Ralph—one of the volunteers working at Memorial. I was sitting in the recreation room, watching patients taking an art class—and daydreaming about myself becoming an artist instead of an actor—when I heard, 'Are you John Corbalis?' I look around and see this guy in the volunteers' blue jacket, saying, 'I'm Ralph, I came to see you because I'm the same thing you are—a neck breather.'

"I was fascinated by this man. He spoke through his throat, as Elaine had described it, by taking in air and regurgitating it. This was a lot better than that poor guy on the train with his mechanical squawk. But to be perfectly frank, I didn't like it. It didn't sound human, it was too much like E.T.

"I later learned that was why Dr. Shah doesn't like his patients to hear this form of speech before an operation. It can never resemble the original

voice, so it's bound to have this effect. Nor did I know how accomplished Ralph is—and how dedicated he is in helping people like me.

"Another one came, sent by Elaine—Sanford Meisner, who's director of the Neighborhood Playhouse in New York. Bless that woman. She knew my theatrical bent and got this busy man to come—another laryngectomee. He said, 'John, you don't have to give up all your dreams. You can still act in some roles, and be involved in lots of other ways.' Very nice guy.

"The next one was really impressive—Ron MacIntosh, a banker. He spoke very distinctly, without the thumping sound of burping out injected air. Very smooth. I thought, 'This is my role model.' "

I started with Elaine a month later—after going home and after a relapse that sent me into a terrible depression, a really bad time. I guess I didn't believe I could ever escape from that prison of silence, those humiliating attempts at dialogue on the Mickey Mouse magic slates or on little bits of paper—scrawls like gasps, like people who can never communicate with each other in a Samuel Beckett play. *(Pauses.)* Try it sometime. Try to say nothing in a group of people, and see how desperate it can become. The faces hang there, waiting for some reply. You write half a dozen words, and that's it. Instant social death.

That's when I started breaking dates with Linda. Those desperate scrawls, and her attempts to stay with me when there was no sign of what was really going on. This was driving me insane.

Then those crazy phone signals. She'd call, and I'd pick up the receiver and hit it once, which meant *Yes.* She'd start telling me something, and if I hit the phone twice, it meant *No.* Three times meant *Maybe.* That was it.

LINDA: *(Interrupts)* No, there was one more. If I started to go off the track, and you wanted to stop me, you'd start beating on the phone like mad. That meant, *Hold it, start over.*

JOHN: I retreated into a cave like a hermit. I put on Judy Garland every night, on the Betamax. I have recorded everything of Judy—films, concerts, the works. She's one of my great idols. The other is Liza Minnelli.

Then one day a miracle happened. In the mail, there was a note from Liza. I couldn't believe it, but there it was—beginning with "Dear John," then saying how disturbed she was to hear of my illness, that she was thinking about me and hoping I got better, and it was signed, "Fondly, Liza." Next to her name, she drew a smiling face. I loved it. Somebody must have told her about me and how much I care for her work. I still don't know who it was. But for me, that letter opened up doors all over the world. I called up Linda and began to beat the phone like mad. *(Laughs.)*

LINDA: I thought he'd gone crazy or was dying. Finally, I said, "You sound excited." I got one knock—meaning *Yes*—then a lot more crazy knocks. I finally understood he wanted me to come over. We went out to dinner and had a wonderful evening. He kept asking me if I thought Elaine could teach him to speak again, and I said, "You'll learn fast because you studied voice projection in acting. It'll come naturally to you."

JOHN: Linda and Liza turned me around, they brought me out of my cave.

"I came to Elaine's for the first lesson with a Mickey Mouse slate, and she said, 'Put that away, you don't need it. Speak slowly and clearly, and I'll read your lips.' We were at ICD†—in her office, a quiet place with plants in the windows, and we were sitting in two chairs, facing each other.

"She said, 'John, I want you to belch.' Then she does it for me. She swallows and lets out a nice-sized burp. Then she does it again—burp! I can't believe it, this nice looking lady sitting there and—one-two-three, burp!—all very serious and controlled. I told her, shaping the words for her to read my lips, 'Oh no, I can't do that.' I was too embarrassed to sit there and burp in front of a stranger.

"But Elaine is a very disciplined lady. She knows her business and how to get what she wants from her patients. She said, 'You'd better start doing this, John, because this esophageal belch is going to be your new form of speech. You're going to control it, you'll fluctuate it into words—but you have to get the initial sound out first.'

"So then I started trying to croak out a burp, and suddenly I did it—burp! Then I did another one and ran out a whole series of them. Elaine said, 'You're doing fine, I think you'll learn fast. Now you should try to formulate one-syllable words, like scotch, house, boy, girl.*'*

"I tried it, but it went all over the place—up and down, completely out of control. It was maddening, and Elaine said, 'Relax, John, it's all right. You have to expect that in the beginning because there's no control. You have an esophageal muscle that needs to be exercised. The whole purpose of this initial therapy is to loosen that muscle and to eventually take in enough air to formulate a sentence.' It was enough to drive you crazy—to speak a whole sentence! I thought, 'God! I'll settle on just three simple words!' "

---

† ICD—International Center for the Disabled—is an outpatient rehabilitation facility in New York City, serving 3,500 people annually, with 6,000 evaluations and 30,000 treatments. Elaine Harris, M. Ed., CCC-Sp, is Clinical Supervisor, Post-Laryngectomy Rehabilitation Program, Speech and Hearing Department of ICD.

After that first lesson with Elaine, I was burping like a trooper. But that was all it was. I still couldn't form a single word, but I felt somehow that I was making progress.

LINDA: Going home, he burped all the way through the Holland Tunnel. *(Laughs.)* He kept saying, "Nobody can hear me in here!"

JOHN: It sounded pretty awful, but it was exciting. I was going to make contact with the outside world. Like someone on the moon, you know, sending back, "We got your rocks, can we come home?" *(Laughs.)*

I began to get up at two or three o'clock in the morning, when my parents were asleep and nobody could hear me, to try and croak out a word. I think the first word I ever managed was *one.* Then I got to two words, *one girl.* After that, I'd open a book and try to read a complete sentence on one intake of air, no matter how it sounded. I said, "Gee, I'm speaking!"

But it sounded like a munchkin from *The Wizard of Oz,* and I thought, "Am I going to use this voice with Linda, my family, my friends? Will I be laughed at?"—and, in fact, Linda did laugh the first time.

LINDA: Yes! The phone rang, and I heard the usual knock-knock. I knew it was John, and I was quite angry with him. He'd stood me up again, broken our date. I was going on and on, like: "I sat around all Sunday waiting for you when I could've gone to my mother's. . . ." Then, all of a sudden, John says, "Shut up." I didn't believe it and asked him, "Did you say something?" There was a pause, and it came back again, "Shut up!" I said, "Oh no!"—and began to laugh. The first words couldn't have been, "I love you, Linda." No—just, "Shut up!" *(Laughs.)*

JOHN: Elaine was building me up, from two-syllable words to short sentences. She said I was fabulous, but I kept saying, "Elaine, this sounds terrible." She replied, "John, you are saying words, you are really speaking." I told her, "I find it repulsive. I don't like the sound."

Elaine is very good at this. She said, "John, you may never like the way you sound, but you are not writing, and you are not using an electronic voice box. You can get your message across verbally. In fact, I've rarely heard anyone pick it up so quickly. It's really remarkable." So you see, she was feeding me what I wanted to hear—what I really needed, psychologically.

So was Linda. She began to talk more and more about the office and how Ginny, my boss, kept asking about me. One day, Linda says, "I told Ginny that you're talking again, and she said, 'So why doesn't he come back to work?' " That made me very angry, and we had a big fight. I said, "Ginny's going to phone me at home, and she'll hear how awful I sound.

That will really blow it. You've done it again, Linda, you've invaded my space."

LINDA: *(Quickly)* That made me furious—his stupid old space again. I told him exactly what the others had told him a hundred times—I mean, Elaine and Karen Baker, the rehabilitation counselor at ICD. They explained that you can't hear yourself as others do. Nobody can. What you hear and what other people hear is not the same. I said, "If you heard yourself on the phone, you'd realize you speak clearly enough to be understood." *(Laughs.)* Especially by somebody asking how to get to Hoboken!

JOHN: Then Elaine started bugging me with the same thing. I knew Linda was behind it, but to shut them up I agreed to a tryout. So then Elaine and I spoke on phones from separate offices at ICD. She asked me how to get from one place in New Jersey to another. I was nervous, and she interrupted me. "Speak more slowly, John. Make every breath of air count. Try it again."

I did it once more, and then she played it back. It sounded like somebody with a bad cold, but it was clear enough to be understood. Yet it belonged to a stranger—not me—and I said, "It still sounds like somebody else. It's not me." Elaine said, "Is that going to be an embarrassment? Do you personally know everybody calling in for bus information?" I said, "Okay, you win," and she said, "Now will you go back and give it a try?" I said I would, but mainly to get her off my back.

LINDA: One evening, John calls and says he's going into the office to give it a try on the phones. I said, "Wait for me! I'm coming too!" He says, "Why don't you phone me and ask how to get to Hoboken?" This is supposed to be funny, his idea of a joke. I get in my car and head for the office.

JOHN: I'd called Ginny, and she said to come at night, when there's less traffic. So we agree, and I finally come back. *(Sighs.)* I can't begin to tell you what it was like to walk back into that room again, to sit down at one of my old booths, to swing around on the swivel chair and face the green and orange map of New Jersey and the shelves with bus and train schedules for every county.

I put on the black earphones, I switch myself into the line of waiting calls, and the first one to come in—I'll never forget it—was a woman asking for the next train from Jersey City to Chicago. "It's urgent," she said. "I can't fly, and my daughter's in the hospital." Ginny is monitoring this. Every word is being recorded to see how well I'm doing. But for a moment, I forget all that. I'm thinking, "That poor woman, maybe her daughter has cancer." I tell her to use Amtrak, the national railroad from Penn Station in Newark—and give her connections on how to get there.

After that, there's half a dozen other calls. Then Ginny sends word for me to come into her office. I put down everything in the booth and go back to hear my fate. Ginny says nothing. She just flicks on the recording, and we listen to the playback. I'm waiting for some disastrous garble, some scrambled word. I'm weakest on the *h*'s and the *p*'s that require extra air.

But I'm surprised. Linda and Elaine were right. I sound fine—in fact, much clearer than I had expected. Ginny flicks it off, then turns to me and says, "Welcome back, John." It's too much, just too much for me. I say, "Ginny . . ." and can't say anything more. Then I'm hugging her and trying to blink back the tears before she can see them.

Then Linda comes, and we're leaving together, and I'm not ashamed for her to see them—those tears coming down. I guess they'd been there, waiting for this moment, waiting for me to come back again.

POSTSCRIPT: Six months later, following his participation at a meeting of the International Association of Laryngectomees (IAL) in New Orleans, John Corbalis received from Louisiana State University certification to teach esophageal speech. He now does this in addition to his telephone work for the New Jersey Transit Authority. He writes: "This is a great challenge, and I believe it was my destiny. Everything pointed toward this —the loss of my voice, then regaining my ability to speak. There was a purpose in it, and it came from above. I have to believe this, that it was programmed for me to teach others to speak again, to help them escape from their prisons of silence."

FIVE

SELF

Reality can be lied about, twisted, and tamed by tricks of cultural perception and repression. But anxiety cannot be lied about. Once you face up to it, it reveals the truth of your situation, and only by seeing the truth can you open a new possibility for yourself.

Søren Kierkegaard
The Concept of Dread

Do not go gentle into that good night,
Rage, rage against the dying of the light. . . .

Dylan Thomas
Do Not Go Gentle into That Good Night

The role that self plays in surviving cancer is first described here by two women—two of Memorial's highly experienced nurses. They are distinctly different people, yet their separate stories merge into a similar accounting of what kind of a human being can be most expected to survive cancer and what sort of care is needed for this to happen.

As a result, we appear to be given a psychiatric profile of the long-term survivor, as well as the support system needed to help patients retain their identity, their sense of being a whole person—or to help them recover this if it has been shattered or lost in the initial shock of discovering the illness.

It is the profile of a central figure, linking all the histories of survival in this book. At first, it is not seen in depth, for we are given only a quick sketch. We do discern, however, certain characteristics which we are destined to encounter in various ways among the men and women whose stories follow. In this manner, a fuller portrait eventually emerges—a collective portrait of the many victors.

As in portraits drawn from life, yet filtered through the human eye, it is possible to contain the essence of all without containing all. Yet it is also possible to fail at this, and our work may lack in some ways. It is, nevertheless, a composite portrait of the cancer survivor—and, most importantly, how he or she manages to turn back the disease.

The first survivor we encounter, providing elements for a basic profile of many others, is an IBM executive who refuses to die. As described by the head nurse who cared for him at the time, "He had every complication in the book, every system failure . . . and he was on a respirator for months."

He had, however, something else going for him. Besides his "tremendous will to live, he was very distressed and so ridden with anxiety and suspicion that he couldn't sleep. . . . He knew everything that was going on, he witnessed everything, watched everything, and kept letting us know how he felt. . . . There was something separate and indestructible about that man."

The second nurse describes two other cases which manifest similar coping patterns—sleepless anxiety, high levels of distress, suspicion, occasional hostility.

Similar characteristics and coping mechanisms are found among others in this book. As might be expected, they are consistent with behavioral patterns of other long-term survivors described in studies elsewhere. In one of them—a clinical report from Johns Hopkins University School of Medicine on thirty-five women with metastatic breast cancer—long-term survivors were found to be "distressed and had measurable elevations in levels of anxiety and a sense of alienation; they were unhappy and showed it in their moods; they were communicative about their distress . . . [whereas] short-term survivors had a particular lack of hostile symptoms, and generally higher levels of positive mood states, but lower levels of vigor."*

This suggests there is some benefit to be had in refusing to relinquish control of one's self, with the consequential emotions and behavior of someone under attack. It does not mean, of course, that anxiety or distress is desired or needed to overcome cancer. On the contrary, extreme anxiety, grief, or emotional trauma are generally believed to weaken our natural defenses against the disease. This was noted by the Greek physician Galen some 2,000 years ago, and there is now a vast body of medical literature describing the influence of emotional stress on the course of neoplastic disease.†

---

* *Derogatis-Abeloff-Melisartos, Psychological Coping Mechanism and Survival Time in Metastatic Breast Cancer, JAMA,* October 5, 1979. Among twenty-five studies cited with related findings was the classic inquiry by Caroline B. Thomas, a psychologist at Johns Hopkins, whose interviews with over 1,300 students since the 1940s reveal a distinct profile for those who later developed cancer. They lacked closeness with parents, seldom showed strong emotions, and had a lower frequency of negative affect symptoms (depression, anxiety, anger) than other students.

† Among many pertinent studies: Grendon in 1701 cites the "disasters of life that occasion much trouble and grief" as a cause of cancer; Burrows in 1783, sees it as "the uneasy passions of the mind with which the patient is strongly affected for a long time"; Walter Hyle Walshe in 1846 finds "mental misery, sudden reverses of fortunes, and habitual gloominess of temper [to affect] the disposition of carcinomatous matter"; Sir James Paget in 1870: "We can hardly doubt that mental depression is a weighty additive to other influences favouring development of the cancerous constitution"; Elida Evans in 1926 *(A Psychological Study of Cancer* with introduction by Carl Jung) found many cancer patients had invested their identity in one role or object (job, person, property) instead of developing their own sense of selfhood. When the supporting role or object was removed, the patient was without resources for coping. Dr. Lawrence LeShan's study of the life history

It is not the presence of distress or grief—human reactions to be expected in this illness—but rather the ability of patients to unload their stress loads, to open up and release anxiety or hostility, which distinguishes them from others who cannot do so and have a lower survival capacity. It is precisely here that the role of self becomes a real force in recovery.

It is fascinating, for in this we seem to be observing the working valves of creation. It is the inner self claiming its separate identity, rather than remaining a subject to its failing body—doing this variously through cries of alarm, through a constant alert that forbids sleep or self-indulgence or any unbuckling of personal armor.

It also has its corollary force, for as the self rejects the inward course of negative emotions, with these patients it rejects the invasive cancer cells. This is a natural way of reacting to it, using the body's biological coping mechanism—probably, in part at least, going through the visceral brain, the limbic system, to the hypothalamus, which in turn sends messages to the pituitary gland and so into the endocrine system while simultaneously boosting the immune system, the body's natural defense against foreign invaders.

Whether or not this is the way our biological mechanism actually works here, we do witness something unusual about these people. They appear to have the ability to throw off native despair while also turning back the foreign cell.

We read on, sifting their testimony to find some explanation for this dual ability. We note, as others have done, that they seem to have more vigor, more strength of being, and to be less dependent upon a supporting object or person. Yet this does not wholly explain it, and we are left to wonder about their special source of power. Why do they have this more than others? From what deep roots does it draw its strength?

Eventually the stories give us clues, and we begin to determine what allows these men and women their special coping mechanism. In simple terms, they appear to be in closer dialogue with their inner selves, to be more consciously aware that this is actually their essential self. Their body might be invaded, perhaps sick unto death, but the inner self has the

---

of 500 patients *(You Can Fight For Your Life; Emotional Factors in the Causation of Cancer)* contains similar findings, including the characteristic of these patients to close off their despair. Similar to other patients, they felt hurt, anger, despair, hostility, but were unable to let it out. As a result, people misread their outer appearances and believed them to be at peace, to be of a sweet and saintly nature. LeShan summarizes: "The benign quality, the 'goodness' of these people was in fact a sign of their failure to believe in themselves sufficiently, and their lack of hope."

power to save them—if only to hold off death until they perpetuate themselves in some way that will not die with them.

As we know, our inner self came with the myth of the Fall. Adam, who
was created as one, became split into a union of opposites—infinite self-
knowledge within a finite body. It instantly separated him from the animals, who are bound by instinctive yet thoughtless action. It made man a
creature whose mind could bring him to dance on the moon, perceive
infinity in an atom, speak of angels, and embrace the cosmos—yet with a
mind forever bound to a body destined to extinction.

It is a terrifying dilemma for most of us, and as others have noted, we
built our lives to be spared of it as much as possible—using illusion, myth,
and especially our own expenditure in self-perpetuation. For this, our du-
alistic nature provides two possible avenues: the body which is standard-
ized and biologically programmed, and the mind which has the capacity to
be distinctly personal, a creation of our individual spectrum and spirit.

Through the body, man leaves behind a biological near replica of self in
offspring. Through the mind, since the beginning of time, he has sought to
perpetuate himself on a higher plane, beyond the cycle of life and earth.
He paints the shapes of animals on cave walls. He builds monuments to
unseen gods. He sings ballads where memory overrides death. And using
the forbidden gift from the Garden, he is able to create, within the finite
cycle of his time, a semblance of the infinity he once lost.

This drive to save and perpetuate the inner self—or the soul, either
through the body or the mind or both—seems to be very strong among the
survivors in this book. It would appear to account for their high levels of
anxiety, and their distress upon finding that the inner self with all its
promises is suddenly trapped within a collapsing form, a sickened body
threatened with death. The suspicion that others attending to their needs
do not sufficiently comprehend this terrifying dilemma would also account
for flashes of hostility or personal withdrawal. It would explain further the
impression of Nurse Pat Mazzola: "There was something separate and
indestructible about that man." We can only imagine the dreams within
that IBM executive—dreams from his inner self which would not allow
him to die.

So we witness in this section, and elsewhere in the book, how many
people have clung to their inner selves to help them perpetuate a dream
which they believe will outlast the cycle of their lives:

A woman golfer, weakened by chemotherapy following a mastectomy,
manages a fusion of mind and body which raises the level of her game to
challenge the best women golfers in the United States. A young man,
facing apparent impotence from testicular cancer, leaves deposits in a

sperm bank, does sexual acrobatics—anything rather than allow his wife to accept impregnation from another man—finally managing to have a child of his own. A boy, emerging from a four-year battle against lymphoma, realizes he was saved to help his minority brothers in a ghetto neighborhood. A business executive, cured of lung cancer, returns on Sundays to Memorial to work as a volunteer—seeking to give back to other patients the courage and help he received when a patient there. A young woman, after a leg amputation and four lung operations, is ostracized at school as a freak, yet becomes a famous fashion photographer.

On the importance of listening to her inner self, the photographer, Barbra Walz, says, "You have to believe in dreams, and it's much easier to believe in your own."

I learned very early that you can't tell when a person is going to live or die —even the ones that appear to have no chance. All of a sudden, the patient takes a turn for the better and just won't die. I've seen such horrendous cases here, you would never believe they could make it. Yet they walk out the door and go back to normal lives.

Patricia Mazzola, director of Memorial's 713 nurses, turns to a mysterious yet frequently observed phenomenon among cancer patients: the role that character, or mind or spirit, plays in survival—often defeating the disease when it appears to be invincible. *

We are having coffee in her office on the nineteenth floor of the hospital, with a splendid view of the East River, its passing boats, and a brisk wind on the water.

Sometimes people come in with such a tremendous will to live that it seems to hold off and even turn back the dying. When we were over at Ewing, I learned my lesson well. We had this patient in the intensive care unit, a very young man, a good-looking man, an executive with IBM—and he had every complication in the book. I don't remember what the primary diagnosis was, but he had every system failure. He went into renal failure, was septic, and everything else you can imagine. Finally, he had respiratory failure and was on a respirator for months.

When you are putting a patient through so much, and it seems increasingly clear that he will never make it, you always have a feeling in your head that there has to be a time to say stop. That's how I felt about this poor man. Enough is enough. Well, that man walked out of the unit. He went back to work, and I followed him for another five years, until he was considered clinically cured. So you really can't tell. I don't make those end-of-life judgments anymore.

Sometimes this tremendous will to live can work against them. They can fight too much, too hard for their own good. With this particular man, I remember we had to finally knock him out with drugs. He was very distressed, and so ridden with anxiety and suspicion that he couldn't sleep for fear of losing the battle. He knew everything that was going on, he questioned everything, watched everything, and he kept letting us know

* For a personal close-up, and her view on the inevitability of emotional involvement in caring for cancer patients, see p. 121.

how he felt. At one point he was up twenty-four hours a day. If you know intensive care units, the lights are on all the time, the stress is incredible—and the man really had to have some rest. He was one of the first patients we ever used a sodium pentothal drip on. If we hadn't, he would never have had the strength to make it out of there.

There was something separate and indestructible about that man, his incredible will, his anxiety and refusal to even close his eyes. Then you have the other extreme—those who feel they have lost the battle. The shock of learning they have cancer leaves them psychologically out of breath—stunned, defenseless. In order to fight back, to have the courage to make the long struggle with all the suffering from chemotherapy and radiation, they need to regain control of themselves, to believe they can make it, to have a real hope of recovery.

The family can't go it alone. The patient needs a doctor he can believe in, and he or she needs a hospital like Memorial which has the most advanced therapy and a very high atmosphere of hope. I learned how important this was when my brother was brought here as a cancer patient.† Part of the therapy here is just that—creating this climate of hope, so you have a sense of being your whole self with an ability to deal with this as a whole person.

You cannot do that for the patient if he feels like he's meeting strangers all the time. Once he comes into the hospital, he has to feel secure, that we are going to take care of him as though he was with his own family, transferred to a more technical, professional level—yet also caring for him, even loving him. The psychology of this, of making him feel his whole self, his own person is very important.

Everyone must contribute to this—the medical side, the surgeons, the social worker, the clergy. But the brunt of it is on the nursing staff. We are closest to the patient in taking care of his physical needs, in the laying on of hands, in answering his urgent, intimate calls. Our nurses here care, they care so damn much, it means so much to them that they will take it all with little question—the late hours, the dirty work, the humiliations from angry, sick people, the infuriating lack of comprehension from some doctors. All of this, believe me, is compensated for by the patient who manages to say, "Thank you." In other words, our nurses are really out on a limb psychologically, and they are very, very long in their belief of the worth of human life.

We can't fully support the patient this way unless we are allowed to care for him from the moment he is admitted—until he leaves. It wasn't always

---

† See first Mazzola interview, p. 121.

that way. When I went down to the operating room five years ago, the nurses were reporting to the Department of Anesthesia—not to the Division of Nursing. So we never knew what happened to our patients when they went down to the OR. We dropped them off at the door and didn't see them again until they were postop, in the Recovery Room. The OR nurses were isolated from the rest of the hospital. My objective, as director of OR Nursing, was to bring them back under the Division of Nursing, so they could take a good look at what happens to the whole patient and get involved in all aspects of nursing at Memorial.

They are so highly technical in the operating room. It's another world, and it takes a particular type of person. I never, never thought I would end up there.

"In college, I was majoring in chemistry and biology, but I didn't want to sit behind a microscope for the rest of my life. I wanted to become a nurse. My father was an obstetrician/gynecologist, and he said, 'I'll show you what nursing is all about.' He took me to the operating room and had me watch while he did a vaginal hysterectomy. I watched the blood, and I fainted in the OR. The last thing I heard was my father's voice: 'Get that kid out of here.' " (Laughs.) *"I landed in the recovery room, and they were absolutely delightful to me. But I got right up and said, 'I want to go and see another procedure.' I went back and watched more of the operation, and again I was sick to my stomach, but I stuck it out. I told my father, 'Nursing can't be just this, and I still want to do it, I want to be a nurse.' He said, 'If you want to go to nursing school, I want you here in the city, so the only place you're going is Cornell University.' That's what I did. I went to Cornell, but with no idea that I'd end up in fifteen operating rooms."* (Laughs.)

After working with OR nursing, I was even more certain that the nursing service in Memorial's operating rooms had to cease being a separate world. Preop nursing care had to follow the patient into the OR, and the OR nurses had to know more about the patients before they came to them, as well as the results of their effort.

To understand the importance of this for the patient, you have to have some idea of the critical role that nurses now play throughout a surgical intervention, especially here at Memorial in dealing with cancer.

We have eleven surgical services where the nurses must be able to fill both functions of circulating and scrubbing—working under sterile conditions with the surgeon. Our circulating duties are phenomenal. The circulator nurse is responsible for identifying the patients as they come in, checking the signed consent and making sure it's proper. She is also responsible for the instrument count. In surgery, it's a discard technique, so there's a large number of instruments, needles, sponges. She has to ensure they're all there. You can't discover suddenly at the end of an operation that you are missing an instrument or a sponge. There are numerous surgical specimens that must be properly cared for by both scrub nurse and circulator.

So the circulator coordinates all the activity that's going on in the room around the patient, and she's an incredible patient advocate throughout the whole procedure. If the physician wants to do something that is not permitted on the consent form, it's the circulating nurse's responsibility to make sure it's not done—and to report the problem to the director. Sometimes you may have a surgeon who is insistent on going ahead, convinced it's for the patient's benefit. But you have to stop him until medical-legal issues are addressed.

For instance, they'll do a breast biopsy. If it's malignant, they have to have the signed consent before proceeding to do a mastectomy. If they don't, it's no way. Or they might say, "Oh, here's a mole. We'll take this off while we're here." This is not permitted unless the patient has consented to it beforehand. At Memorial, the surgeons are very careful about this, and the nurse acts as a further control.

So you can see the OR is a very technical world and very pressurized. Each surgical intervention is a violation of nature, you may be risking a life if you make an error. In this environment there is always the risk of forgetting the patient as an individual. In the day-to-day handling of fifty or more patients, one after another, who are draped except for the wound area, who can't speak or otherwise reveal their identity—with all this, a conscious effort must be made to maintain the dignity of the patient as a whole.

There's one thing I can't stand, and that's someone saying, "Oh, the gallbladder is finished." I say, "Hey, wait a minute, that's not a gallbladder. It's Mrs. So-and-So. It's a person."

Well, for the most part I stopped hearing that sort of thing, the organ or limb used as an identity, when we began sending nurses out of the OR, up to the patient's rooms to talk with patients preoperatively. They asked about particular problems which an OR nurse would know to be important. Does the patient have any back problems, which we need to know about in positioning the patient on the OR table? With their arms or neck? Whatever. The nurses then came back to the OR, saying, "This patient has a particular problem with this or that." Also they were aware that this wasn't just an operation but a total person they had known, however briefly.

These preop visits helped the patients in another way, giving them immense psychological relief. They now knew someone who was going to be there, by their side, when they were asleep undergoing their operation. This was a healing, helping friend, a surrogate of the floor nurse who was also a friend.

So there we achieved a continuity of care, helping the patient participate as much as possible in what was happening to him, to realize he had caring people around him all the way and so retain a sense of his whole person, his total self.

I had two people down there, two veteran OR nurses, who were so interested in this that they developed a program we now call the Surgical Nurse Coordinating Program—bringing us even closer to the patient and the family. These two nurses make preoperative rounds, seeing patients and their families, instructing them in what to expect on the day of surgery. They follow them all the way through—to the OR, the recovery room, and then back to their own room. They make rounds every two hours and report to waiting families in the lobby on the patient's progress and location.

They also see the families during the surgery, which is a great relief for these people. I'm sure you've seen them, the huge number of people sitting around the hospital lobby, waiting to hear what's going on. They used to somehow wander up to the second floor. I'd come out of the OR at seven or eight in the evening and see these people drifting around outside, saying, "I've had no information, I don't know what's going on." So I'd go inside—we have fifteen operating rooms—and get the information and come back to at least inform them of what was going on.

So now that's taken care of. If you look at the information desk in the lobby, there's a sign-in sheet for family and friends of patients going into surgery. The surgical coordinator comes down and gives them a two hourly bulletin on what's happening. If there's been a delay and the patient is in the holding area, they can tell them their loved one is still outside the operating room. For example, they'll say, "Your wife is not asleep yet." Or, if it's going to take another couple hours, they'll say, "Go out and get something to eat, then come back. I'll see you and give you an update later."

The coordinator makes rounds in the operating rooms to find out if there's anything the surgeon wants to relay to the family. If the surgeon thinks they're going to have a problem with the patient, he might tell the coordinator, "Will you meet me downstairs in an hour and a half?"— meaning he will tell the family at that time. The coordinator doesn't relay anything specific without the physician telling her what to say. For example, if the family knows it's a possible radical mastectomy, he may say,

"Go ahead and tell the family it's a radical." Otherwise, the coordinator merely tells them the time and location of the patient, like "They're still in the operating room, they're doing well." Just telling them where their loved one is really helps relieve the tension, like, "They'll be in the recovery room another two hours, then they'll go back to their room upstairs."

Another place where we need to follow the patient, where they are subject to sudden, unexpected stress, is in the bed holding area—the waiting station outside the operating rooms, before the patient is brought in and placed on the OR table. The patients are brought down and wait in the area until the surgical team is assembled, to avoid as much delay as possible. There is always a few minutes, and often it is longer for a lot of reasons. However long it is, for the patient waiting there, a few minutes can seem like an eternity. They've been given a narcotic as well as an anticholinergic agent such as atropine, and by the time they get to the holding area, they're feeling the effects of the medication. Their mouths are dry, they have difficulty speaking, and need a good deal of reassurance.

You watch them early in the morning when they arrive. Usually one patient says, "Hey, this is one helluva lineup." You've got fifteen patients waiting because you want to start fifteen rooms at once. Suddenly patients start talking to one another. It's integrated. There's male, female. Everybody's in a little slot.

Some of them are having a good time reassuring each other. "Oh, I've been here three or four times. Don't worry, they're great." Someone else goes, "Well, I've never been in an operation room before." Another says, "Don't worry about it, they'll take good care of you here." It's interesting. Then you get the very young. We often allow the mother to come with the child and wait until everything is ready to bring the child into the OR.

You also get those people who are lying out there, wondering, "How come I'm not asleep?" So you explain, "You're only here until you get onto the table, then you'll go to sleep"—because our policy, of course, states that no one goes to sleep until the attending surgeon is present in the operating room.

Some people have had a bad experience with anesthesia, and they start relaying it to the other patients around them. That's where the coordinators are so valuable. They find out when a patient is apprehensive and then go down with the patient and wait with them. Or someone on the floor will call down and say, "We have a patient that's really apprehensive." Then the circulating nurse will come out of the OR and try to stay with the patient until they bring them into the OR. It's a heavy time.

To reduce this tension and let the patient know we are caring for him all the way down the line, our nursing staff made a preoperative video tape,

which describes exactly what happens to patients from the time they sign
the consent form. It explains that, if you have any questions, the time to
ask them is when you sign the operative permit form. It explains all the
things we eventually will ask them to do, like coughing and deep breathing
postoperatively, leg exercises, the prep that is done preoperatively and so
on. This tape was done by Sheila Watson, who originally had the idea for
the coordinator program, and it takes the patient each step of the way—
down to the OR, out to the recovery room, and what to expect when you
wake up—then back to the room on their floor.

We show this to the patients and their families. It's made an enormous
difference for them. It gives the patient the feeling that he isn't just a
number in a hospital bed but someone whose special problems will be
taken care of. It helps give him the sense that he is somebody, a whole
individual, a separate human being who has his own will, his own sense of
self, his own ability to hold himself and his family together—and to survive this disease.

I think death and dying has been worn out. We should speak about the living and how these people manage to survive and are going out to face life again. I gave a speech to the chaplains at New York Hospital and was completely appalled at some of their attitudes. For them, you have cancer, and that's it. They failed to realize that cancer is not the number one killer. It's heart disease. If you have a massive heart attack or stroke, you're dead in one minute. If you have cancer, you have a chance of three to five years, sometimes ten or twenty. We've got patients who had their breast taken off in 1953 and are still alive. Those chaplains overlooked that or just plain didn't know it. The public, too, is not up on it. They should be.

She's 42, plump and black, with the look of a woman possessing an immense reservoir of strength. She smiles easily, and with laughter, her eyes roll upward, then settle back again into two dark, quiet pools which have reflected the struggles of thousands of human beings winning, and losing, the battle against cancer.

We're having a cup of coffee in the nurse's lounge on the sixth floor at Memorial. "I always wanted to be a nurse, as long as I can remember. I grew up on a farm in South Carolina with three brothers and a sister. All the sick animals and the fowls, I used to take care of them. They called me Dr. Goode. (Laughs.)

"There's nothing I enjoy more than taking care of somebody, especially the oncology patient, because there's so much to be done for them. They're sick, and you know you're really needed. And you want to help them with everything you have. I began working with cancer patients when I was 18. That was after the Dominican nuns took over Calvary* in '58. I was a nurse's aide and technician while going to nursing school, then a registered nurse, supervisor, and ten years ago I came here."

She has fourteen nurses under her. "On this floor, we have a lot of lymphomas and leukemia, also breast cases and those that can't have more surgery. They come here for chemotherapy. When I began, there was almost nothing that saved you from cancer. Now it's a whole different story. Take leukemia, acute lymphoblastic leukemia. Untreated, it has an average survival rate of only two months. Here at Memorial, they've worked out a protocol with chemotherapy that has an average survival rate of five years,

---

* Calvary Hospital—a New York hospice for terminally ill cancer patients.

and it's increasing all the time. Many patients are completely cured as far as
we can tell."

A lot depends on getting the right treatment at the right time, especially
with chemotherapy. But I think the psychological outlook plays a large
part, too, because sometimes the psychological problems can be as big as
the physical ones. If a patient is determined and has the willpower, he can
overcome them. I've seen some of them function on willpower alone, just
by hanging onto themselves.

We had a lady here not long ago—Mrs. Salt. She was so full of cancer
nobody knew how she managed to live. Just willpower. My God, what a
will to live. She'd failed all the chemo protocol, but went on and on and
just wouldn't die.

We had a girl here, Donna Williams, who began a chemo protocol for
leukemia. But after only two courses, she went into liver failure, developed
fever and infection, bacteremia, and she got a large, bleeding ulcer that
could have killed her before the leukemia did. With such complications,
they had to stop treatment and send her home, hoping she'd recover so
they could continue the treatment. Since she hadn't taken enough chemo
to knock out the leukemia, the ulcer and liver had to get better, or she was
going to die.

She told us she wasn't going to die. She said she had a lot of living to do,
and that meant having babies. Well, she got pregnant, and at the same
time, the liver and the ulcer began to improve. The doctors wanted her to
get rid of the baby, so she could continue with her chemo. Otherwise, the
leukemia might grab her again. She got angry with everybody, saying,
"You're not touchin' my baby." Well, she had the baby, and the leukemia
never came back. That was three years ago and that baby's the cutest thing
you ever saw.

So you see what I mean about holding onto yourself. Going at it her
way, being herself, Donna got pregnant, and she got well. She asked God
to help her, and maybe He played a part in it. Whether He did or not,
there's a difference between a patient who has a religion and one who
hasn't. If you have something to reach out to, for a spiritual lift, it helps.
The others get lost in space, because they have nothing to reach out to.
They expect mankind to fill all those special needs, which is sometimes
impossible.

A couple of years ago, there was a young kid here, Stephen Zweiz, who
was really a vegetable case with Hodgkin's disease. He couldn't walk, he
was so full of edema. But he refused to give up, and he drove everyone
crazy by saying how bad he was feeling but how he was going to lick it
sooner or later. Finally, they sent him off to Calvary to die. When they

took him away on a stretcher, he was full of fluid and three times his normal size. He didn't want to go, and he was very angry—saying we were sending him off to die, but he was going to recover and come back. About seven months later, he just walked right in on us, saying, "Look at me, I did it." His disease had disappeared, and he was off on a trip around the world.

You want to save all of them, but sometimes there's just no possible way. It hurts to see them go, right under your eyes. I don't feel so badly if the person is 80 or 90 because they've had a good life or a chance at a good life. But when you lose patients that are 16 or 17, it hurts real bad.

Yes, we get emotionally involved with some patients. You can't help it if you take care of someone every day. You write their day-to-day struggle on the chart, and you follow them all along, from the time they come in. Don't forget our patients keep coming back, over and over again. So there's definitely an attachment there.

Nursing has changed greatly in recent years, especially at a center like Memorial. "We're not just Florence Nightingales anymore. We draw blood, hang blood, give some kinds of chemo, change various pieces of equipment, control patients on monitors, put them on respirators, the MA-1, and we do a lot of teaching. In a general hospital, you don't see that on the floor. We also have an ongoing educational program on the mental, psychological, and physical care of patients. How to avoid them getting bruised, early signs of infection, what to look for in monitoring, side effects of chemo or other drugs, and how to intervene when indicated. You have to know when to act on your own and when not to act, whether the doctor's been called or not."

If you're just there for the paycheck, then you can forget about how effective you're going to be with patients. You have to be stuck in here *(points to heart)* and there has to be a high interest and motivation. You *want* to do all you can for a patient, no matter who the individual is, or what he says or does. Because definitely, you're going to get difficult patients. You just can't write them off as a pest or as hostile. There's got to be a reason why someone's that way.

So you find out what the problem is, you work with the patient on the problem, and try to solve it. Or at least, make him amenable to what's going on, because it's very difficult for the cancer patient to cope with his disease's process. Especially with the young, you almost never find acceptance of the disease. You have to locate the young in their development level, what period they're at in their life, and that's a constant crisis in itself. You know, Eric Erikson's eight stages of man? You get a young man, and you have to know what stage he's in, what should be happening to him in his growth, what he should be doing—except now, he's unable to do it. Is the aid we're giving him causing modifications in his life? If so, he has a reason to be angry and hostile.

You can't look at a patient in a fragmented sense. You know, just walk into a room and come back out and write, "Mr. So-and-So was very quiet today." You find out *why* Mr. So-and-So was quiet. What is really bothering the patient? Is it a psychological problem? A socioeconomic problem? If he doesn't talk, there's gotta be a reason why. You understand what I mean? There's got to be *something* there, a reason why he's acting like that, so withdrawn. Does he have a family? How close are his family ties? What support system does he have? What can we do to enhance that support? There's many stimuli here to motivate you. If you become lethargic, you start saying, "Oh, I don't have nothin' to do." But there's no such thing. It doesn't exist.

I don't have to pry information out of patients. For some unknown reason, most of the time they'll automatically talk to me. I don't know if it's the mold of my face *(laughs)* or what it is. It's considered a talent of mine. Because if I sit down for a while, even if the patient is extremely hostile, and I offer him a chance to relieve himself of the problem, he'll tell me what's botherin' him.

Last Sunday morning, I was taking care of a patient in one bed while the patient in the next bed was restless. So I asked him, "What's the matter?" He says, "Oh, nothin'." So I went back to taking care of the first patient, but I keep my eye on the other one. It'd been some time since his chemo treatment, but he was still vomiting. I said, "Why you vomiting so much? It's supposed to be wearing off now. There's gotta be sometin' else botherin' you. I know, I can tell from the way you're behavin'." He said, "Well, there is something bothering me, but why should I tell you my problems?" I said, "Why shouldn't you? Why shouldn't I know it? Maybe I'd be able to help you." He said, "I don't know if you can. This is a family problem." I said, "Does it hurt too much, is it too personal?" He said, "No." I said, "Well, then tell me about it."

So he started to tell me about his parents. His mother and father believed in materialistic things. They weren't giving him the love that he needed. They wouldn't even keep the kids when his wife came to see him. So she had to leave them down in the lobby. There'd been a fight between the wife and the mother, and he didn't know how to handle it. They were going to come and see him later that day.

I said, "Why don't you tell them just how you feel? Tell them to leave your wife alone, 'cause you have other things to think about than this garbage." He said, "Well, that's gonna really upset them because I've never spoken to them like that." I said, "All right, I'll ask your doctor to allow you a Valium, so you'll be perfectly calm and not worry when they come. That way, you can tell them exactly what you want them to do and how you feel about their behavior."

He did that, and it worked. It helped him but also me. It's good for me. I have to do that. I like that.

I don't know if a mental attitude alone can lick cancer, but I'm sure it has a lot to do with it. There was a seventy percent chance I wouldn't be clean of it, and the same odds that I'd be sterile. Maybe it was just being dumb, or young or cocky, but I said, "It's not going to overtake me. I'm going to walk away from this clean—and with my manhood." Well, I walked away clean. I was playing tennis three weeks after the operation. But getting my sex strength back wasn't so easy. When we tried to have a baby and kept failing, I knew I had to hold onto that belief in myself—or I'd never have a son of my own.

He's 29, six feet tall, blue eyes, and is wearing a white and green Adidas warm-up suit. We are seated in the living room of the Spiegel home in Livingston, New Jersey. His wife, Gail, sits in an opposite sofa chair. She is a slender, tense woman with brown hair and blue eyes similar to her husband's. A former schoolteacher, she listens with occasional nods as David begins: "I was a tennis instructor, and I'd just bought my tennis shop in Livingston, putting everything I owned into it, plus a bank loan, when this thing hit me."

It was June, six years ago. I started experiencing pain in my left testicle. You know, when you're a kid playing baseball and you get hit in the groin with the ball or something? I had that kind of aching. It sort of subsided, except I was having strange sensations I can't really describe. Then a couple of days later, in the shower, I felt a hard spot on the testicle.

Our family doctor at first thought it might be an infection, like epididymitis. So we tried medication for a week or two. When it didn't get better, he sent me to a urologist who took one look and said, "I'm sorry, but we have to remove this immediately."

It was done by Dr. Read at Mountainside Hospital in Montclair. He removed my testicle on July third, the day before my second wedding anniversary. Some anniversary present, right? I went home after four days and assumed that was it. They told me I could still have children with only one testicle, and they had inserted a prosthesis in place of the one they took away. So I'm fine. We joked about it: "One down and one to go." *(Laughs.)*

When I went to have the stitches out a week later, Dr. Read said they had examined the testicle, and it was malignant. He said, "I want you to go see Dr. Whitmore at Memorial Hospital.* You probably need another operation." He didn't elaborate or say it was going to be real bad. I remember asking, "How big a cut? How big a scar?" But he didn't tell me everything because he wanted Dr. Whitmore to do it his way. Fortunately, he knew Whitmore, and I got a consultation within a couple of days.

After my examination, Dr. Whitmore sees me in his office. He must have just come from the operating room because he's wearing green surgical dress. He's very low-keyed and laid back, but I can tell from the way he moves that he's very fast, very coordinated, and I get the feeling this guy's going to fix me up, no matter what. He explains they have to do a radical nodal resection, which is to remove the lymph glands in the area in case the cancer had spread.

I asked him the odds of getting it clean, and he said, "About fifty-fifty." Then I got a worse blow. There was also a fifty-fifty chance that I'd be sterile. Afterward, I learned it was closer to seventy-thirty, but he didn't say so then.

GAIL: *(Interrupts)* I remember his saying, "There's the possibility that you will never have children." I was with my mom, and David was with his dad. I ran out of there hysterical, crying, right into the ladies' room, and my mother came after me. She realized how I felt, but she told me, "Gail, look at what David's going through. You have a choice. Are you going to think about having kids at the moment, or are you going to think about having a husband? That's where it's at now." After that, I pulled myself together and went back in and dealt with it.

DAVID: So I'm stunned. My wife and I are married two years, we're very children-oriented, and we'd been waiting to be financially ready for a child. I'd just bought the tennis shop, and we were planning to have our first baby as soon as I'd paid back part of the bank loan.

Whitmore explains why the odds are so high against me, and I try to listen. During the operation, they can't help but sever nerves which are not visible. They know where they are, they try to save as many as possible, and often they are successful. If not, there is either no ejaculation, or it is retrograde—that is, all the semen does not emerge. Some comes out, the rest goes up into the bladder. He said, "If the nerves regenerate, it'll happen within four to six months." I remember he smiled, he had a nice smile, and said, "You're young and in good shape. You'll probably make it fine." But as a backup, just in case, he suggested I go to Idant, a medical outfit which collects and stores sperm. "You have about ten days before

---

* Willet F. Whitmore, Jr., M.D., attending surgeon, chief of Urology Service, Department of Surgery, Memorial Hospital.

the operation," he said. "At your age, you can leave some there. If you need it later, you can use it."

"I went to Idant. It's in midtown Manhattan and one of the largest centers for frozen sperm in the country. They mainly collect donor sperm for artificial insemination, then ship it out to doctors everywhere. But they also collect it from people threatened with sterility, like men who work with radiation or in chemical plants or who have to undergo surgery that might destroy their ability to reproduce.

"Gail and a friend of ours, Frankie, went with me. We had a great time. I mean, if you can believe anybody can have a good time at Idant. It goes like this. You go into a room with reclining chairs, and there's a coffee table with copies of Playboy *and* Penthouse *to help you. Gail, of course, had to wait outside. You masturbate into a little container. They take it from you and liquefy it further with glycerol, then draw it up into little strawlike tubes which are frozen in tanks with liquid nitrogen. One ejaculate is split into three straws, more or less, so each time you get enough for three inseminations. I went three times, so I had nine chances if I ever needed to use them.*

"When I came out, Frankie said I'd made it in sixty seconds, an all-time Idant record." (Laughs.) *"We goofed around about the whole thing, which I guess was the most healthy way to deal with it. Frankie was really great in helping us laugh at it. I just wish we could've kept on laughing."*

The operation went off fine. Whitmore is supposed to be one of the best men in the world for this. My only complaint is that no one told me what to expect when you wake up in the recovery room, with tubes up the nose, down the throat, and a catheter in the penis. I didn't mind the catheter, but I thought I would choke to death from the tubes. I beat the bed rail with my wedding band until some nurse came and helped me. She was very nice. In fact, they're all incredible there.

Whitmore had said if the nerves regenerated at all, it would occur within four to six months. About four months later, mine came back, and I began to have emissions. It was great, and we began to try having a baby, but nothing happened. Whitmore said I was experiencing retrograde ejaculation. Part of the semen was going backwards, up into the bladder, but he didn't rule out my eventually making it. I told Gail not to worry, but she was already very uptight about it.

GAIL: *(Stiffly)* Was I? I thought I was very cooperative. Except we were on a different time schedule. You acted as if we had all our lives to do it, while all our friends were having babies, and we had none.

DAVID: Yes. Well, I didn't see any reason to panic, especially since we were still young, and also we had the frozen sperm. So we began to go into

Manhattan for Gail to receive it. Idant sent it to her gynecologist, who inserted it, but nothing happened. My count was too low.† So they tried to build it up by combining two or more straws, but it was still no dice.

GAIL: That's when you also got desperate.

DAVID: *(Shakes his head)* Then we went to Dr. Mort Cohen, a young urologist in New York, who specializes in male infertility. He gave me female hormones, HCG, a course of twenty injections. It's supposed to pick you up, and each time he'd measure my count to see how I was doing.

GAIL: *(Interrupts)* Maybe you weren't desperate, but for a while you weren't so hot on going to the doctor, remember?

DAVID: Well, Gail, I got a little tired of masturbating each time. You can whack your puppy only so long. Then, you know, it gets really tough. But I stayed with it, and at first, it really seemed to pick up my count. Then, all of a sudden, the next time around there was nothing there again. Like, all dead sperm. Dr. Cohen was totally baffled. I was the first case like that he'd ever seen, and, in fact, he didn't charge me.

But I wasn't ready to give up, and neither was Gail. By this time, she was going to some female fertility specialists, although the problem wasn't hers. They were just helping her along. During a checkup, I told Whitmore what was happening, and he said, "Why don't you go to these guys, Dr. Amelar and Dr. Dubin? They're tip-top people in this profession." So I went to them, in Manhattan, and they were baffled, too. Dr. Amelar said, "Dr. Cohen gave you the course of injections?" I said, "Yes." He said, "That's really all that I can do. Let's just wait awhile and see what happens." He asked me not to smoke pot because chronic use can reduce your sperm count. I wasn't a chronic user, but I stopped anyway. No big sacrifice. But that's when it got a bit tense between us.

---

† The average sperm count of young donors at Idant is 100 million per ejaculate. The count of most married men—due to tobacco, alcohol, and stress—is closer to 60 million. At that figure, conception usually occurs within three to six months. Males below that count are considered semisterile, capable of reproducing only in 200 to 400 attempts. Any number below 20 million is usually sterile. Idant has had success, however, with a count of only 5 million—in a Hodgkin's case from Memorial Hospital—mainly due to a special-stage freezing technology, available only in its New York Center.

Sperm is counted by a Coulter electronic counter with semen samples projected onto a TV-type grid screen. Shapes and direction of sperm flow are closely observed. Virile sperm swim straight up and are eventually drawn into the ovum. Less virile ones circle about in an aimless fashion. David Spiegel's count left him semisterile, and a critical number of his reanimated sperm circled about, as if lost. Tight undergarments—such as jockey briefs rather than boxer shorts—also lessen sperm count, since testicles should be at a lower temperature than the body.

GAIL: You kept saying let nature take its course. But nature wasn't doing anything. Why shouldn't I get tense?

DAVID: I was optimistic. I felt we'd eventually make it, and I said, "Let's leave it alone, and see what happens in six months or so." But Gail was always insisting, "Let's do something now." That was always her response—*now*. Every single month was crucial. At one point, in the middle of the worst snowstorm we'd ever had, she was due to go to the gynecologist in New York. I was in the store, and she called, saying, "I'm going to the doctor." I said, "Gail, you're out of your mind. It's God-awful out and too dangerous. There's no way you're getting on those roads just to see the doctor. It's not that important." She said, "Not for you, but for me it is." Nothing would stop her. So I go to take her in, and the car stalls in the snowstorm. I get out, and I'm under the hood, trying to dry off the wires from the snow slush, when another car plows into us from the rear. My car hit me in the face—literally—and the bumper rammed into my knee. I ended up in the hospital with plastic surgery, torn knee cartilage, and dislocated shoulder.

GAIL: I got to the point where I was really bunked out about the whole situation. I guess I was just down about everything, and David was always optimistic. But we were nearly four years married and I really felt it was just never going to happen. Also, my friends would call. Like our dear friends, David and Dale. When Dale got pregnant, she called to tell me, and I couldn't even talk to her. I said, "Hold the line a minute," and put David on. Here she was, my best friend so happy, and I was hysterical, crying. I just couldn't deal with it. We'd been trying for three years, and they tried only three months. You know, that kind of thing.

Then we'd sit around with friends, and they'd talk about their little children, how they're doing, and you'd say to yourself, "I want that to be me, I want to be experiencing these things." Then you'd wonder, "Why are they being so cruel? These are our friends, dammit, why don't they shut up?"

Then I began to think about artificial insemination, but David wouldn't hear of it.

DAVID: *(Interrupts)* We had a lot of conversations. Gail always wanted to talk about it, but at one point I didn't want to talk about it anymore. There was no way that I wanted to have a child by artificial insemination using someone else's sperm. I felt I would have nothing to do with that child, genetically or otherwise. Also, I was not that desperate. I was still optimistic. We were only 28. I figured I might give up when I'm 35, say, when we're really out of the box—but not now.

So I said, "Gail, I still love you. We have each other. If we remain childless for the rest of our lives, that's not the end of the world, not the worst thing that could happen to us. I'm alive and healthy, with no more cancer, you're alive and healthy, we should be thankful and not go crazy if we are childless."

GAIL: Yeah, but I really wanted a child.

DAVID: So did I, but I felt the most important thing about having a child is really to have your own. Whether it's selfish or not, good or not, my opinion is that it's an extension of yourself. You want to see whether what you produce looks like Gail, looks like me, whether it looks like both of us, whether it has Gail's intelligence or stupidity or sense of humor or mine. All those things. That's really why people want to have children. It may be considered selfish or needful or whatever by some, but that's why people initially say, "Yeah, let's have children. I love you, you love me, let's see what we can produce." That's why I said, "If this can't happen, then I don't want it to happen any other way."

GAIL: Except insemination would've been an extension of *me*, which you could not consider. It would have come from at least one of us, which would've been better than adopting a child who would have nothing of either of us.

DAVID: *(Shakes head)* It would have been her child by another man, not mine. Further down the road, in our thirties maybe, I would have been for adoption, but never for another man's child out of Gail. Even if I didn't know who he was, I would be thinking about it, seeing that man in my child. No, no—no way.

GAIL: Our marriage was definitely threatened. At one point, a woman we knew went through the same thing. Something was wrong with her husband, she couldn't have children. So she divorced him and married another guy. I don't think I would have.

DAVID: *(Interrupts)* I think I might have.

GAIL: *(Startled)* Because you couldn't stand me?

DAVID: I might have pushed for divorce at some point because you were so depressed, so melancholy. I was trying so hard, but there was no way, nothing helped. Finally, I was saying, "Look, Gail, you have to realize that I'm not going through life depressed, period." As I said before, I'm an optimist, and I'll go on trying, no matter what.

"Look, my father had polio when he was 3; now he has two artificial hips, but he plays squash every day. He had cancer three times, including once in the testicle, was treated with radiation therapy, and today he's healthy as a bull. He's a chemical scientist, and he says, 'There's always another solution; you don't give up.' And that's how I feel."

One day, looking for the solution, I went back to Dr. Amelar. He said, "I'm glad to see you. I happened to read an article that might solve your problem. It's an obscure study by a German doctor on retrograde ejaculation. He claims if you have intercourse with a full bladder—and, if possible, even standing up—the fluid that would ordinarily go into the bladder will be forced out the right way."

I knew immediately that was the solution. I went out and had a couple of beers, then came back with a full bladder and gave him a specimen doing it that way. Sure enough, the sperm count was much better.

I went home knowing it would work. It was so logical. A simple, basic thing. We tried it, and eventually Gail conceived.

GAIL: I thought I was pregnant and went right into town for a blood test. Then I went shopping with my sister at one of the malls, and I called David and said, "I'm sure I'm pregnant, I feel it's happening. . . ."

DAVID: (Interrupts) I called the lab, and they didn't want to tell me anything. I said, "Look, it's just a pregnancy test." Then I thought, "What am I saying? Just a pregnancy test?" Finally he said, "I'm not supposed to give results to anyone except the doctor—but, yes, your wife's pregnant." Then Gail called me back, and I told her, "It's happened Gail, you're going to have a baby."

GAIL: I was in Livingston Mall, and I sat there and cried. (Laughs.) My sister is jumping up and down screaming, and I'm sitting there crying. Crazy.

DAVID: That whole day in the store was an incredible high. Everybody had been on pins and needles for us, and we called every single friend and our parents ten times. My mother, wonderful woman that she is, said, "Keep cool, don't say it because you shouldn't say anything." She came to this country from Poland where it was an old Jewish tradition, you don't say anything for three or four months. Later she felt badly because her words came true when Gail miscarried. It was the biggest tragedy of our life.

GAIL: It happened on my birthday. Before going to work that morning, I went to the bathroom, and I was spotting. I didn't tell anybody, and I went to school—I was teaching grade school Spanish then—and I said to the nurse, "I have to go home, I'm spotting." She said, "Gail, calm down." I was shaking, and I called David, and he said, "Calm down, just go home." So I drove home and called the doctor. He said, "Stay in bed for a while and see what happens." It didn't get any better, and later in the afternoon, I went in to the doctor, and he did a D&C in the office . . . (pauses) and that was it, my birthday present.

I had a bad summer, but I kept it inside me. I went to the club, I went swimming, I kept it all closed up. And then, like a miracle, it happened again. I was one day late, my temperature was up, and I said, "I know I'm pregnant." I went for a test, and it came back borderline. I said, "Borderline, baloney. I'm over the border." *(Laughs.)* I had to wait another two days to repeat the test, but then I still hadn't gotten my period, so I knew for sure I was pregnant. Finally, my friend Pat in the doctor's office called me, screaming, "Congratulations!" *(laughs)* and the doctor told me the same.

This time I was much lower-keyed. I was real nervous after miscarrying the first time. But it worked out fine. I had Matthew, who's a dream child. It was the best year we ever had, and it's been great ever since.

DAVID: *(Smiles at Gail, but shakes head)* Like I was saying about my father, you get a longer view or maybe a better hold on life from all this. Yes, we finally have Matthew. We are blessed by a son. But the way I see it, I'm also twice blessed by this cancer experience and everything that came with it.

Look, when I say I believe in positive attitudes, it's not feeling that you will get well, or that you aren't really sick, so you can't die. It's also feeling aware and appreciating life. You know what I mean?

It's funny that I don't know how to say this because it's the most important part. I mean, how it comes to you with this experience when you realize that you have a mortality. Especially me, at my age. Suddenly at 25, I realized that I could conceivably die very soon. I could have died on the table. I could still die of this disease. Not of what I had, because I'm cured. But I have no guarantee that I won't have another outcropping of this somewhere else. I like to think that I won't. But I don't know. Once you become aware of that, you start to be grateful. You say, "I'm well now, and I've been well for seven years. And not only that, I've licked the fertility problem and have a beautiful boy."

Then you begin to appreciate every day you're alive, every day you are pain-free, and able to go about your daily business. That's what I mean by being twice blessed. It's having a son but also being aware of how really great and beautiful it is to be alive.

POSTSCRIPT: A last-minute letter from David contained joyous news: "We are all well and happy, especially with the newest addition—our second child! Jordyn Amy Spiegel was born in September. Our family is now truly complete and my ordeal is fading into the past. . . ."

I had a very nice body, I loved my breasts, I never wore a bra. That's how I went around. Then I lost one breast and, six months later, the other one developed the same thing—medullary carcinoma. So I had two modified radicals, and it left me with no breasts at all.† I had even less than a man has—just skin over the ribs.

I was really lost without them, and I wanted a breast reconstruction. But then I discovered my husband didn't want me to do anything about it because this made me less attractive to other men. That's when I knew I was in a crazy house. I had to do something about it if I ever wanted to feel like a woman again.

She's 29, light blue-gray eyes, long dark hair, and a face so loved by the Greeks that they gave it to their goddesses—the long straight line of the nose between high cheekbones, and a rich, sensual mouth with a full chin. A golden pendant resembling a bull's horn is visible in the opening of her blouse, resting between the twin slopes of her reconstructed breasts.

She's a schoolteacher. "I studied Russian at Queens College and for a while taught bilingual Russian at Canarsie and Meadows Junior High. There was a whole slew of Russians living right on Brighton Beach. Then, after my marriage broke up, I was laid off from my job. But since I also had a lot of math credits, I got another license to teach in junior high schools."

We are in her high-rise apartment at Far Rockaway. From the studio window, the long stretch of the beach is visible with its white-crested waves under a gray sky. The sun is just breaking through the clouds.

Let me tell you how it happened, otherwise you might think I overreacted to this. After my second mastectomy, I went home and started healing. I was doing exercises and started getting better. But I was very depressed, needless to say. I felt disconnected, I didn't like the way I looked, and it affected my life.

---

* Identities of patient and husband have been altered.

† Breast removal, the most common treatment for breast cancer, is called mastectomy. There are four general types: (1) *radical*—removal of entire breast, chest muscles, and lymph nodes in armpit; (2) *modified radical*—removal of breast and lymph nodes, but with chest muscles left intact; (3) *total* or *simple*—removal of breast but not lymph nodes or chest muscles; (4) *partial* or *segmental* (also called lumpectomy, tylectomy, or local incision)—removal of part of the breast containing the cancer with surrounding margin of breast tissue. Some doctors follow partial surgery with radiation therapy and removal of armpit lymph nodes. Increasingly, others seek to use radiation alone, without surgery.

I wouldn't watch television because I would see bra commercials and start crying. I wouldn't buy magazines because that would mean fashions and lingerie articles, and I couldn't wear them. I had to have separate clothes. I wouldn't go to dinner with friends because I didn't want pity or to talk about it. Also some of them didn't know what I had. They thought it was pneumonia, and I left it there.

I was being impossible, I know it. But I've since talked to a lot of women, and this can really put you under, there's no question about it. Me, I never take pills, and I was taking Valium. I felt disconnected from myself and everyone else, including my husband. I needed help from him —sympathy, understanding—but I got nothing. Besides the sex, you expect your husband to also be a friend, to give you help. But Richard is not a giving or generous man. He's an endodontist, a dentist specializing in root canal work, and I think that's all he understands about people—the roots of their teeth. (Smiles.)

So our marriage wasn't going too well before this happened. The problems were there, only now they became intensified. The nonsupport, the nongiving in a crisis situation made it overwhelming. Then I discovered something so incredible, so horrible that it changed everything. I should have suspected it, but I didn't.

He wanted me, he insisted on making love even when I didn't want it. When I cried, he said he didn't mind me without breasts. I said, "Just the same, I miss them, I want to have reconstruction." He said, "I like it this way, don't do anything about it, leave it alone." At first, I thought he was finally trying to be kind to me. But then he told my stepmother, "You know, in a way it's good because now other men won't look at her. She'll be less independent, more dependent on me." When I asked him how he could ever say such a thing, he told me he was trying to see the positive side of it, and I had to do the same.

I knew he was sick, he was under psychiatric care, but I never knew how sick he was. This was a sort of *Gaslight* nightmare. He wanted me deformed, mutilated, the better to keep me, like those tribes in Africa that cut out a woman's clitoris so she won't enjoy it or be tempted to try it with somebody else. For me, that was the end. I told myself, "Either you're going to die, or you're going to do something about this."

I started researching breast reconstruction, I went to lectures, I met a lot of the top guys in the field. I got surgical books, I read articles, and I made up a list of questions before going into consultations. Then I saw Dr. Chaglassian on television.‡ He was on *Health Line,* Channel Thirteen.

---

‡ Toros A. Chaglassian, M.D., associate attending surgeon, chief of Plastic & Reconstructive Surgical Service, Department of Surgery, Memorial Hospital.

There was something about him that I liked, and I went to him for consultation with my whole list of questions. He was very patient and went through the whole thing with me.

"I'll tell you what he said, including the basics I already knew. Any woman can have a reconstruction, starting three months after her mastectomy, provided she's cancer-free, not having chemotherapy, or being subjected to heavy radiation on the chest wall. If a plastic surgeon and breast surgeon work together, or agree on a procedure, it's easier to reconstruct later. Also it helps a patient mentally as she's going into the operating room, knowing she can have it done later if she wants it.

"If a woman did not have a plastic surgeon involved—like me, for instance—it can still be done, even though there's less skin flap to work with. He said, 'If there's no plastic surgeon, the woman should tell the breast surgeon to please close the wound so she can have reconstruction later if she wants it. That means closing it in a cosmetic fashion, using fine sutures, fine instruments. It takes ten minutes more, but it leaves only a line instead of a thick scar.'

"Then he showed me the prosthesis they use. It feels just like any breast. It has a silicone center, sealed in a saline solution. They've been using them for fifteen years, they're leak-proof, and there's no fear of cancer from them. I'd heard they can become hard after a while, and he said, 'The implant remains soft, but in some cases the body forms a natural scar around it. When that happens, you can squeeze the chest wall and break the scar. It's easy and painless, and we do it in the office.' I asked about the nipple, if he was going to take it from my vagina. He said, 'We now take it from the inner thigh. The skin is lighter, but it works better.' I asked if my health care, Blue Cross, would pay for it and he said, 'It depends on the doctor, but usually it covers most of it.' "

I like Ted Chaglassian. I think I'm like a lot of other women with mastectomies. I don't just want a good surgeon. I want someone who can deal with me psychologically so I can trust them and feel comfortable. I asked if I could see some photographs of his work. He not only showed me some, but he gave me the phone number of a woman my age he'd done in New Jersey. I called her up and asked, "Would you mind if I come to see you? I'm interested in reconstruction." I told her my story, and she said, "Come on over." It's very interesting. Women who have gone through this are very supportive. I went to New Jersey, saw her, and I liked what he did. It looked really good.

So I made my decision to have Dr. Chaglassian do it, and I checked into Memorial Hospital. Counting two biopsies and the mastectomies, this is now my fifth operation. It's easier than all the others because my mind is at ease, I trust my surgeon, and I know where I'm going.

It's April, and he puts in the implants. Then, in June, he took skin grafts from the upper thigh and made the areolas, and then a month or so later, he took ear cartilage and made the erect center piece. There are three basic sizes of implants—A, B, and C. I wanted a big B or even a small C, but I hadn't been prepared for it when I had my mastectomies. So Ted gave me a regular B. You can only go so far, and that's it. After all, this is just skin over your ribs, and it can be stretched only so much.

It really looks pretty good. It's not going to look absolutely normal, there are scars there. But it looks great in a bra, and actually I don't have to wear a bra. They are perfect without it. So it's normal and just right for me.

A lot of women don't want any more trauma or operations after the loss of their breasts, so they don't go for reconstruction. They say their husbands don't mind, and after a while they get used to slapping on a prosthesis and let it go at that. I think age has a lot to do with it, also your love life. An older person might feel different, especially if they've been married a long time.

"The work done on me always amazes people, even those who say they don't want it for themselves. I began to get calls to talk to women. They want to see it, so I show them. I bring different types of bras to show them, since you can't wear all types. It has to be basically just stretch material, because these breasts don't fit into a cup. So I bring different types just to show them that you can find nice things. They ask me about clothes, and I tell them you can wear anything you want. I show them how it looks with nothing, and I'll have them touch it so they can feel it's soft and natural.

"They ask me about sensitivity, and I tell them that there is touch sensation. It's not the erotic sensation that used to be there because the nerves are all cut. Sometimes I feel it more than other times, so I guess it's psychological. I don't care, but it's nice anyway.

"I'm not saying you can't see the scars across the top because you do— even though they're getting lighter all the time. I've had people say to me, one man said to me, 'What's that?' I said, 'I had some surgery.' He said, 'What happened?' I said, 'I had some cysts removed.' That was it. If I don't tell them, they don't know. I choose who I share it with. Some don't say anything. I guess they don't know what to say, they don't want to hurt my feelings or anything."

So everything fell into place finally, and it gave me the power to get out of my marriage. My husband knew my plans, I had talked to him about it many times, but he wasn't listening. He kept saying it would get better, but it only got worse. Something was broken, there was no more trust, I guess, and nothing could bring it back.

The day after school ended in July, I filed for divorce. He was furious, like it was all of a sudden a surprise, a dirty plot against him. He said, "I'm not giving you a cent, just wait, you'll regret this the rest of your life." It was an ugly scene, he was trying to scare me—anything to hobble me, to keep me from being free of him. I expected it, but not with such terrible anger, so many threats. Part of his psychiatric care deals with his obsession for money. But his analysis didn't help, because he was convinced that if he had to give me alimony, he'd lose whatever manhood he had left. So he counterfiled, claiming I was cruel and inhuman. *(Laughs dryly.)* Me! Can you believe it?

We went to trial. There was just the judge, the stenographer, and the lawyers. I was very nervous, Richard had said he was going to destroy me, and he had a high-priced lawyer to do it. But I didn't see how they were going to do it until we had presented our case. We didn't call any witnesses because my lawyer said it was not necessary. He said that Richard wouldn't have any, either.

Well, my husband pulled out five witnesses, one after the other—friends of ours, doctors even, that lied. It was incredible. I was pictured as an insane, hysterical, and even dangerous woman. I had fits of rage, and I had punched Richard several times in the face. He even testified to this, one lie after another. I looked at him, at his friends lying about me, and I knew I was going to lose the case. I asked my lawyer how he could allow this, but he only shook his head and said, "I'm sorry." That's all he said as he threw the case.

My husband won, and the judge not only decided against me—meaning I'd get no alimony—but he gave Richard our home, which we jointly owned, a lovely estate home on the Island. It was supposed to be a bifurcated trial—first the divorce, then the property settlement. But it wasn't. My lawyer had lied to me there, too. I had worked all summer, getting the records of payments, checks—everything I'd also spent. But it wasn't used. Richard got it all at once.

On top of that, my lawyer slapped me with a nine thousand dollar fee. I'd already paid a thousand and told him I didn't have much more, so he'd promised to file for counsel fees in the trial. But he didn't do that, either, and now he wanted it all from me. I said, "I don't have it." He said, "Then get it, or I'll take you to court. You can't sue a lawyer, don't you know that?"

I didn't know what to do and was very depressed. I'd gotten rid of one monster, and now I was being chased by another one, this horrible lawyer asking for his pound of flesh. Everything had been going fine with my new breasts, my ability to help other women, my plans for a new life. Only now it was a mess with this man sending me letters, threatening me if I didn't pay him. I didn't have it, I felt betrayed, and I began to distrust everybody.

Then one day at school a big black guy in a denim jacket came to see me. I thought he was one of the parents, and I got to talking to him. He said, "I'm really upset." I figured it was about one of the kids that I left back. I said, "What's your problem?" He said, "I'm a process server." My tears started, and he said, "Don't cry, don't get upset. I'm really sorry, I hate to do it." He said, "Go someplace and read it." I went to the bathroom, and it was like pages and pages for that nine thousand dollars. I came back and said, "You wouldn't believe what this lawyer did to me."

So I'm telling him the story, how this man lied and tricked me, and the black man says, "You know, I also used that firm. My wife split and took everything out of the apartment—kids, furniture, everything." I said, "Then you should have won the case on grounds of abandonment." He said, "That's right, but I had the same lawyer you had. He pulled a fast one and ruined it for me. So now I'm paying my wife who's living with another man."

It was incredible. They just happened to give him that law firm to serve, and he happened to get this same lawyer. He's angry about that, and also he said, "You know, they were talking about your case in the office, they were laughing about it, they thought it was a big joke. I didn't think that was very nice." So I guess it was the ethical part, too. It bothered him that they were ripping me. The paper also spoke about my mastectomies, the surgeries—all of it. I guess anybody reading that part couldn't help but feel some sympathy.

He took the paper back and said, "How many days you have left teaching school?" I said, "Only five." He said, "Do they know where you live?" I'd just moved, and I said, "No." He said, "Usually I get twenty-five dollars, but they offered me forty to serve you. I don't care, I'm going to take it back."

I was ready to cry. Just when I was feeling I couldn't trust anybody, along comes this beautiful man. I hugged him, and he gave me his name and address if I needed any help. He said, "Get yourself a good lawyer, an honest one, who'll fight this guy. If he's honest, he won't go to trial because he'll look stupid. If he's a crook, he won't risk it either, and he'll probably settle out of court."

That's what I did. I found a very decent lawyer who stopped them from pursuing me. He thinks we have a good chance of reducing the fee. I can't wait for the day. I'll finally be a free woman again to begin my new life.

POSTSCRIPT: Six months later, a note arrived from Elizabeth. She was ecstatic: "Everything's going wonderfully. My lawyer settled the case. He negotiated the fee down to $1,350, payable at $50 a month for twenty-seven months. I can't complain. Thank God, it's over!!!

"But here's the best news. I met a delicious man whom I'm in love with. He's sensitive, affectionate, kind and caring. He makes me very happy. And he loves my new tits! He even wrote a poem about them!!"

The poem was enclosed:

> *Two man-created orbs*
> *delicately smooth and round,*
> *loosely freeing themselves*
> *from your bikini top*
> *as you lie on your back,*
> *straining themselves to reach*
> *the sunlight.*
> *Straining themselves for my*
> *lips,*
> *so majestic in their beauty,*
> *so magnificent in their taste.*
>   M.R.

About this mysterious night visitor that came to take me away, I haven't talked much—not even to my father. It was right after my first operation. They'd put me in an oxygen tent for the night, and I was having cold sweats, a terrible time, and couldn't sleep.

I called the nurse several times, asking to please give me some shots in my IV or something, you know, to put me to sleep. She said it was forbidden because I'd just come out of anesthesia. "Try real hard, and if you can't sleep, I'll contact the doctor."

I tried, but I wasn't about to fall asleep by myself, so about an hour later she came back with a needle syringe which I didn't expect. I'd thought she would inject something through one of the IVs, you know, but she said, "Roll over, it has to be intramuscular." I'd had enough holes in me, I didn't want any more, so I just said, "Never mind." Then she said, "I'll leave the syringe here, and if you want it, just call me."

I remember seeing the syringe and just laying back, trying to figure out how to get some sleep. Then, all of a sudden, I'm not feeling any pain anymore, my neck didn't hurt, the IVs didn't hurt—nothing.

I was sort of raised up on my elbow in the oxygen tent. It was like I could see myself laying there, and I looked really bad. My hair had not been cleaned for days, the cold sweat made it all oily and, ugh, I had a terrible stench about me. My clothes were all sopped with sweat, my IVs were running, my arms were bruised with holes, my eyes were sunk in, I was pale like a ghost—and then I saw this man sitting next to me.

The man, I don't know what he was, but there was something about him that was easy to like. People have told me they see that in me, like an attraction for other people. But something about this man, wow, and then he just came out and said, "Would you like to come with me?" That's all, and I'm not even sure he said it that way. But he was looking at me, and I knew he wanted me to go with him. It was my choice, if I wanted to go or not, and somehow I knew if I had gone with him, I would have died that night.

I said to myself, "No one dies at my age. Who dies at 14?" I wanted to die older, so I showed him that I didn't want to go with him, and it was something that more or less surprised me.

He's 18 now, a slender, light brown youth with a broad nose, eyes like almonds, dark curly hair, and a pleasant smile. His mother is Korean. His father is black, mixed with Cherokee and Irish. We are drinking beer in a bar on Manhattan's Lower East Side, near his old neighborhood.

This was in the beginning, when they took me to Flower Hospital on Fifth Avenue for a cough that was going on and on. They'd found something in the X rays, a lump in my throat and another one in my chest, like a small-sized fist between my heart and my lungs. So they operated, going up under my left arm to my throat.

The chest mass was too big, too close to the heart to mess around with, so they closed me up and sent me back to my room where I encountered that late night visitor. That's what's so scary about this. I didn't know how sick I was, you know, like I was going to die unless something was done somewhere else—because here they'd given up on me. So I guess that visitor, you know, he probably didn't go very far away, like he was just waiting there to see if he was going to have to come back again. *(Laughs.)*

The next morning my mother's there, and the doctor takes her out of the room. Then she comes back all red-eyed, and I said, "Wow! What happened?" She's all choked up, and I say, "Wait a minute, Mom, is something wrong?" She went, "Oh no, Baby, it's not that." Then she goes, "Just let me hear you say you're going to be all right." I say, "But is it bad, Mom?" And she goes, "Oh no, Baby, but just let me hear you say those words."

The doctor had told my parents that I had lymphoma. That's a cancer of the lymph gland system. It's the non-Hodgkin's type, called lymphosarcoma. It had got loose and was running wild in my body, so I didn't have much chance to live more than a few weeks or months, maybe. Luckily, there was a consultant doctor there who had trained under Dr. Wollner.* As I understand it, he told my father, "Your only chance to save your son is Dr. Wollner. If anybody can do it, she can." Then they phoned her, and she told my father to get all the X rays and tests and bring me to Memorial as soon as possible.

When they let me go, I still had a fever, and my father wrapped me in a blanket and took me in his car to Memorial. That's when I found out I wasn't all alone with this. There were kids all over her floor in the hospital. Little kids and big ones—all kinds. Some without hair, some without a leg, or just sitting there, all hunched over in a wheelchair.

They were outpatients, you know, coming in for their blood count, weight measure, and the chemo shots—but I didn't know about that then. I thought it was like some kind of club of brothers, with so many wearing baseball caps or cowboy hats to cover their bald heads. The parents sat

---

* Norma Wollner, M.D., director, Pediatric Day Hospital and attending pediatrician, Department of Pediatrics, Memorial Hospital.

there, all sad-looking, and most of the kids were standing separate from them, like they were going to run away if they got a chance.

"Dr. Wollner was very busy, so they put me on a table in a room to wait for her. Then she came in and began to look at the X rays, the tests, and then examined me. She's got those thick glasses, you know, and I remember looking at her and seeing her eyes real big and blue like the sky. She's bent over me, looking at me closely, like she's come down from another planet, like some science fiction doctor, to just look at me, and I thought, 'Wow! She's got me now, I'm going to have to do what she says, no matter what.' Then she said, 'All right, you can get up, we know what to do.'

"So I sit up, and I'm really shocked to see she's smaller than I am. And me, I'm only 14 then! (Laughs.) You know what she looks like? Like a kid that's grown old with white hair. There's other doctors there who know a lot about pediatrics. But for us kids, nobody knows more than Dr. Wollner. Only it just isn't knowing. It's feeling, and all that, like she came along, telling our parents, 'Just you move over now, 'cause I'm coming into the family, too.' Like we were all her kids, and she wasn't about to lose one of us. And we don't want to lose her, either, because if you walk into her office, you'll see photos and cards with loving words from kids all over the world."

Right away, that same night in my room, I got cytotoxan—my first chemotherapy. My mother was in the room with me, and I slept the whole night and the next day. So you miss a whole lot of days, like I missed St. Patrick's Day.

That's how it began, the chemo treatment and the radiation that was supposed to shrink that cancer they said was like a fist next to my heart. Only I didn't know it was cancer then. My father says they told me, but I don't remember. Dr. Wollner says it's very common that you won't ever hear the word "cancer" until you're ready to accept it. Anyway, I remember finding out by myself.

I was in Dr. Wollner's office with Lee—she was the secretary back then —and I went up to her. I remember seeing the word "cancer" on odd papers, like Memorial Hospital for Cancer. I just asked her, "Do I have cancer?" And she said, "Yes." I wasn't surprised or anything. I said, "Okay," and went out the door. That's the first time I said to myself, "David, you got cancer, you got to fight it and get out of here."

My roommates, they put a big load on me. The first one, Michael, he had the same lymphoma I had, and he was dying from it. Michael lived in Philadelphia, and at first his family got money through the church to take him to California to get treatments. California couldn't give him any help, and by the time they got to Memorial it was too late, the cancer had spread too far. I knew he was going to die because they gave him injections every four hours, just to keep him alive some more.

One night, I was on the phone, and he was yelling at me about being quiet, screaming for help and awful things. His mother, she apologized to me, which I found very touching. She said, "I'm sorry about the way Michael is, but the drugs and disease and all is affecting his mind to some degree, so a lot of times when he yells or screams, it's not his fault." I felt very bad, because really, I never complained about him screaming. I said, "I don't mind too much," but his mother said, "You don't have to suffer because of my son." So she moved him to a room by himself, and that's the last I saw of him.

The next one was a South American. This dude went for an operation, and he came back with his leg gone. He was in such a deep depression, and I thought, "Well, I can't blame him, his leg's gone." Then he said to me, "Nobody told me they were going to do this to me when I was asleep." You see, his mother felt like she was sparing him something by not telling him, so now he wasn't talking to anybody, not even his mother—nobody except me. "We have to get out of here," he said, "before they cut off all our arms and legs."

So I got a lot of stories that were real scary. I asked Dr. Wollner if I was to have another operation, and she said, "I hope not, David, but we don't know. We'll try real hard, and you try, too." Well, they gave me chemotherapy and radiation therapy really heavy so my weight was down to ninety, and my hair was always dying. You know how your hair falls out and your eyebrows, too? Everything falls off. I was really pale, and I had these little red marks to mark the radiation area. Another thing about hospitals, they don't have mirrors in them, they don't want you to know what you look like. I found one hidden in a locker and, ugh, I looked like some kind of weirdo from outer space.

After a month, maybe more, Dr. Wollner came to me and said I had to have another operation. She said, "That swelling you have, we've shrunk it to like a little walnut, but it won't get any smaller." So they were going to have to cut me open and take it out, only I didn't know how close it was to my heart, how serious this was. I was shocked to find out later that everyone thought I might die because Dr. Wollner wasn't sure I was going to survive it. I didn't know that.

"I was waiting for them to roll me into the operating room, and I was making a kind of prayer, saying, 'Please, please, just don't make this thing hurt at all'—though I don't know why God would listen to me, even if he heard me. I never prayed much or went to church a lot. Me and my brothers, we acknowledge there's a God in existence, but we never developed too

much closeness to Him because our church, St. Anthony's, has a twelve-foot barbed wire fence around it. You can't get in unless it's Sunday. We get upset because a church should always be open, and there's nothing inside that place that needs barbed wire on top."

I remember being in the operating room and waking up in bed, and I had tubes in me coming out every way you could think about. I looked around, wondering if the night visitor was back again, sitting next to me, but he wasn't there. There was just my mother and a special nurse, and they were both asleep, so I went, "This is great!" *(Laughs.)*

They told me I'm one of the first ones in the world to survive an operation like that.† They'd taken that cancer fist away from my heart and my lung so now I was like heading toward freedom, getting out of the hospital. Dr. Wollner, she was very happy. Through all this, my temperature had been constantly about a hundred and three, but now it was down to normal, everything was good, and she was going to let me go home in a week. I wasn't in remission yet, they hadn't knocked out all the cancer cells hiding in parts of my body, so I still had to do a lot more chemotherapy. But I could go home and come back during the day as an outpatient.

"Soon after I came home, my brother Ronnie took me for a walk down to the East River. I really liked to look at the boats, which I never did before. You know, after being in the hospital for a long time, your values change. Before, I'd always been looking real close, like at my neighborhood and my friends. Now I was looking out, staring at those ships like I just knew I was going somewhere in life. I felt so good, I wanted to yell at them, 'Hey! Let me come aboard!' One of them was named Canada Sue. *I remember thinking, 'Wow! What a lovely boat!' Who was* Canada Sue? *Maybe a pretty girl my age, like the captain's daughter. (Laughs.) Then, you know, somebody with long hair came out on deck. It looked like a girl, and I waved to her, but I guess she didn't see me.*

"We stayed so long, when I got home my mother was crying because she thought we'd run away. Funny thing is, I had kind of run away. (Laughs.) Like in my head, I was running to get out of the ghetto where I grew up, to go to Canada maybe, to go to a good college, to make my life mean some-

---

† The "fist" next to David Smith's heart was actually a fist-sized tumor, attached to the upper great vein leading into the heart (vena cava) and the lining of the heart itself (pericardium). The mass was extended to the neighboring surfaces of the lungs on both sides. It was totally removed, after four hours of surgery, by Dr. Philip R. Exelby, B.M., B. Ch., chief attending surgeon of Memorial's Pediatric Surgical Service.

thing. But first, I had to get into remission, get rid of the cancer cells left in me."

At first, for my maintenance therapy at Memorial, I had to go every day for three months. Then it gradually got less, but it dragged on and on for two years. I was always very good about taking the treatments, no matter how sick they made me. I felt little kids should be seen and not heard, so I said, "Whatever the grown-ups want is going to be all right, I'm not going to complain." Then I found out they took advantage of it. If there was a new doctor coming in, they would always give him to me first because I wouldn't complain like a lot of other kids did.

"There was this guy, Rod Warren, and we were good friends. He had the same disease I had—except he was just the opposite of me, complaining all the time, giving the doctors a hard time. To stop this hassle, Dr. Wollner matched me with Rod, so when I came in for my shots, he came in, too. The drugs he got, I got beforehand. His main excuse to the doctors and nurses was always, 'You don't know what I'm going through.' He tried that on me a couple times after I'd just had my shot and was feeling real woozy and bad and about to start throwing up. It got me mad, and I'd say something like, 'Look, you dog, I just got the shot, I feel real ill from it, and you'll get it sooner or later, so I don't want to hear your mouth no more.' After that, he always took the shot because none of his arguments worked on me. I'm glad it helped him because he got through it, he's off treatment now and doing fine."

It's amazing how I went through all this, and still kept up with my high school work. My life was mainly school, home, hospital. My social life was nothing for two years—zilch, zip. When I did get into it again, when I went off treatment and went back to my friends, I was exactly two years behind everyone else. You know, like all the kids experiment with drugs and everything else in adolescence. They had long gone through all that.

So I found out that with my normal high school crowd, I was an outsider. When I was with them, I wasn't able to join in any longer. I couldn't get close because there was a lot of things I hadn't been through. That left me alone, and kind of lonely. Then Dr. Wollner said, "David, did you ever think that maybe you're older than they are now?"

She meant I was older because of what I'd been through with my disease, the way I'd come close to dying two times, how I'd met the dark man of death and sent him away, how I'd gone through two years of them shooting poison into my veins to kill the cancer—all that. It was true, you know, I did feel older than all of them, like I'd been pushed ahead in years and like they were still kids playing in the street where I couldn't play anymore.

I said to her, "Why did this have to happen to me, why was I made to be separate and different?" She said something like, "Everyone is marked in some way. You've got a special marking." I said, "What am I supposed to do with it?" She said, "That's up to you, David. You have to get to know your own mark, make it your friend, make it work for you."

Maybe Dr. Wollner tells that to all her kids, because they all lose time and get mixed up like I was then. Whatever, I remember that day I walked home along the river. I was trying to get it all straight, you know, about having a special mark. Maybe I had it because I felt I had something, but I didn't know what it was yet. Like I didn't even know what race I was because I was all four races in one body. Then I thought about all those people like Dr. Wollner who'd fought so hard to save my life and how I was living now. So there had to be some reason for it, you know, like maybe there was a sort of mission for me and my special mark.

I remember the river, how empty it was except for some faraway boats sounding their horns, like they were real lonely, too. I wondered whatever happened to the *Canada Sue,* the beautiful boat with the captain's daughter . . . *(laughs)* because that's the way it came to me. Then all of a sudden, I remember I was running, running as fast as I could. I didn't know why, just running.

This mark of mine, I got to know it better when I went to college. I got into Cornell University through the EOP, the Educational Opportunity Program. It takes minorities out of ghetto neighborhoods and puts them into Ivy League schools.

I had enough minorities in me to qualify for four schools. *(Laughs.)* In one discussion class, they were trying to stereotype me, what race I was, what ethnic background. I named all my races—father black, but also American Indian which is red, plus Irish white, and my mother, Oriental yellow. They gave up on me. They said I was "confused chromosomes." *(Laughs.)*

So far, I can cope with this sort of thing and with my work, and also I'm president of the chess club. But most of my minority friends can't cope with this Ivy League pressure and everything else. A lot of minorities come from the ghetto neighborhoods, and they've brought with them some things that they can't stop, that they haven't outgrown. One example would be stealing. I found out that a lot of my minority friends steal, and I'm not sure they can stop.

I used to steal earlier, but I slowly cut down on my system, and now I don't anymore. It was the neighborhood I was brought up in, you learned to do that. But I also learned you can't do that because it holds you back, it makes you a constant loser. Not just the stealing, but everything that goes with it, you know, what it does to your mind and how you relate to people.

I found out a lot of these people in college are not going anywhere because that habit holds them back forever. I'm trying my best to tell them that, to make them aware you don't have to steal anymore. It makes the big difference, it makes you into a real losing minority.

Everything you want in life—if you can think what it is—can be yours. You can work for it and get it. Like if you live in a ghetto neighborhood, it's very hard to get out of it, almost impossible. But you can do it, you can get out if you try hard enough. Sometimes I think maybe that's part of my special mark, why I was allowed to live—to someway help these brothers of mine.

I'll never forget my first patient at Memorial Hospital. She was an elderly lady from Brooklyn. The first time I met her, she had just been told that she had a massive, inoperable tumor. I arrived on the scene, and we talked about it, about her fear of dying. I couldn't believe that she opened up that way on the first interview. I was away for a couple of days, and when I got back, I began to pick up where we had left off—where she was in crisis. Of course, she would have none of it. She turned on me angrily: "What do you mean, I have a tumor? What do you mean, I'm dying?"

In the coffee shop at Memorial Hospital, Sister Rosemary continues to relate her experiences with patients in the battle to survive cancer.

I was in training then and did not yet understand this was a normal need to protect oneself and avoid overwhelming trauma, a withdrawal from an outer reality into a protected, inner image of self. I was too inexperienced to see it for what it was—a way of defending herself. In her struggle, this lady was going all out. Not only did she no longer feel that she was dying imminently, but I was also a major threat. She said, "Why must you be so cruel? I always believed you were supposed to be kind to people who are sick." She was so angry, she reported me to the nursing staff, to the doctors, and to the rabbi. I was devastated. I didn't know what to do, and I went to my supervisor in tears. She said, "You've got to go back into that room and talk this out." She explained to me the dynamics of what had happened.

Well, it took me all day, eight hours, to go back into that room. I was embarrassed in front of the nurses. I was terrified of the patient. I just about crawled into the room. It was a six-bed room in the old Ewing Hospital, and I felt the other five patients were sitting there waiting to see what was going to happen.

I can still see her. I walked in, and I said, "I guess I made a mistake." She nodded, and I said, "You know, I'm sorry if I hurt you. Maybe I just wasn't hearing. I came in with my own agenda." Then she calmed down and said, "Well, you sit down, and let's talk about it." She had already taken charge, which made her feel better. So I dutifully sat down, and she talked to me a few minutes. She told me she was very concerned. She didn't understand my being a Catholic sister. Where was my religious dress, and why was I assigned to her? We talked it all out, that I was a social worker on the service, and that not all sisters wore a religious habit.

Gradually, she became more comfortable. Finally, we decided that each morning I would say, "How are you?" If she didn't feel like talking, she would say, "Oh, it's a nice day. I'll see you tomorrow." If she did feel like talking, she would say, "Sit down." So with that arrangement, I saw her for a year, and we became very fond of each other.

After being sent home, she came in regularly as an outpatient, and I would always see her. Toward the end of my year of training, I began separating from my patients. In a therapeutic relationship, you start doing that about six weeks before leaving, to give people time to get angry and work it out. She said to me, "All year you've seen me, and I don't know anything about you." As a student, I had followed the letter of the law: never reveal a thing about yourself. I thought, "Is this right? What am I supposed to do?" On one level, it was normal to share such information. But I was unclear as to whether it would be therapeutic. Would it really help her or would it make separation more difficult? I was too inexperienced to know the difference. She asked, "Do you have a family?" and I wondered if she thought I was hatched under a rock or something. So we talked about the fact that I had parents, and when I said my sister was getting married, her eyes lit up. "Married . . . a wedding? Will you go to the wedding?" I said, "Yes." She said, "Will you dance at the wedding?" I said, "Oh yes."

This was a new link between us, and I was worried. I remember writing to my supervisor, "Did I do the right thing?" Now I realize that she was bridging her life through me. There was a difference. *Would I dance?* also meant: *Would I dance for her?* After more than a year, she was still emotionally distanced from the seriousness of her illness and the threat of impending death. She still clung to her desire to return to normal health and to live out her dreams. She was still in the dance of life and had no intention of withdrawing until the absolute end. Before the wedding, she said, "Will you let me know about it?" I was already leaving and said I would let her know.

I wrote her a letter and told her about the wedding and the dress my sister wore. She died shortly after that. I knew she got the letter, but never knew what happened until I came back to work here. I can't say how much was due to chemotherapy, or how much was due to her tenacious hold on life, but she did manage to more than double her expected life span.

You meet these people, you find nuances, but you don't really have enough to go on, to develop valid hypotheses. I mean, we know there are benefits in setting personal goals, in having a positive mental image of yourself, and in using various mind control and meditation exercises. We see cases where these are really positive forces in survival. But we also see another kind of strength, in overcoming human fears, in sharing deeply with others.

There was another woman—very articulate and very precise. If I put a book down on her table, she would pick it up and put it a few inches away, in a more precise corner. That rigid. Couldn't develop any close relationships in her life. But basically a very productive person and very caring, from a successful family.

One weekend, she had terrible hallucinations. She reached up and grabbed my hand. She had fever, and her eyes were bright. "Tell me something," she said, "why weren't they nice hallucinations? Why not of heaven and good things? Why were they so angry?"

It was the first time I'd ever had any real contact with her. She had been distant in our contacts—and now, suddenly, this opening. She continued to hold me. "This is the first time I've ever been afraid. The first time I'm aware of the fact that I don't want to die."

She was sharing, for a few moments, her terror of pain, her fear of what was coming. "I've asked my sister to come up," she said, ". . . for my death."

She was giving up the tight control of her life. I told her no matter what happened, we the staff would be with her. But then, this openness vanished. After she had articulated her fear, which she had never shown to anyone, and after she was relieved, she closed up again. "Thank you very much," she said—and that was it, with no further talk about it.

It was a moment of strength that came through. She was able to overcome her desperate fear and accept a human contact. Overcome her need to defend and protect herself and relate in a more intimate way. People can open up like that when they are being threatened in a way that they've never experienced before. What you see is something brought on by an unexpected situation—a moment of awareness, a moment of being able to accept and share, a moment of ultimate humanness.

You know, one of the things I've found here is that I'm less negative about behavior or ideas that differ from mine. In fact, I have no question anymore about the relationship between God and the individual. And I'm not necessarily speaking as a sister. I'm speaking as a person working here at Memorial. There's no question for me as to why God loves human beings, why there is a love relationship there. If you don't want to use the word "love," then let's call it a close relationship on both sides, which we often tend to ignore.

Human beings come into this hospital, and we see them suffering from pain, from emotional distress, from injustice, from fear. We see the impact of this on people. But when all this can be contained and set aside, you often find a whole, wonderful person underneath. You find a lot of gentle lovability, a tremendous amount of goodness. Then you are dealing with the basic person—free to be what they wish, free from their deepest pain, deepest fear—and you find a common thread of greatness. When they don't have to be something they are not, you are dealing with people who have a deep desire to be human and who find great value in just this.

There are inevitable personality differences and medical crises, so it doesn't happen all the time—perhaps once or twice with a patient, and not with every one. Nor does it last. Once the patient is removed from the threat of death, when they go into remission or get well, they gird themselves to return to everyday life struggles. The deepest feelings, the previous real inner self, gets protected again. Then they're back in life once more, with all the necessary defenses for the real world.

So at the moment near death, or when threatened by it, they experience a rebirth, a second innocence. Then, upon getting well, they lose it again. Do they ever tell you they regret having lost it?

I often hear from people. They don't remember or don't want to relive what we talked about. But if they forget what we talked about, they don't forget the feelings that came with it. It happens when I walk into the outpatient department, and they see me—and respond. With all this, the timing of such contact is important. But what we had shared once, what we experienced at the time they sensed they were dying, is usually gone. The interior that was exposed, the awareness they found, is now covered up again. They are left, I believe, with a memory of the feelings they experienced and a greater sense of security. The words, the acts, the openness are gone—for a while, at least.

Listen, I know I can come back. I can still achieve some success out there. The first time I had this, I fought to make a comeback. I can do it again. . . .

It is two days after her third cancer operation, this time for a second mastectomy. Talking on the phone to a sports reporter, she waves her hand as if to wipe away any thought of never again playing competitive golf. She is 34, with green Irish eyes, bobbed brown hair, and the trim figure of an athlete. We are alone in her room at Memorial, but her many friends and supporters are manifest in scattered letters, cards, telegrams, flowers—and a copy of Newsweek *with a Pete Axthelm column: "In a business where athletes make a living with healthy female bodies, Kathy—weakened and mutilated by cancer—has become an inspirational legend. Modern sports are full of people who bring out the worst elements of greed, selfishness, or chicanery in our would-be heroes. What she has done is bring out the best instincts in her friends."**

The phone continues to ring until she pulls a blue robe about her, saying, "Let's get out of here, or we'll never talk." We walk to the patient's lounge on the fifteenth floor—a comfortable, sunlit, spacious area. A young male patient is at a piano, playing Gershwin. Further along, a group of patients are taking a drawing class, others sit in lounge chairs, reading, talking.

Before sitting down, Kathy shows how it is after the loss of her second breast. She lifts the left arm slowly, barely reaching shoulder height before the pain shows in her eyes. Then she raises her right arm without effort and whips it down forcefully, as if hitting a golf ball. She smiles.

This one lacks the pectorals. *(Flexes right arm.)* They removed them in the first mastectomy because it had spread to the lymph nodes. But this time *(touches left chest)* they left them. So I don't think this operation will limit me or make me less qualified. It's more disfigurement, yes. But it doesn't affect the vital organs or muscles. So I'm sort of walking through it, like any other competitive challenge.

I've always been very competitive by nature. Not with people but with

---

* Friends cited: Amy Alcott: "We throw around the idea of willpower in sports, but it took Kathy to show us the real thing . . . the human spirit at its best." Beth Stone: "She's handled her problems in a way that makes you feel good to be near her." Catherine Duggan: "She's an example for anyone with sickness or other major problems. She can take the worst thing that might happen and show you how to make fun of it, or smile through it."

myself—trying to do things as well as I could do them. I probably studied math to serve my analytical nature. *(She has a masters in mathematics from the University of Wisconsin.)* I've always wanted to know the variables I have to work with. What's the framework I have to operate in? Tell me that, and I'll go ahead and try to solve the problem. I believe this constant awareness has tuned me into the kind of life I have.

She faced her first cancer in 1972 with removal of lymph nodes from the left leg. It struck again six years later—her first mastectomy—during a third year with the Ladies Professional Golf Association tour, "just when I was becoming competitive." Determined to make a comeback, she built up her strength and adjusted her game to re-join the 1980 LPGA tour. Without her right pectoral muscles, however, she lacked the driving power of her competitors. Short-hitting Kathy was usually hammering a fairway wood while her rivals, near the green, were reaching for seven irons. But with remarkable control, she overcame this by skillful approach shots—chipping, pitching, putting.

It was then, in the middle of her comeback and while taking a shower, that Kathy once again discovered the dreaded symptom—a swollen node in her left arm.

I knew I was in trouble. I probably had cancer again for the third time, now on my left side. If so, I might even lose my other breast. I also knew that this had to be examined and to delay it was dangerous. But if I quit the tour now, I'd lose everything I'd worked for.

So I decided to stay with the tour until it ended in Birmingham. Until then, I would continue taking my regular chemotherapy treatments for the first mastectomy. I would go on, playing the best I could, and maybe even raise the level of my game. I was in the running, but not in the top group where I felt I belonged.

I found myself in the range of those people who make the cut and miss money. What I mean is this. One hundred and twenty players start a tournament. After two days, the playing field is cut to seventy players. Of those, sixty get money. The last ten don't. That's where I was—beating fifty players with sixty others beating me. That wasn't too bad in terms of competition and ranking, but in terms of making money, which is the name of the game, I wasn't doing very well. All I needed was just a little more improvement, and I'd be drawing checks constantly.

Yet when the tour played at Raleigh, Kathy made the cut and missed the money again—for the fifth time. She felt "kind of downhearted," and wondered if she would ever be able to lift her game to the winning level. When

*the tour moved on to Orlando, Florida, she stopped off briefly at her parents'
home in Tequesta. "The golf pro, Bob Cook, at the Turtle Creek Club, is an
old friend. He took some movies of my swing, and we saw an error that I'd
had perhaps all my life, without realizing it. The club face on the takeaway
was in a closed instead of a square position, causing it to be off at the top of
the backswing. To get the club head applied properly to the ball on the swing
through, my body went out of position, with a loss of power."*

I went to Orlando, and I hit the ball much better than before—but not
straight, and I was in sand traps to the left and right of the green. Also, I
didn't do as well in my pitching and putting. And, I missed a close cup,
which normally I would never do. That aggravated me because I had
finally corrected a major error, only to lose whatever else I had going for
me.

I realized then that my mental side was defeating me. Birmingham was
next—the end of the tour—and I told myself, "Whatever happens this
week, don't let your mind defeat you. Get in there and evaluate every shot
for what it is and don't let a missed shot bother you." That's important
because if you think about any other moment, any other shot during the
day, it's only going to detract from your ability to perform at that moment. So I did not allow my mind to go forwards or backwards, or even to
absorb the full impact of the level of competition I suddenly found myself
in.

*On the first day, Kathy shot a sensational 69—3 under par—to lead the
tournament. It was the second-best competitive round of her pro career. It
meant she was to play the following day with the last group—the tournament leaders who are of greatest interest to the gallery. Now she was in the
tense, winning arena with television cameras on her and crowds watching
each shot.*

*Yet more intently than cameras or crowds, her teammates watched, hop-
ing for spunky Kathy to give her best on the long, damp course. They all
knew she was in the middle of a month-long cycle of chemotherapy treatments, and this was a critical week with the maximum of nausea and side
effects. "I knew I had only so much energy to channel into four hours each
day. The rest was pure adrenalin, and I rode on it the whole week."*

*The wave of excitement for Kathy extended to the locker room, where
dozens of players followed her on television, cheering each shot. This was the
Kathy they had grown to love and admire. They had cheered her in another
way after her first mastectomy with the "Linney Line"—a newsletter which
kept her informed of real and imaginary events on the circuit. Dozens of
players contributed, making it appear that Kathy was still there, playing in*

their midst. And now, she was out there, on the tough, wet Birmingham course, confirming their belief in her.

I tried not to think about being in the midst of where it was happening. It's not so much a blocking out as a positive thing of focusing on something, putting something in your mind so that, whatever is going to destroy you can't get in there. You keep your mind filled with the right things, so the wrong things can't work on you. I concentrated on the environment, the wind conditions and the weather, my own self, my own psyche, and tried to do only those things that would put me in the best possible state of mind to perform.

Looking back at it now, I think there's a certain amount of tuning-in to the inner self, almost standing outside yourself, watching what's going on, so that you're not affected by things that could ruin what you're trying to do.

I'm talking to myself the whole way around. Sometimes it's a friendly chat, sometimes it's very harsh. On a four-hour golf round, the mood changes. You can't maintain the same level of personality through the whole thing because you have different levels of adversity coming at you. You have to gear up for some of them, and you kind of just laugh at the others. Each golf ball is a new adventure. Each swing could create anything, and you've got to be ready for it. Some of them will give you tremendous joy, and some will give you tremendous anguish. You have to kind of buffer your emotional reaction to what's going on—or else you'll lose track of yourself.

So buffered and talking to herself, Kathy turned in a 72 the second day of the Birmingham event, with another 72 the following day, finishing fourth behind Barbara Barrow. But she was greeted as the real winner when she came into the clubhouse. Flushed and excited, she bought beers for the occasion, even though she was broke and had to cash a check to pay for it. The tour was over, and she had finished with the best women players in the United States.

It was a great high, but I could not have reached it without encouragement from my teammates. I responded to them, and together we kind of motivated each other. This was never discussed or anything. I was just out there trying. But I did notice that when I'd shoot a seventy-two, people would be quite happy for me. Everyone likes the underdog sort of thing. Then I'd have an eighty-one the next day, which means that I'd blown it, and they'd say, "That's too bad, Kathy, but don't give up!" That helped, and I think it kind of snowballed. It's not especially anything I did, or anything they did, but together we became something more than we are individually.

Beside their wanting to help, I think many of the girls realized there's not much difference between me and them. They could also be going through this. I'm sure a lot of them have breast lumps and things to worry about, and they think: "If it ever happens to me, there's a hope, there's a chance my career won't be ended." So there's a real effort to do for me what they would like to have done for them.

That makes me feel particularly fortunate because a lot of people go through a lifetime and never have something that serves as an emotional trigger, as this illness has, to get people to express their feelings. Those girls and my friends and my family have expressed how much they care about me, how much they're rooting for me. This has helped me to express myself in return, and, in experiencing this, you find a far greater joy in living.

It's helped me especially now, after they've taken off my other breast. *(Laughs.)* Maybe there's a parallel between playing golf and going through these cancer surgeries, when the present moment is all you can handle and all that really matters. If you thought about all the "whys" and "ifs," you would just torment yourself, you would lose the tournament and any enjoyment of the present moment.

The quality of life is made from that—a series of present moments, whether you like them or not. To have the highest quality that life can assume is to be happy the greatest number of possible moments. That doesn't exclude the future at all. In fact, it incorporates it, because if you see a lot of hope there, if you set your mind on the good that might happen, you enhance the present moment.

That's what I'm trying to do. I don't succeed all the time, of course. But if that's your goal, you can keep it in hand by saying, "Okay, I didn't handle it very well today, but I have another chance tomorrow, and I'll try a little harder."

POSTSCRIPT: Mary Katherine Linney died at home of cancer metastases March 15, 1982. She is retained in this book as a survivor because she was just that—turning back cancer three times in ten years. There is much more, however. In a very natural way, she combined all the qualities that make for survival and make for champions. As we have seen here, she was capable of fusing a beautifully spatial mind with a broken body to win on the playing fields of champions. At the same time, she won the hearts of millions who will never forget her. Of all the men and women in this book, she is one who will perhaps survive longest in a way that both explains the meaning of survival and does tribute to all the others.

You're laying on a table that you've never laid on before in your life. You're looking at a floor you've never stepped on in your life. You're thinking, "Wait a minute, what the hell's going on here?"

Then you remember that you have to do this to live. They tell you there are five million people out there, walking the streets, who've been where you are—on the table, staring at the floor, at the light in the ceiling, into the eye of the doctor, also wondering, "What the hell am I doing here? Yesterday I was playing golf, I was in bed with my wife, I was a million miles away."

You tell yourself, "They were all here, five million of them. They all had cancer and they survived—so can I." But it's not true. A lot of people say that and don't make it.

They simply die, and I think it's like those people from the concentration camps. You see them in the papers, at Holocaust reunions, looking fat and normal, except for something in the eyes. Then you see a photo of them, close to death in a striped uniform, with those same eyes, like openings into the soul. You ask yourself, "How did they do it? How did they make it when others died like flies? What did they have?"

That's what this is all about for me—more than just saving my leg or my life. It's about everything in people—legs, arms, hearts, hopes—that helps them survive and how, in the concentration camp of cancer, you have to hold onto something inside yourself if you want to stay alive.

He's 24, a dark, handsome youth with broad cheekbones, large jaw, full lips, and long black hair pulled back behind the ears—traces of Indian ancestry in his father's family from St. Croix. "He gave me my body and strength. My Irish mother made me smart in the street, she taught me how to survive."

He worked while going to school—beginning with a paper route at 12— and competed in a variety of high school sports. "I was into everything— wrestling, baseball, football, ice hockey." From a mail clerk for a major printing equipment firm—Mergenthaler Linotype—he became a specialist in computer graphics. "It's a new field. The computer draws what you design."

We're in an apartment built into the basement of his father's home at Bay Shore, Long Island, where Bob Challenor grew up. With us is his wife, Josephine, a stunning blue-eyed blond of 19. "We built this place, Josie and I. As newlyweds, we needed to save money, so I said to my dad, 'Gimme a hammer and a saw.' Everything is perfect, except the wall behind you is one-

half inch off." He laughs. "Josie was great. She's gone every step of the way with me—including the trip into cancer."

My first feeling that something was wrong came when I was running along the beach at Acapulco during a vacation. Sand weighs your feet down, but I knew I could run a lot faster, and afterward I felt a gnawing pain on the outside of my left calf. I thought I'd pulled a muscle and didn't think anything of it, until the next morning, when I put my foot on the cold tile floor and felt the pain again.

I think the second time was at Josie's house, going up the stairs to her bedroom to wake her up. There's about thirteen steps, and I got halfway up when suddenly there was nobody home—the leg couldn't bear my weight, and I just fell on the stairs. Plop. Straight down. The pain came back, and I suspected I'd done something to it in Acapulco, running along the sand—a ligament or something like that.

At that time, I had to do a lot of walking at work—down corridors, up and down stairs—and I started to feel tired in that one leg. Then, one day coming down the stairs at work, pouncing on the leg, I felt the pain again. Since it was getting no better, I stopped in the personnel office to tell them I was going to have it checked out.

That was on a Friday, and we played golf Saturday. By the time I got to the seventeenth hole, the pain was back—a lot more this time. I turned to my father and said, "This leg is killing me. I can hardly walk on it." It made me angry, and I said, "It's probably bone cancer or something like that" as if I somehow already knew it was inside me.

Monday I went to Arthur Quackenbush, our regular physician. He sat me up on the table and began to feel both legs at the same time. We were talking about golf, but when he got down to the lower area, his conversational tone changed. He said, "I want you to go and get an X ray of this leg." He pointed to the spot. "Right here, nowhere else."

It was in the middle of the fibula. At the time, I didn't know which bone was which. I didn't even know I had a bone back there. For me, there was just the shin bone and muscle. Later that day, I had the X rays done, and they said they'd send the results to my physician.

The next day, my mother had to go back to Quackenbush with my sister. So I called her from work and asked, "What did the X rays show?" My mother was afraid to tell me what the doctor had told her, so she said she didn't know anything.

After work, I went over to Josie's house and called again. This time I got my father, and he said, "Listen, they found something. They want you to see Dr. O'Connor, the orthopedist. It looks like a cyst of some sort, and they might have to remove it."

JOSIE: *(Interjects)* I remember I was sitting in the rocking chair when he hung up the phone. He was stunned, and he said, "Oh my God, I've got cancer." My heart just dropped, like going over a roller coaster.

BOB: The next day, I go with my father to Dr. O'Connor. He has the X rays, and he asks me to stand on my tippy toes against the wall, then lie flat on a table. He pries my left leg as far back as he could, squeezing it while looking at the X rays. "Does that hurt?" I said, "No, not really." Then he moved his fingers a little bit, and I'll never forget when he squeezed again. "That hurts, yes?" Fire came to my eyes, and I said, "Yeah, that hurts a lot." Then he said, "That's all, you can get dressed."

My father was in the room with me when he turned around and said, "Listen, I think Robert has to go to New York, to Memorial Hospital." We looked at him, both surprised, and my father said, "Is it that serious?" O'Connor said, "Maybe not, but I'd rather we check it out with their specialists. It's a growth of some sort. It could be a massive benign tumor or a calcium deficiency. . . ." He went on in medical terms. Then he said, "I'd like nothing more than for them to say, 'Who's that quack that sent you here?' But you have to go immediately. Maybe we can get you in this weekend."

Leaving there, my father tried to make it easy for me, saying, "I'm sure it's benign and nothing to worry about." I remember how angry I was. I smacked the front door going out, telling him, "What's this benign bullshit? Why the hell don't you face the facts? He knows it's bone cancer, and I know it." I kicked the door and ran out, and went to Josie's house.

JOSIE: He didn't say anything at first. He just sat there, but I knew what he was thinking. The leg. He might lose it. I think I said I'd love him no matter what happened, and he picked it right up, saying, "A one-legged lover, is that what you mean?" I didn't know what to say, but I think I realized that this was going to be the most difficult part—this kind of rejection.

BOB: *(Interrupts)* I don't remember that. It came later—not then, because I still didn't know that I was facing amputation.

JOSIE: *(Quickly)* Well, your mother and your family knew it. Maybe they had reasons for keeping it from you—but not from me. When they said nothing to me, I felt like I was being rejected by the family.

They had met at a neighborhood street carnival. Josie recalls: "I'd won this stuffed animal, and he stole it from me. I was walking with my girlfriend, and I asked this guy I knew—Dave—for a match. While I was getting the match, Bob took my stuffed animal and started running toward his car. I screamed, 'Gimme back my animal!'" Bob interjects: "She was foxy. She was pretty." Josie: "I was only 15, and I wanted my little animal. It was a blue banana with eyes on it." Bob: "I got in my car, and she came in after me, just as I figured. So I slammed the door and drove off." Josie: "I'm hysterical, wondering who is this crazy guy?" Bob: "She's yelling, 'If you don't stop, I'm going to start screaming rape!' So I slammed on the brakes and let her out. I was only trying to have some fun." Josie: "Fun? Jesus! (Laughs.) I found out he was a cook down the block at a pancake house, so we'd stop there on the way home from school. I had a penny bank, and I'd roll the pennies into fifty-cent wrappers to get two quarters from the pharmacy across the street. Then with my girlfriend we'd get a table and order French fries and a small Coke. He used to look from the kitchen and watch us. I was really shy, and I'd say, 'I don't want to eat while he's watching me.' After that, he started coming over to my house, and one night I told my father I was going out to this movie, and I didn't get home until six a.m. the next morning. When he pulled up, my father was in his car waiting for us. He yanked me out of Bob's car and yelled, 'Stay away from my daughter or I'll kill you!' He's a real Italian, my father." Bob: "He said he'd shoot me with a shotgun, and I knew he meant it. But he had a second job, as a security guard, so I'd wait around the corner at night, and when I saw him pull out around midnight, I'd go to Josie during the late hours. I had to be at work early, so I was getting only two or three hours sleep. (Laughs.) Lemme tell you, you gotta be crazy or really in love to keep that up for very long." Josie (laughing): "I wrote my father a letter, saying if he didn't let me see Bob, I was going to run away with him. I remember sitting one day in my bathroom, blow-drying my hair, and my father comes in and says, 'I hate to tell you this, but I don't want you to think you're going to marry this guy.' I just laughed and said, 'But I am.' I've never loved anyone else. I was a virgin when I went to him, and I've never wanted another man."

BOB: I learned I faced amputation after I got into Memorial. Dr. Lane told me.* He was my surgeon, and the first time I see him is in the operating room when they are about to open up my leg for the first biopsy, to see just what I have.

When you're on the table like that, faces come rolling up and over you like waves, and all of a sudden he's over me, saying, "Hello, Robert, please forgive me for not coming to see you sooner. After this, we'll have more time. This is rushed now for your sake—to do the best for you." He had his mask on and glasses, but I could see he was very young, and I thought, "Jesus, they've sent a kid to cut me up."

---

* Joseph M. Lane, M.D., attending surgeon, chief, Orthopedic Service, Department of Surgery, Memorial Hospital.

After that, they had to do another biopsy and a couple of days later I'm bouncing around the place on crutches, waiting for the results. I was in the solarium, looking at TV and having a cigarette, when suddenly the white jacket was standing on my left. I look up, and it's Dr. Lane. "C'mon," he says, "Come with me." Saying good-bye to all my friends, I jump onto the crutches and start walking down the hall. We were near the nurses' station when he said, "We got the results back from your biopsy." I said, "Yeah? Was it bad or what?" He shook his head, and I said, "How bad?" He said, "Well, it's pretty bad." I said, "What are you going to do?"

I'm walking on crutches, talking to him like this, and each time he says "bad" I lose more strength in my arms until I feel like I'm going to fall off the crutches and say, "All right, you win. Let me go home now." Then he said, "I don't want to talk in the hall, let's go in the room."

He walked ahead of me and was waiting in the room when I got there, saying, "Sit down." I got on the bed, and the nurse began pulling the curtains like she knew this was going to be bad. I felt like I was going to pass out with tinglings in my head. He said, "Lay back, relax." I could feel my body starting to shake, and he said, "It's in the bone, but it's on a small part of your bone. With your permission, I'd like to try a resection— that is, taking only a piece of the bone out, trying to get it all without amputating." I thought, "Jesus help us, this man is going to save my leg."

Then he said, "There's a problem, however. The tumor appears to en-compass two main arteries to your leg. We can cut one, but not both. So you're going to have to have an arteriogram, for your blood flow, to deter-mine if this is possible or not. So keep your fingers crossed, kid."

He called me "kid" because I was only 17 when I came into the hospi-tal, and they'd put me in the pediatric unit under Dr. Rosen.†

JOSIE: But you turned 18 right after that.

BOB: Yeah, that's right—18. I was at the age where you're old enough to vote, old enough to drink, old enough to enter the army, or do just about anything. But you also still want to be young enough to run home and cry on somebody else's shoulder. I wondered, "Which course do I take? Do I fall down and crumble up like a leaf? Or do I stand up and try to be a man in the family?" I chose to be a man—or try to be one. I think it was a good decision because it gave me the strength for the soap opera that was about to begin on whether they were going to let me keep my leg or take it off.

---

† Gerald Rosen, M.D., attending pediatrician, associate chairman, Solid Tumors, Depart-ment of Pediatrics, and attending physician, Solid Tumor Service, Department of Medi-cine, Memorial Hospital.

"It began with eight weeks of chemotherapy to shrink the tumor. Dr. Rosen explained the arteriogram showed the tumor entangled with my two main leg arteries—just like Dr. Lane suspected. He said, 'Robert, we think we can free one artery with chemo treatments. As long as one is free, there will be enough blood for your leg to survive.' By this time, I'd heard they had not had much luck with these resections to save legs, but Rosen said, 'I think it'll work with you.' I asked him why, and he said, 'Because you have a great spirit, and you're a fighter—you bounce back.' Little words like that, they mean so much. They stay in your head, and you keep grabbing hold of them.

"So they shove me into eight weeks of chemo treatments, eight weeks of shooting me with poisons that take you to death's door, then let you go. Methotrexate and cytotoxan. I'd take cytotoxan over anything. It's the worst, but it's the easiest and fastest. It's like, 'How're you going to die?' So you say, 'Well . . . (Snaps fingers.) Shoot me in the brain, don't chop me to death.'

"It knocks out the cancer, but it also knocks you to pieces. It tears up the house you live in. You lose all your hair, you lose everything. Armpits, pubic, eyebrows—everything you can think of. Even the legs. You have to constantly fight it, especially little things you least expect. You look at your cock, and there's no hair. Things like that just blow people's minds. They flip out. They say, 'Look at me, I'm a little boy again.'

"You get tolerance. You get madder, but you build up tolerance. You say, 'This isn't going to get me. You're going to whip me one more time? C'mon, whip me again.' That's the kind of attitude you must have. It's like standing against a pole and letting them lash you. They can lash you until you drop, and you have to be pulled up again, until they're done beating you, and they take the ropes off and let you walk out the door."

It was an unreal place, especially for me under Dr. Rosen's care in pediatrics, since I was just under the age limit for adult chemotherapy. So sometimes I was lying next to kids 2 and 3 years old—me, old enough to have one of them! *(Laughs.)*

I can understand how soldiers get very cold in war and don't like to make friends because that's exactly what happened to me. I got friendly with a lot of people, kids of all ages, but in the long run I turned my back on seeing them get violently ill from the drugs, because everyone was sick that way. Everyone was ill, and you more or less just took care of yourself.

If anybody's going to get an award for the year, it should be the mothers and fathers with their children up on the chemotherapy wards. Because some kids don't have mothers or fathers, or their parents are at work, and they're left alone in those wards. They get violently ill, I mean they're off the side of the bed and onto the floor. The mothers with their own kids, they've got the burden of their own babies, it's so sad. Yet they care so much, they walk across the floor and pick up this child who isn't theirs and put him back in bed and give him a box of napkins and a barf tray— that's chemo slang for vomit tray. They won't call the nurse and say, 'Pick up the kid,' they'll pick up the kid first.

They could be sitting there reading a newspaper, and their kid is asleep, but another kid will get sick, and they'll get up. I said to myself, "It's the same women all the time who are up here, and they keep giving themselves to these others. Jesus, isn't it enough pressure that their own kid is laying in bed with leukemia?"

Their faces, week after week, I see them, I'm familiar with them, I say hello. I'm old enough to carry on a conversation with the mother, yet the kid can't even talk. So I talk to the mother, the mother talks back to me. It's the same woman that will go across the floor and pick up another kid. It's bad enough that your house is collapsing, yet you're across the street nailing up some other guy's house. If you spend a week in that ward, I guarantee you won't walk out the same person.

"When you're in a situation like I was, as total as I was, when you're put in one place—in the shoes, or in the bed, or in the pajamas as I was—when it's like that, it's all or nothing. This is the World Series. This is the big thing. You reach out and take all the help you can get.

"I began looking for other answers, in different directions. I didn't believe somebody could knock you on the head—cut you up or give you poison—so you fall down and feel better in the morning. There had to be something else with it, and I started reading Dr. Simonton's Getting Well Again.‡ *You know the book? You're supposed to visualize your cancer cells—to see them in your mind—then attack them and imagine them being destroyed. Many people—even terminal cases, they say—have been saved by this method.*

"I had to find an entrance to get at my cancer, so I figured, 'I'll go through the nostril.' I pictured it like a bullet, a spaceship, and I'm inside it. The hardest part is getting started—the entry. When people first try, they force themselves too much. You have to relax and close your eyes and make believe you're looking at television. It's the easiest way to do it. (Closes eyes, leans back.)

"I'm now inside the capsule. I can see around me, and at the same time,

‡ *Getting Well Again,* O. Carl Simonton, M.D., Stephanie Matthews-Simonton, James L. Creighton (New York: Bantam Books, 1980).

I can talk to people who are on the ship with me—like you are, at this moment. We're now going down through the throat, we can see ourselves in it, we can see ourselves going through the intestines, down all the way to the groin area. Now we're going through an artery, down into my leg and then we come out of the artery and—finally!—we can see the inside of the leg. Did you ever see a side of beef lying somewhere? The bone and the redness of the meat? That's what we see at first, the healthy leg and its bone with veins straggling down.

"Then we see the cancer and say, 'There it is! Right there!'—a gray-blue mass, with tiny gray and blue particles on the bone because we can see the freshly cut place where Dr. Lane made the biopsy. So then we get ourselves in position with the laser beam, and I cry, 'Fire! . . . FIRE!' We shoot into the mass with the laser, and you can see it deteriorating, chewing and charring down to nothing, shriveling up from my powerful forces—and it works! The cancer has disappeared! (Deep sigh, opens eyes, smiling.)

"I did that constantly, and I do it now, any time I lay down and feel a need for it, to make sure the leg stays clean. It's a form of meditation that you can teach yourself. You can use it for anything. Josie has bad migraines and gets rid of them that way—visualizing herself inside her head."

Then came the big disaster—the day my chemotherapy was finished. Dr. Lane wants to see me in his clinic to discuss the operation.

I went with my parents, and when he had us inside a little room, he says, "Well, I've been studying the case, and I'm sorry to say that I now think we must amputate."

We didn't believe it. My father is especially shocked. His father died of cancer, this is really laying on him now, and he lashes out at Dr. Lane: "Wait a minute. We've been telling everybody in the family and all across the U.S., that this kid's going to have an operation so he can survive, and still walk. Now you're cutting our hopes just like his leg."

Dr. Lane is trying to be nice about it. He says, "I know how you must feel, but I must be frank. The X rays show the tumor has shrunk, but not enough. I don't think we can do what we wanted to do." We stand there stunned. We can't believe what we're hearing. Then he says, "I want Robert to take a couple more weeks of chemotherapy. Then we will perform the operation."*

---

* The tumor had spread to both major leg arteries—the anterior and posterior tibial—as well as both bones of the leg—the fibula and tibia. It had also invaded the muscle area with possible metastasis. At this point, Dr. Lane reluctantly saw no other prognosis than amputation. He ordered two additional weeks of chemotherapy, however, hoping this might critically alter "a situation that was touch and go from the beginning."

So from an optimistic ride to the hospital and a friendly doctor, we now ride home from a doctor we see as a foe. Those forty-five-minute rides, in and out, were terrible. How many times can you stare at the white lines of the road, the trees, and abandoned cars that have been stripped? It wanders through your mind. That's when it started to really affect me—that day. An awful lot of tension had been building up for a kid my age. I sat in the back of the car with this thing choking me, and I was cut off from my parents, the world, everything.

My father tried to say something to help, but I shut him up. My mother reached out to touch me, and I pulled away from her. Nobody could help me now. This was it—D-Day, the end of everything. The leg was going and everything else with it: football, baseball, ice hockey, running, golf—even Josie.

Josie would say it didn't matter, but what the hell could she know about it? I wouldn't even be able to mow the lawn, let alone handle a woman in bed. I thought of Jane Fonda mounting Jon Voight in *Coming Home* and wanted to vomit. I saw us at the beach, me with a stump, and Josie running down to the water with other guys looking at her. How the hell would I get to the water? On crutches some kids would steal? Or I'd just lay there, and each time Josie looked at some guy with two legs, I'd go crazy wondering what she was thinking. I wanted to jump out of the car.

When we got home, Josie came over. I knew my mother had called her because I could tell from her face that she knew about it before I could tell her, and that made me angry. She kissed me without saying anything, and that made it worse. I felt I was getting pity, and I didn't want it—not from her, especially.

JOSIE: *(Interjects)* It was love, not pity. That's what upset me, how you just assumed I would stop loving you. I'd see some guy on the beach with two legs and run off with him.

BOB: I didn't know what was going to happen to me. So how could you? You were only a kid.

JOSIE: A kid? *(Smiles.)* That all depends. I was 17, yes, but I was working in a convent for senile nuns. I was on a medical floor with geriatric cancer patients. I used to see amputations come and go. I had the best relationship with these people because, without the leg or whatever, they weren't—I don't know how to explain it—they were just themselves. Not having the other leg to walk on didn't mean they thought less highly of themselves. People take their bodies for granted. You're supposed to have two feet. So when Bob was saying, "What am I going to do without them?" I was saying, "You can do a lot."

Not that he shouldn't be angry. I expected that, and I told myself, "You have to take all his anger, anything he gives you, because underneath he doesn't mean it. He's testing you, he wants to feel your steadiness, even when he tells you to leave for another man.

BOB: *(Interrupting)* I never told you to leave for another man—never. I gave you your freedom, if you wanted to go.

JOSIE: *(Interrupts)* Exactly! And that made me really mad. I didn't need your approval, believe me. If I'd wanted to leave, I would have left whether you did or did not approve.

BOB: *(Defensively)* I was trying to make it easy for you.

JOSIE: Easy? I'd loved you for two years, you were the only man I'd ever known. *(Smiles brightly.)* I *liked* it with you, and I thought, "If they take his leg, it won't change anything, it won't stop us from being happy together." So when you said to me, "Go out with other guys if you want," that really hurt. I asked you, "How can you say that?" You said, "How will you ever be happy with a one-legged man? Can you see yourself in bed with a stump?" That hurt, too, but I knew you didn't mean it.

BOB: *(Nods)* That's true, and it's a terrible situation. There's something that's close to you, but you're mixed up, you don't want it to come any closer. So you just kick it away and hope it goes far away. But even if it does, you want to feel it's very, very close to you. *(Pauses, looks at floor.)* This is horrible to say, but maybe I was jealous of you, of everybody who had two good legs, and didn't realize how much they could mean. I was thinking, "They should know what it's like. They should be in bed with me."

JOSIE: *(Brightly)* I was—even in the hospital. Remember?

BOB: *(Smiles uneasily)* All right, but that's not what I meant. My friends were calling up, saying I was crazy, "Why are you treating Josie that way?" I just didn't know what I was doing. My mother said, "Robert, you treated that girl Josie so badly, it's a miracle she stuck by you. Most girls would've run off. But she stuck it out, side by side. I hope you marry her someday." *(Pauses.)* That was only a few weeks before she died—like she knew it was coming . . . like God had heard her. *(Breaks off.)*

JOSIE: This happened when we first heard Bob had cancer, and we didn't know if he was going to live or die. We were down in the basement —the two of us and his parents.

BOB: *(Interrupts)* My mother was very upset and got carried away. She slapped her hand on the table, like she was making a covenant with God, and said, "Listen! This is my son, he's too young to go. Take me instead!" I got chills down my back, and my father said, "Maybe God didn't hear her, down here in the cellar." *(Pauses.)* My father should've known better.

God may be blind sometimes—who knows?—but He's never deaf. He heard her all right. He proved it later on.

"It was going to be a traumatic change in my life. I wasn't sure if I was ready to accept it, but I'd be damned and dipped in shit if I would let them do it, just like that, without putting up a fight.

"I did everything I could to beat it, especially during those last two weeks of chemotherapy before I was due in for my amputation. Three times a day, I got into my imaginary rocket ship and went down through my body to my leg, to blast away at that blue-gray mass, destroying it with my laser beam.

"Then a friend of mine sent me to this pastor out at Port Jefferson— Pastor Knapp, a Baptist not a Catholic. I went to his Sunday service and got embarrassed when he called me up on the stage before five hundred people. I was on crutches, and I'd lost my hair from chemo. Josie was there, watching me.

"The pastor said, 'This young man needs help. He has a growth in his leg, and they want to cut it off. But now we are going to pray that it never happens and that he be healed.'

"He called up one of his people from the audience, a follower, who took my hand while the pastor held my other hand. Then he asked everyone to bow their heads while this gentleman prayed. He went on for about five minutes, and our clenched hands became tighter and tighter until I noticed the pigment of the skin was white from being crushed against the knuckles. I didn't mind the pain. I felt great strength coming into me, and when it was over, I embraced the gentleman who prayed and also the pastor.

"They sang a hymn, and I was told a woman prayed that my hair would grow back. It did later, but she didn't ask for the right color. I'd been a redhead, and it came back a dark auburn! (Laughs.)

"The Sunday before my operation, the whole congregation prayed for me. They sent me flowers and gave me a modern day version of the New Testament. I'd gone to Catholic school, but didn't realize how little I knew about the Bible. I started reading this book and couldn't let it go. This frightened me. I said, 'This is like throwing a lit match into a can of gasoline. I'm so much in this, it can take me with it.' I knew God gave me this problem. Maybe it was only a warning, maybe He was going to call me in. No matter, I'm now turning face-to-face with him, saying, 'I'm listening to you, I'm talking to you, and I'm going to ask questions all the way to the end—no matter what it is.' "

When I go back into the hospital for the operation, my fate is on the line, and I'm asking a lot more questions there, too.

The first one is for Dr. Lane, asking if I can have another arteriogram. I said, "I think there's been a change in my tumor. It's not only the two weeks of chemotherapy. There have been other forces at work." He asked me, "What forces?" I said, "Lots of things. I don't think you need to amputate anymore." He laughed and said, "That's the spirit, Robert. I hope you're right." Then he agreed to the arteriogram, saying he'd planned it anyway, to determine just where we were at this point, before going into the leg.

The night before my operation, two of Dr. Lane's assistants come in with consent forms for me to sign—including one for the amputation. I say, "Hey, what about the arteriogram? What'd it show?" They tell me that Lane is coming, and I tell them, "Okay, I'll sign the papers when I see him." They are not too happy and leave.

Half an hour later, the door kicks open, and Dr. Lane comes in, his white jacket flying, and behind him are six other Dr. Lanes. He's moving so fast, he just spins around, saying, "Okay, it's good news. We're going to try and save your leg." I thought, "Thank God, we're back on that old plateau of hope. We fell off—but we're back up there again."

Lane throws the consent papers onto the bed table and says, "This is the deal. We're going to try for the resection. But if we can't do it, we'll proceed immediately to amputate." That didn't sound too good, and I waited for him to explain. "The arteriogram and the last X rays show the original tumor has shrunk from the size of a lemon to that of a peach nut. It's a slightly better margin, and it may be crucial." He's leaning on the windowsill and talking for my benefit, but the other doctors are listening as if it's a classroom. "We don't know how much we'll have to cut until we get in there. As we go along, we'll send specimens up to the pathology lab for a reading on whether we are clear or not of the disease. We'll probably have to sacrifice one of your two major leg arteries. If we find we have to cut the second one, we will stop—and amputate."

He pauses long enough to make sure I've understood. I nod, and he nods back—like a handshake. Then he says, "If we can keep going until the pathology lab tells us the outer perimeters are clean, then we'll try for a bone resection—okay?" I say, "Okay"—and sign the consent forms.

As he's leaving, he says the same old thing to me: "Keep your fingers crossed, kid." That meant we were back on the plateau, but only on the edge, and we could fall off at any moment. I thought, "Fuck it, we're not falling anywhere." So I said to him, "It's a piece of cake." He turned around and asked me, "How do you know?"

There was no way to tell him about my spaceship and the laser beam. No way to tell him about Pastor Knapp and all his people praying for my leg, and that lady going for my hair. No way to explain how I was now tangled up with the word of God. No way to explain how I had to continue in sports and continue to love Josie as I was loving her now.

I heard him ask it again, "How do you know?"—and I just shook my head.

Before I could tell my mother the good news, she comes into the hospital and bumps into the Oriental doctor who is training there under Dr. Lane. At this point, Mom is very nervous. She has gone with me all the way, like my father has. She knows I've been saying this will not happen. They will not amputate—and she believes me. But still, the doctors haven't said so, and we're now approaching zero hour.

So she asks this doctor about me. He doesn't know about Dr. Lane's last-minute decision, and he can't speak English very good. So he points to his leg, extends one arm, and with the other indicates he's sawing it off. This goes against everything we've been saying and hoping—and she gets violently upset. She runs out of the hospital. I'm in my room and have no idea of what's going on.

JOSIE: I was with her, and she was hysterical. She ran out into the middle of the street. You know New York, how people do crazy things. So cars are just going around her while she's standing there, screaming, "No, it can't happen! No, no, no! My son, oh my God! Please take me instead!" We had to finally drag her off to the car.

BOB: This time it wasn't said in a cellar. It was out on the street, and my father knew—we all knew—that this time God heard her. This one fixed it up. *(Deep breath).* She died five months later, after a hysterectomy at Good Samaritan Hospital. Can you believe it? She was only 43 and still very beautiful. She had blond hair and green eyes, and when she was young, she looked like Susan Hayward. *(Another pause.)* It just doesn't add up. Who dies in recovery after an operation like that? *(Shakes head.)* There's no other answer. God held her to her word. He called in the contract she'd made. I was to live, I was to walk again, I was to be free of cancer—and she was to take my place. . . . *(Breaks off.)*

JOSIE: The same day she died, everything fell off the wall downstairs. Pictures and glass were being smashed, everything was breaking. When they went to look at it, there was the odor of fresh flowers.

BOB: The next day, my sister Allison walks in the front door, and from the dining room window, she sees our mother in the swimming pool. She is sitting on the float, kicking her feet very slowly. Allison goes up to the window, looks out very carefully, and there's Mom wearing a bathing suit.

She runs out the side door to the pool, but there is nobody there, and the water is perfectly still. My sister Debbie comes, and they begin looking for that bathing suit—a pink one with a flower on it. They go through all of Mom's things, they tear the place apart, but they can't find it. Three days later, it shows up on the shower curtain—wet. No one put it there.

JOSIE: And your Aunt Lillian . . .

BOB: Yes, she's riding on the Long Island Railroad, and all of a sudden, she looks out the window and sees my mother's face outside the train, trying to tell her something. *(Pauses.)* I believe I'll know what it is some-day. I believe my mother will be the first person to greet me when I go through the long, dark tunnel.

"Shortly after Dr. Lane leaves with my consent to amputate if necessary, a young man comes in to shave my leg. Then another one arrives with a pencil marker and makes a series of X's on my knee and leg, to indicate the operating area.

"After that, a young priest turns up, asking, 'How do you feel about your operation?' I didn't want to talk about it or even think about it, and I wanted him to leave. But the poor guy was only trying to be a good priest, to get as near to me as possible. So I began talking about the Yankee-Met game: 'What do you think about Steve Henderson's homer?' He seemed very nervous, and I said, 'Relax, sit down—take it easy.' Finally he gave me his blessing and pulled back the curtain to tell my folks, 'He's fine, he'll do all right.' It was his way of getting out of there. But you know, as he left, I felt sorry for him. How many dying people, how many impossible guys like me did he have to tangle with each day? I started to feel sorry for both of us—but stopped. I wasn't about to let myself go—not yet.

"Josie began to say good night, kissing me and holding on, and I gave her the old routine Bacall gave Bogart: 'If you need me, whistle. You know how to whistle, baby?' Josie says, 'Oh come on, stop it.' I say, 'Stop what? I'll see you in the morning. No problems.' She says, 'Are you sure?' I say, 'Sure, babe, it's a piece of cake.' I wasn't about to let go with her, either—not with any of them."

The next morning, they wheel me down to what I call the MASH unit. It's the waiting area outside the operating rooms. You're put in there with all the other bodies, like a green parking lot. I'm wheeled into my little spot, and suddenly we're all getting acquainted. A third person down the line says, "I'm in for a prostate, how about you?" And you say, "I have a leg." Some other guy says he's a colon or a lung—or whatever. We're getting real intimate, and you say to the body next to you, "Sorry, ma'am, would you mind lowering your knee a little so I can see my friend, the prostate?" This is drawing everybody closer until suddenly one of us is pulled away, and we say, "Let's give him a hand! Give 'em hell!"

People are being dragged away, left and right, and then they're pulling

me into the OR. We roll in there with all the bright lights, and there's Dr.
Lane again. I've been there twice before—for two biopsies—and it's beginning to feel like a soap opera. I lift up my hand, fingers crossed, and say,
"How long do I have to keep them this way? I'm getting a cramp." He
laughs and says, "You can let go now, Robert." Then he says, "Okay, put
him under."

The anesthetist bends over me and says, "Do you want to count from
ninety-nine up or down? Take your choice." I say, "I'll go up," and I
begin: *Ninety-nine, one-hundred, one-hundred and one . . .* Have you
ever been put under? It's an amazing feeling. The room starts to get condensed, and you feel your head is being proportionately condensed, until
the blackness comes over you—but not all of a sudden. It trickles through.
You seem to lose your senses, but you really don't. You can no longer go
on thinking about one thing, or counting numbers, but you sense what's
going on around you.

Next thing, I wake up in the recovery room, and it's very peculiar. My
hands and feet are all blurry, but I can read the clock clear across the
room—three o'clock. I don't know if that means morning or afternoon,
and I really don't care, because I'm still floating in and out of time.

Suddenly, I think, "The leg . . . the leg!" I try to move it and can't feel
a thing. I feel the right one, but not the left. It's like there's a sudden
crashing all around me, inside me, and I'm thinking, "No, it's not possible.
No, dear God, no, no. Jesus, no, they didn't take it. The bastards, they had
no right."

I try and look down and gradually see a mound where my leg should be
—something rising up under the sheet and a rocket fires through my
brain: "Holy shit—a STUMP!!"

I see a nurse and try to yell at her, but nothing comes out except a
quack like a duck. I start waving like a lunatic, and finally she sees me and
comes over. Now I'm in full panic. I'm afraid to ask her if they've cut off
my leg. I'm trying to hold onto the idea of it still being there. I try to talk,
but I'm just quacking away, and she puts her head close to me. Finally I
manage to ask her, "Is there a pulse in my foot?"

She nods that she understands, and I see her going down along my leg
to the foot, then bending over, but I still can't feel anything—nothing. My
heart is going, *Boom! Boom! Boom!* Then she comes back up toward me
and, leaning over, says, "Your foot pulse is plupping like a chicken." I
heard that word—*plupping*—and I asked her, "Are you sure?" She said,
"Yes, you've got a good strong pulse down there."

I knew then that the operation was successful, and I thought, "Hey! Here we go!"†

After that, Dr. Lane came around, making a thumbs-up salute, like we'd won the Olympic Games. He said, "You're a lucky boy, Robert. We were able to save it—just barely. Now you owe me one." I asked him, "Like what?" He said, "Like becoming a golf champion. Can you do it?" I said, "Sure, it's already in the works."

Then he said, "But we haven't finished yet. We still have to do more chemotherapy to clean up any small cells that might be left behind." I could have killed him. "You must be kidding," I said. "How can I ever be a golf champion with you as my coach?"

"Today, bone resection patients get less chemo than I did four years ago. Mine was one of the first ones, and Dr. Lane was doubly careful. I hated going back on the chemo, but I can't complain now. The leg is doing great." Seated on the living room sofa, he pulls up his left jeans leg, then his right. The left calf is one half the size of the well-developed right calf. "You can see there's still a difference in size and always will be. But I can still run the fifty yard dash in less than five seconds. I play competitive golf in the high seventies. I bowl, play tennis, and dance—anything I want. The leg does everything except wag. They had to cut a nerve, and there's no side action." With both legs extended, he moves the feet of both legs up and down. The right foot then wags sideways, while the left remains inert. "Lane says he can fix that, too. Hook up a piece of the working muscle from the side and tie it to the front. It's an old polio operation."

When you're on chemo, month after month—losing your hair, throwing up in the car, waking up at night to take a pill—you start counting the days to the end. Then it becomes like a graduating class.

You start off with maybe fifty people lying in beds around you. They're from Philadelphia, Michigan, Wyoming, California—everywhere. After a while, they aren't patients anymore. They aren't family, either. They're like students, classmates, going for that last chemo treatment, which is

---

† Skillfully preserving as many nerves and blood vessels as possible, Dr. Lane excised a central portion of the calf muscle, ligated one anterior tibial artery, resected most of the fibula and a small part of the proximal (upper) tibia—leaving sufficient residual tibia for it to reconstitute itself over a three-month period while the patient was supported by a leg brace. To protect against possible microscopic metastasis, further chemotherapy was prescribed. The four-hour intervention that preserved the limb was an advanced surgical procedure at the time—May 1979. The leg would normally have been amputated above the knee, and this form of surgical treatment is the usual mode of therapy even today.

graduation day. Then you brave it up, like "This is my last treatment, man. I'm going to take this one standing up."

On my last day of chemo, my sister Debbie came to take me home. I jumped in the car and said, "Let's go, kiddo! Let's barrel out of here before they change their minds!" She pulled away from Memorial blowing her horn. We were laughing like crazy. She blew it all the way up the East River and over the Triborough Bridge. Then she pulled over and I got out to say good-bye to what I was leaving—forever, I hoped.

I looked across the river toward Memorial and thought, "I came to that place two years ago. They saved my leg, but I lost two years of my life there." You don't blame the hospital. You don't blame God or the doctors —or yourself. But that's a lot of time when you're 18 or 19, when your friends are going to school, going away for weekends, and you're sick at home or in a hospital bed. Losing two years at that age is like taking a ruler and cutting out the fifth and sixth inches.

You can become very bitter about it. Or you can become very radical, and race as fast as you can to make up for lost time. But neither way works. The only way is to accept it. You grab the two closest poles, ask which way is forward, dig them into the ground—and shove off.

Then you discover something else. You've lost a lot, yes. You're not aware of what went on in Iran with the hostages, or even what's happened in your own neighborhood. But you've returned with something that's precious, that most of the others don't have. You're aware that life is a lot more important than you ever realized, that you must learn to deal with it in your own way, on your own terms. So you care for it, and you enjoy it a lot more. You know . . . *(laughs)* it's like you've found the secret to eternal youth.

I believe all cancer survivors should get the Congressional Medal of Honor—or something like that. But I also believe that we the victors should help others coming after us. We should turn about and take three steps backward and pick up at least two people on their way out of the cancer concentration camp. Those two should take more steps backward and pick up two others, so that it becomes an ever-extending chain of people helping each other. In that way, no one will be alone.

It's not a dream. It's a natural instinct, like those women in the chemo ward picking up the kids of other women. That's how it can be—like one total human body, with thousands or millions of hearts and legs and arms, but only one collective soul or spirit or karma or whatever, saying, "No they shall not have me, I will overcome, I will live again—more than ever before."

EPILOGUE

There can be no ending to this book, any more than one can slice off a segment of a river. Cancer will continue to run its course through human life until it is stopped at its source by blocking the first grouping of runaway cells which refuse to obey the biological laws of the body's republic —growing and multiplying until they destroy the life which nourishes them.

The people in this book are from the great river of those so afflicted. In the United States, it sweeps up one human being every seventy seconds— members of our families, a neighbor next door, and distant relatives everywhere. Many of these victims recover and their stories are inevitably similar to those of the men, women, and children who have been selected here, out of a total of 100 cases, to tell of their victories over the most prevalent forms of human cancer.

That was the first major problem in structuring this book: to obtain from a comprehensive cancer center a varied yet representative number of cases that had been successfully treated by the most advanced techniques available at the time.

A second and far more difficult task was to get these survivors to relive their ordeal, step by step, as they had experienced it anywhere from three to thirty years ago. In a new life free of the disease, the mind tends to block out past doubts, fears, panic, the loss of vision—essentials to the intimate drama of survival. Forgotten moments of despair, buried levels of hate and terror, the unexpected moments of prayer, of laughter, of hope, of renewed strength—all of these had to be recalled and relived.

As a result, these stories were not obtained by the usual sort of interview. Instead, they were assembled from a studied, methodical search into the past. In transcribing a tape, the inflection of a voice, an unexplained pause, a sudden turning away from the mainstream of events would often indicate that something had been forgotten or purposefully left unsaid.

Sometimes it was a key emotion or event which would release a sudden flood of memory. Inevitably, this required returning for a second—or third or fourth—encounter. In this way, some transcripts exceeded 300 pages—extensive life stories which had to be edited down to fit within the book.

Inevitably, some splendid episodes had to be dropped, as did many inspiring stories among the many patients. They included Alfred Ciciulla, a man of extraordinary courage and love; Judith Morrison, a magnificent woman and mother; and Harold Noll, who possesses the bravery and humor of a folk hero.

It is painful to merely mention the names of these remarkable people without being able to relate their stories or those of others. It is also difficult to explain this emotion, how heavy it seems to be at this moment of parting. For over the past five years, there has developed an intense feeling of close identity with all of these people. I became aware of it, of how it was seizing me, in a very simple and unexpected manner.

It occurred at a desperate moment during the first year when I was going each day to Memorial Hospital—to the operating rooms, the radiation and chemotherapy units, and to the private hospital rooms—trying to learn the run of the hospital, and to come as close as possible to the cancer patient.

It was necessary to do this—to understand the process of the disease from its inception, through clinical trials, and into each form of treatment —in order to conduct in-depth interviews with the long-term survivors. To follow them into the past, to live through each phase of the disease, the interviewer had to understand not only its clinical course, but also its effect upon the mind and spirit—or, as Sabina Cunningham describes it, cancer's assault upon the body's biological innocence.

I had free run of the hospital. After the MSKCC board had approved my book project—without support or restrictions—I was given an identity badge with the theoretical right to go anywhere. In practice, however, I could go nowhere—that is, I could not proceed in any depth until I had obtained the personal confidence of each single surgeon, doctor, or staff member. In this sense, the hospital is built like a submarine. If you manage to penetrate one section, there are still more insulating bulkheads separating you from all other sections. Also, my acceptance was similar to what could be expected from combat-weary troops: they looked, they nodded— and they waited to see if I was worth it.

This constant testing—while I was also studying elements of biology, medicine, surgery, and the latest in chemotherapy—left me increasingly alone, with a growing sense of awe and wonder and fear of what lay before me. Increasingly, I felt buried within the hospital's twenty-one floors of patients, surgeons, doctors, nurses, social workers, clergy, technicians, research fellows, and, winding through it, into the most remote corridors and hidden rooms, those desolate remnants of families, broken families now, following one or another of their members through this vast labyrinth of the sick and the dying, the medicators and the mediators, while somewhere about us were those who at this moment were managing to survive, patients who would perhaps give me some answer, or help me find my way—but I never knew for certain where they were or, indeed, that any of them would survive.

As the months went by, I became plunged into a deep crisis. All around me, the risks of life were so high, the personal involvement so total, the possibility of error so evident on every hand, that I realized this medical search had to also be seen and experienced in ethical and religious terms. As such, it raised personal and moral questions which I could not fully answer.

What right did I have, in the name of God or science or public health, to invade the lives of these people who were stranded, as my brother had been, on the other side of the great abyss separating those with cancer from all others? My brother had waited for me as I struggled over to him. Yet where was it written—other than in my book outline—that I could make the crossing over to these men, women, and children at Memorial? If anyone had a right, if anyone possessed the moral truth to look and judge, it was these people looking at me—not me, at them.

At my very best, as an inspired instrument, even as a tiny pencil of God, I could only hope to observe them, to listen and then, somewhere within the recesses of my mind and spirit, perhaps catch one small truth, one narrow ray of light that came from their far side.

Before all this, I was totally humbled. I had reported wars, the elections of popes, the making of saints, the rise and fall of nations. Yet all these were visible, or they possessed signs and symbols which could be read for some acceptable reality. Yet here was something else. Here we were dealing with an unknown enemy in an ongoing war that had not yet been totally won, a disease with the configuration of a crab that worked ceaselessly within every human organism, even in a child from the moment of its conception.

I began to feel helpless. Worse, I was threatened in a most fundamental and frightening way. Each one of us harbors a sheltered innocence which has not been violated, an inviolate chamber, a secret self—the source of courage, of physical stamina, of patience, of security, and of personal grace. Without it, we are defenseless and so perpetually threatened in a way that makes ordinary living and creative work impossible.

So it was with me after that first, fruitless year at Memorial. I walked the corridors and made the appointed rounds, yet I felt increasingly lost. I had begun this assignment with a belief, explored in previous books, that life in any form is sacred—from start to finish. A reverence for its worth is not measured alone by a capacity for extension of self in procreation or in creative labor. It is contained, rather more, within the unfolding process of life itself, within its innermost recesses, within the working of each single cell. It is there—in the individual cell's ability to communicate with itself, then to adjacent cells by secretion, and eventually with many cells through the nervous system—that we appear to discern the mystery, and possibly some hidden meaning, of all creation. So it had seemed to me, and I had pursued this work with the hope that it might bring me closer to understanding that mystery and its possible meaning.

On this particular day, I went to a chemotherapy ward, entering a small room where patients were sitting in armrest chairs while being medicated. Each one had a needle in the forearm with a feedline which administered a saline solution to cleanse the introductory vein or a prescribed drug capable of killing cancer cells to the limit of the body's endurance.

There was an empty seat and, as I sat down, everyone stared at me. You entered this clubroom with the forearm bared, ready for a needle. I wore a business suit and a hospital name tag—without the white jacket of a specialist or a doctor. Clearly, I was not a patient, and they wondered what I was doing there.

In front of me, against the opposite wall, sat a thin gray-haired man, wearing a red and green sport jacket and reading the *Racing Form* while receiving his medication. Beside him was a black woman in a print dress of palm leaves that bent and rolled with her folding flesh. Next to her, a young man in a blue warmup suit and baseball cap took his injection while listening to music through an earphone.

Beside me, I noticed a woman's arm that had the rose-colored, translucent quality which Renoir loved and painted from women whose "flesh drew the light." The arm was well shaped and its hand, long and delicate, lay open and inert as the needle conducted its medication into her vein.

"Is this your first time?"

She was about 45, with the looks of someone who once had a special beauty—delicate features, high cheekbones, the eyes brown and flecked with green. She pointed to my arm and said, "You should roll up your sleeve."

I explained I was writing about cancer survival and had come merely to observe patients taking chemotherapy treatment.

"Really?" she said. "Well, let me tell you, it's not always so easy. Like today, they told me that after this treatment I might lose my hair. Would you believe it?"

I glanced at a brown wave of her hair coming over her brow, then framing her delicate neckline—and I frowned to indicate disbelief.

"Oh yes," she said, trying to smile. "But you know what? I've got a wig that's fabulous. Hair just like my own. You wouldn't know the difference."

She glanced anxiously around the room, aware that everyone was listening.

"You see, I'm a waitress in a real fancy place, and if it gets out that I've got cancer, they'll fire me. Sounds real lousy, right? It's a dirty trick. But you have to face it. The customers just don't want a woman with cancer and no hair touching their food—no way. Except they won't know about me. Nobody knows other than my daughter and her husband. My boss thinks it's some kind of woman trouble."

She paused to see if I agreed.

"Of course," I replied. "Nobody will know, especially if you have a good-quality wig."

"Oh, it's the best! Real hair, they told me, from young girls who became nuns. And you know what? Look!"

She pulled back her hair to reveal recently pierced earlobes, with inserted post-earrings, the opening ready for its pendants.

"I'll wear big, flashy ones," she said. "So people won't look at the wig!"

"That's a great idea," I said.

"Yes, yes!" she cried happily.

Everyone in the room showed their support by nodding and smiling, and she lifted her head high in triumph.

"Then you know what? I'm going to buy wigs of all different colors to wear on my days off, and I'll get outfits to go with them. That way, I can be different people, depending on how I feel and what kind of date I want. It'll be wild!"

She laughed, a marvelous laugh, and everyone else laughed with her, as though she was going to fool the entire world with her wig and earrings, she was going to triumph over her disease, and she was going to change herself into anybody she wanted to be, depending upon her desires.

Our eyes met and in that instant I felt there was no barrier between us. I had somehow crossed the abyss to reach the other side, to be with this woman. She apparently also sensed this, for she looked at me carefully.

"I have a feeling that you understand, that you know how it is and how I feel." She paused and touched my arm. "But how can you?"

How could I tell her, or even indicate my loneliness and despair, my sense of frustration and humility before her—before all of them in that room? I saw the face of my dying brother as he lay in my arms, I saw my own face in a barroom mirror, looking for an answer, and I shook my head, unable to explain it. Then I noticed her glancing around the room, smiling at the others who were sitting before me now as a jury, nodding their approval.

At that moment, I saw myself in the face of my brother. I saw myself in this woman next to me, and in all the others in the room—the old man, the black woman, the young man. All of us were one total life, one believing mind, one faltering yet recovering spirit. All of us were part of one anthropomorphic figure where we could all be found, as an island is inevitably part of the continent.

Another patient entered, needing my chair, and I took her hand to say good-bye.

"My name's Eileen," she said. "Could you talk about the earrings in your book? Maybe it would help other girls like me."

She was smiling so bravely, and I wanted to take her into my arms, to hold her close, to tell her how precious she was. But I had no words for it, or how I felt.

Looking back now, I realize I should have told her that I was grateful for her trust, for giving me the strength to go on and so meet others like her—until this book became a reality.

Perhaps, also, I should have said something more, closer to the truth as I understand it now. I should have said, "Eileen, I love you as I love all the others like you, and as you are loved by those caring for you . . . men and women in this hospital who are giving you their lives in one way or another to help you live. So this is not a good-bye, for there can never be a parting between us."

                                                                    C.B.P.

Acknowledgments

This book derives from former cancer patients who have consented to tell their stories of survival so that others may take courage and realize how cancer may be defeated. My debt to them, and my intimate involvement with them, is described in the Epilogue.

I am grateful to Memorial Sloan-Kettering Cancer Center for allowing me to research this book through its hospital. In particular, I wish to thank Lewis Thomas, M.D., for his initial support and wise counsel. Samuel Babbit should also be thanked for helping to get this underway, and for caring about it all the way down the line. I am especially indebted to Dr. Paul A. Marks, whose appreciation of this book—and all that went into it —is but a small reflection of how deeply this doctor and scientist cares about human lives and, eventually, defeating all forms of cancer.

The counsel of Robert D. Seely, M.D.—as a physician and a man of letters—was invaluable. His intense critical surveillance, his unremitting care and concern were beyond any measure, as is my gratitude to him for all that he has shared with me in this undertaking.

All the others who appear in this book—the doctors, surgeons, nurses, social workers, and volunteers at Memorial—also helped in essential ways and, as a consequence, were also invaluable collaborators.

Dr. William G. Cahan was especially considerate and helpful, particularly during the first bewildering year of research. Often when I faltered, he was there—offering friendship and advice. Other doctors and surgeons to whom I am especially indebted include Jerome B. Posner, Joseph G. Fortner, Edward J. Beattie, Jr., Norma Wollner, Joseph M. Galicich, Philip R. Exelby, Man H. Shiu, Carl M. Pinsky, Nael Martini, Willet F. Whitmore, Elliot W. Strong, Walter B. Jones, Zalmen Arlin, Hiroyuki Ashikari, Joseph M. Lane, Ralph C. Marcove, Jatin Shah, John H. Raaf, Richard J. Gralla—all at Memorial—and Fred Plum at New York Hospital.

Suzanne Rauffenbart's understanding and support of this work was critical in extending its logistical range and its message of hope. As she did this, it became clear that she belonged in spirit with the book itself—with the lives of all those in it.

A special note of gratitude should be made for Memorial's medical secretaries, an unsung tribe of heroic, overworked souls who I suspect are a secret force that holds the hospital together. Most of them were kind and understanding, even when pressed, and I am especially indebted to Bea Arbaiza. Jerry Delaney generously shared his experience at Memorial, teaching me the run of the hospital, as did Mary Chebotar, Adele Slocum, Denise Wood, and Pat Molino.

I am grateful to Robert Markel for helping to initiate this project and for his patience and friendship along the way. Julian Bach—more than agent, more than friend—helped immensely, as he has many times across the years. Michael Remer, a consummate helmsman at law, steered a daring and brilliant course through high legal seas.

I am most fortunate to have had Tom Guinzburg as an editor, assisted by Felecia Abbadessa. Many thanks are also due to Shaye Areheart and Ann Finlayson for sensitive, skillful line and copy editing. I am also grateful to Elizabeth St. John and Marianne McKeon for helping me and the victors to reach the media on so many distant shores.

I wish to thank Marvin Bell, whose inspired lines from his poem *The Nest*—appearing as an epigraph to the introduction—so perfectly embody the new spirit, the sense of wonder and joy experienced by many of these survivors.*

James Galvin and Jorie Graham came to my side many times, bearing their splendid literary gifts. Many others should not be forgotten, including Jerry Leiber for providing a writing sanctuary, and Dorsey Waxter who generously helped in transcribing tapes. Carole Wahl was invaluable in typing endless scripts, as were Dan Clark and Scott Sudano in preparing the final manuscript.

Beverly Pepper contributed in countless ways. Her judgments and suggestions were invariably astute and constructive. They helped make this a better book, as her love and support made it possible.

                                                                              C.B.P.

---

* Reprinted by permission: © 1983 Marvin Bell. Originally in *The New Yorker*.

INDEX